# Why Mothers Die 1997–1999

## The fifth report
of the Confidential Enquiries into
Maternal Deaths in the United Kingdom

Director and Editor
**Gwyneth Lewis** MSc MRCGP FFPHM FRCOG

Clinical Director
**James Drife** MD FRCOG FRCPEd FRCSEd

**Central Assessors and Other Authors**

**Beverley Botting** BSc HonMFPHM

**Christine Carson** SRN SRM PGDip MSc

**Griselda Cooper** FRCA

**Marion Hall** MD FRCOG

**Catherine McCormick** RN RM

**James Neilson** MD FRCOG

**Margaret Oates** FRCPsych

**Robert Shaw** MD FRCSEd FRCOG

**Michael de Swiet** MD FRCP

**Harry Millward-Sadler** FRCPath MHSM

**Trevor Thomas** FRCA

**William Thompson** MD FRCOG

**Sheila Willatts** MD FRCA FRCP

First published December 2001

© Confidential Enquiries Into Maternal Deaths 2001

ISBN 1-900364-65-4

Published by the **RCOG Press** at the
Royal College of Obstetricians and Gynaecologists
27 Sussex Place
Regent's Park
London
NW1 4RG

Registered Charity No. 213280

Design: Tony Crowley, RCOG Press; Typesetting: FiSH Books, London
Printing: Henry Ling Ltd, The Dorset Press, Dorchester DT1 1HD

All correspondence with regard to the content of this Report should be addressed to:
Dr Gwyneth Lewis
Room 520, Wellington House
133–155 Waterloo Road
London SE1 8UG
Tel: 020 7972 4345

Copies of this Report can be obtained from:

**RCOG Bookshop**
Tel:             +44 (0)20 7772 6275
Fax:             +44 (0)20 7724 5991
Email:           bookshop@rcog.org.uk
Online bookshop: www.rcog.org.uk

pdf files of this Report and of the Executive Summary are available at: www.cemd.org.uk

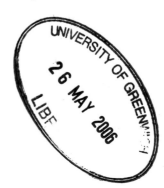

Cover photo: FORMAT/Judy Harrison

# CONTENTS

# PREFACE

Each case in this Report represents an individual tragedy. In some, a woman died despite exemplary care but in others the fatal outcome might have been avoided. The 'Maternal Mortality Reports' represent a sustained effort by professionals to learn lessons from sad case-histories which may otherwise go unreported or even unexamined. It is not an easy task for those personally involved in a maternal death to describe it to us in detail and to comment on how they might have done better. Nor is it pleasant for the local and national assessors to imagine themselves at the scene and then to make a judgement on whether or not care was substandard.

The large numbers of professionals involved in producing these Reports are driven by a desire to improve care. Fifty years ago, when this project began as a collaboration between the Royal College of Obstetricians and Gynaecologists (RCOG) and the Ministry of Health (as it then was), doctors knew that some women were dying unnecessarily. Today, the authors of this Report can still feel anger at the way the system continues to fail some vulnerable young women.

As well as highlighting problems the Report also illuminates successes. Great improvements have taken place over the years in, for example, the safety of obstetric anaesthesia and the treatment of hypertensive disease. The present Report records a remarkably low death rate from obstetric haemorrhage and a dramatic fall in deaths from thromboembolism after caesarean section, following publication of RCOG guidelines. After a decade in which further reduction of maternal mortality seemed elusive, the latter breakthrough shows how improvements in practice can still be made and can still save lives.

The scope of the Enquiries continues to broaden. The new and wider public health focus shows starkly what many of us have long suspected but never proved: that maternal mortality rates are higher among the most disadvantaged groups of our society. What we did not expect was to find a twenty-fold difference in the risk of death. This finding alone underpins our recommendations for changes in the delivery of antenatal care. Also, the number of women who had self-disclosed domestic violence points to another, hidden, issue of concern for maternal and child health.

Indirect deaths now outnumber Direct deaths and this Report reveals, for the first time, a distressing number of suicides within the first year after childbirth. While it is essential to continue scrutinising the well-known Direct causes of maternal death, it is also important to take a fresh look at emerging problems. Only such an observational study as this can do this.

In the UK, as in other developed countries, maternal mortality rates are low. Globally, however, over 600,000 women die each year of pregnancy-related causes. The authors of this Report frequently discuss its findings with colleagues from other countries and we are repeatedly reminded that these Maternal Mortality Reports have an importance well beyond the UK.

For nearly five decades these Reports have underpinned obstetric practice in the UK. In this Report we make far-reaching recommendations for the provision of sensitive, flexible antenatal care which should not only help reduce the maternal mortality rate but also improve the quality of care for pregnant and recently delivered women and their babies, particularly those affected by social exclusion, mental illness and domestic violence. Clinically, the challenge now is to ensure that relevant findings also inform other specialties and indeed agencies outside medicine. We believe that our recommendations offer an opportunity for all of us involved in planning services and caring for pregnant and recently delivered women to make a real and lasting difference to their lives and those of their families.

We also want to acknowledge the invaluable contribution of a number of people who are not often thanked in reports of this kind. We owe a huge debt of gratitude to Natalie Wilmot, the part-time secretary to this Enquiry, whose sensitive and sympathetic manner is greatly appreciated by all who need her help. We thank Sanjay Patel for his IT skills, without which much of the public health data could not have been analysed. Lesz Lancucki and Mary Grinstead, statisticians in the Department of Health, have provided invaluable data, as has Nigel Physick of the Office for National Statistics. Carol Abrahams, also of ONS, developed and piloted the invaluable record-linkage study that will be used by this Enquiry to great effect in future. And without the coding clerks at Great Titchfield Street, the social deprivation analysis would not have been possible. We also wish to acknowledge the wise advice given to the authors by Eleri Wones.

We owe an immense debt of gratitude to the late Professor Channi Kumar, the first psychiatric assessor to this Enquiry, who sadly died last year. Channi was the driving force behind the expansion of this Enquiry into deaths from mental illness and he set in train the mechanisms for this increasingly important aspect of our work. He was keenly involved in trying to improve the perinatal psychiatric services for the women of this country and was still making suggestions to us a few days before he died. We believe that he would be proud of the fruits of this work, now carried on by his chosen successor Margaret Oates.

Most of all we wish to thank all the health professionals who assisted with the individual cases. With your help, this Enquiry remains an outstanding example of professional self-audit and will continue to improve the care provided to pregnant and recently delivered women and their families.

Gwyneth Lewis

James Drife

Directors of the Confidential Enquiries into Maternal Deaths

December 2001

# Introduction and key findings     Section

# 1

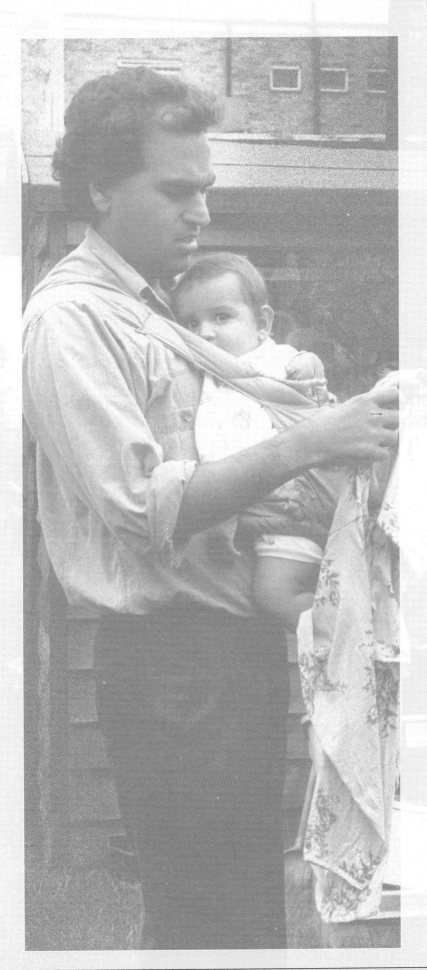

# AIMS OF THE ENQUIRY AND ITS ROLE IN CLINICAL GOVERNANCE

## Aims and objectives of the Confidential Enquiry into Maternal Deaths (CEMD)

The aim of the CEMD is to form part of the Government's agenda for clinical governance to help ensure that all pregnant and recently delivered women receive the best possible care delivered in appropriate settings and taking account of their individual needs.

The objectives are:

- to assess the main causes of and trends in maternal deaths; to identify any avoidable or substandard factors; to promulgate these findings to all relevant health care professionals

- to improve the care that pregnant and recently delivered women receive and to reduce maternal mortality and morbidity rates still further, as well as the proportion of deaths due to substandard care

- to make recommendations concerning the improvement of clinical care and service provision, including local audit, to purchasers of obstetric services and professionals involved in caring for pregnant women

- to suggest directions for future areas for research and audit at a local and national level

- to produce a triennial Report on behalf of the CEMD in England and Wales for the National Institute of Clinical Excellence, on behalf of the Scottish Programme for Clinical Effectiveness in Reproductive Health acting for the Scottish Executive Health Department and on behalf of the Department of Health, Social Services and Public Safety for Northern Ireland.

## The Enquiry's role in clinical governance

The Confidential Enquiry into Maternal Deaths, which now forms part of the work programme of the National Institute of Clinical Excellence, the Scottish Programme for Clinical Effectiveness in Reproductive Health acting on behalf of the Chief Medical Officer of the Scottish Executive Health Department and the Department of Health, Social Services and Public Safety for Northern Ireland, is the longest running example of national professional self-evaluation in the world. While much has changed since its inception in 1952, the lessons to be learned remain as valid now as in the past. While the CEMD has always had the support of professionals involved in caring for pregnant or recently delivered women, it is now a Government requirement that all maternal deaths should be subject to this Confidential Enquiry and all health professionals have a duty to provide the information required. This represents, to a large part, a continuation of current practice. The Health Departments of all the four countries who participate in this

Enquiry have a clear commitment to clinical governance.[1,2,3,4] In England, *A First Class Service: Quality in the NHS*,[1] states that:

- the responsibilities of NHS Trusts and Primary Care Trusts have been reinforced by a new statutory duty in respect of the quality of the services they provide

- all relevant hospital professionals and other health professionals must participate in the Confidential Enquiries

- the findings are to be given greater clarity and coherence and fed into NICE or equivalent guidelines

- the findings are an important part of clinical practice locally.

In April 2001, the Department of Health for England published *Building a Safer NHS for Patients*[5] which built on the findings of *An Organisation with a Memory*,[6] which recognised that there has been little systematic learning from adverse events and service failures in the NHS in the past. *Building a Safer NHS* sets out the arrangements for a new national adverse event reporting system under the auspices of a new body, the National Patient Safety Agency,[7] which will incorporate the findings of the CEMD. The lessons learned will be shared to effect change at local and national level, so that risk can be reduced and recurrence prevented through changes in practice and in service organisation and delivery.

In addition, *Building a Safer NHS* sets a target 'to reduce by 25% the number of instances of harm in the field of obstetrics and gynaecology which result in litigation by 2005'. A comprehensive programme is being developed by the Department of Health in England to help achieve this target and the implementation of the recommendations in this Report should help to achieve this.

References for similar or relevant Government initiatives for Scotland, Wales and Northern Ireland are given at the end of this section.

In participating in this Enquiry, the **professionals** concerned are asked for two things:

- to provide a full and accurate account of the circumstances leading up to the woman's death, with supporting records

- to reflect on any clinical or other lessons that have been learned, either personally or as part of the wider institution, and what action may have followed as a result.

At a **local level,** the Trust uses the findings of the CEMD to:

- ensure that all *Direct* deaths are subject to a local review and critical incident report

- develop or regularly update multidisciplinary guidelines for the management of complications in or after pregnancy

- review and modify, where necessary, the existing arrangements for the provision of maternity or obstetric care

- promote local audit and clinical governance.

At a **national** level in England and Wales, the findings of the CEMD are or will also be used:

- as part of the new national adverse events reporting systems to improve patient care

- to help inform Government policy

- to inform NICE or other guideline or audit development

- to inform guideline and audit development by the relevant Royal Colleges

- to set minimum standards of care, for example as set out in the criteria for the management of maternity services by the Clinical Negligence Scheme for Trusts (CNST)

- as part of postgraduate training and continuous professional self-development syllabus for all relevant health professionals

- to identify areas for further research.

In Scotland, the findings of the CEMD inform the work of equivalent bodies responsible for national quality initiatives. These include the Clinical Resource and Audit Group (CRAG), the Scottish Intercollegiate Guidelines Network (SIGN), the Clinical Standards Board for Scotland (CSBS) and the Clinical Negligence and Other Risks Indemnity Scheme (CNORIS).

In Northern Ireland, the findings of the CEMD will inform Government policy, the development of local guidelines and audit programmes, the work of the Clinical Resource and Efficiency Support Team (CREST) and the Regional Multiprofessional Audit Group.

## References

1. The Department of Health. *A First Class Service: Quality in the NHS*. London: Department of Health; 1998.
2. The Scottish Office Department of Health. *Clinical Governance. Management Executive Letter No. 29*. Edinburgh: Scottish Office; 1998.
3. Welsh Office. *Quality Care and Clinical Excellence*. Cardiff: Welsh Office; 1998.
4. Department of Health, Social Services and Public Safety, Northern Ireland, *Best Practice, Best Care: A Framework for Setting Standards, Delivering Services and Improving Monitoring and Regulation in the HPSS*. Belfast: Department of Health, Social Services and Public Safety; 2001.
5. Department of Health. *Building a Safer NHS for Patients*. London: Department of Health; 2001. Website address www.doh.gov.uk/buildsafenhs
6 Department of Health. *An Organisation with a Memory*. London: Department of Health; 2000.
7. National Patient Safety Agency, web site address www.npsa.org.uk

## Other relevant publications

Clinical Resource and Audit Group. *Clinical Outcome Indicators*. Edinburgh; 2000.

Scottish Executive Health Department. *A Framework for Maternity Services Scotland*. Edinburgh: Tactica Solutions; 2001.

Scottish Executive Health Department. *Clinical Risk Management Strategy Standards. Clinical Negligence and Other Risks Indemnity Scheme*. Glasgow. Willis; 2001

Scottish Executive Health Department. *Goals for Clinical Effectiveness*. Edinburgh; 1999.

Scottish Executive Health Department. *Management Executive Letter No. 75*. Edinburgh; 2000.

Scottish Executive Health Department. *Non Clinical Risk Management Standards. Clinical Negligence and Other Risks Indemnity Scheme*. Glasgow: Willis; 2001.

Scottish Executive Health Department. *Our National Health: A Plan for Action, A Plan for Change*. Edinburgh; 2001.

Scottish Office Department of Health. *Acute Services Review Report*. Edinburgh: SODOH; 1998.

Scottish Office Department of Health. *Designed to Care: Renewing the National Health Service in Scotland*. White Paper. Edinburgh; 1997.

# DEFINITIONS OF MATERNAL MORTALITY

The ninth revision of the International Classification of Diseases, Injuries and Causes of Death, (ICD9)[1] defines a maternal death as 'the death of a woman while pregnant or within 42 days of delivery, miscarriage or termination of pregnancy, from any cause related to or aggravated by the pregnancy or its management, but not from accidental or incidental causes'. Deaths are subdivided into *Direct*, *Indirect* and *Fortuitous*, but only *Direct* and *Indirect* deaths are counted for statistical purposes. In addition, the latest revision, ICD10, recognises that some women die as a consequence of *Direct* or *Indirect* obstetric causes after this period and has introduced a category for *Late* maternal deaths defined as 'those deaths occurring between 42 days and one year after abortion, miscarriage or delivery that are due to *Direct* or *Indirect* maternal causes'. The previous two Reports included all *Late* deaths occurring up to one year after delivery or abortion, as does this Report. The precise definitions for these are given in Table 1.

For the period covered by this Report, the Office for National Statistics (ONS) continued to use ICD9 coding on death certificates, for the purposes of internal consistency, but this is does not affect the number of deaths described in this Report in any way.

**Table 1**     Definitions of maternal deaths

| | |
|---|---|
| **Maternal deaths**[a] | Deaths of women while pregnant or within 42 days of delivery, miscarriage or termination of pregnancy, from any cause related to or aggravated by the pregnancy or its management, but not from accidental or incidental causes |
| ***Direct***[a] | Deaths resulting from obstetric complications of the pregnant state (pregnancy, labour and puerperium), from interventions, omissions, incorrect treatment or from a chain of events resulting from any of the above |
| ***Indirect***[a] | Deaths resulting from previous existing disease or disease that developed during pregnancy and which was not due to direct obstetric causes, but which was aggravated by the physiologic effects of pregnancy |
| ***Late***[b] | Deaths occurring between 42 days and one year after termination of pregnancy, miscarriage or delivery that are due to *Direct* or *Indirect* maternal causes |
| ***Coincidental*** (***Fortuitous***)[c] | Deaths from unrelated causes which happen to occur in pregnancy or the puerperium |

[a] ICD9
[b] ICD10
[c] ICD9 classifies these deaths as *Fortuitous* but the CEMD prefers to use the term *Coincidental* as it a more accurate description.

## *Fortuitous* deaths are now classified as *Coincidental* deaths

In the opinion of the authors of this Report, the term *Fortuitous* is seen as out-dated, inappropriate and insensitive, its general use in the English language implying a happier unexpected event. Therefore for this and future Reports, the definition will be replaced with the term *Coincidental*. Even this word is an imperfect description for some such maternal deaths, which are related to pregnancy in the wider sense of public health and which may have important implications for appropriate health care delivery.

## Denominator data used for calculating mortality rates

It is impossible to know the exact number of pregnancies that occurred during this or any preceding triennium, since not all pregnancies result in a registrable live or still birth. Because of the unreliability of these data, due to the lack of appropriate denominators, the most common denominator used throughout this and previous Reports is the number of maternities, rather than the total number of pregnancies. Maternities are the number of pregnancies that result in a live birth at any gestation or stillbirths occurring at or after 24 weeks of completed gestation and are required to be notified by law. The total number of maternities for the United Kingdom, 1997–99 was 2,123,614.

### Estimated pregnancies

This denominator is used for calculating the rate of early pregnancy deaths. It is a combination of the number of maternities, together with legal terminations, hospital admissions for spontaneous abortions (at less than 24 weeks of gestation) and ectopic pregnancies, with an adjustment to allow for the period of gestation

---

### Maternal mortality definitions used in this Report

| Maternal mortality definition | Reason for use |
| --- | --- |
| Deaths from obstetric causes per million women aged 15–44 years | This enables comparison with the other causes of deaths in this age group |
| Deaths from obstetric causes per 100,000 maternities | Maternities are the number of mothers delivered of registrable live births at any gestation or stillbirths of 24 weeks of gestation or later, i.e. these are the majority of women at risk of death from obstetric causes |
| Deaths from obstetric causes per 100,000 estimated pregnancies | This denominator is only used when calculating rates of death in early pregnancy, because the data for spontaneous abortions and ectopic pregnancies are unreliable |

Precise details of these, together with background figures and tables for the United Kingdom 1997–99, can be found in Appendix 1 Trends in reproductive epidemiology and women's health.

and maternal ages at conception. The estimate for the United Kingdom 1997–99 was 2,873,300. However, the resulting total is still an underestimate of the actual number of pregnancies, since these figures do not include other pregnancies which miscarry early, those where the woman is not admitted to hospital or, indeed, those where the woman herself may not even know that she is pregnant. Further details are available in Appendix 1.

### Deaths from obstetric causes per million women aged 15–44 years

This denominator assumes that all women of childbearing age are at risk of becoming pregnant. It lacks the rigour of confining the rate calculated to women who actually were pregnant but has the advantage of enabling comparison with other causes of women's deaths.

## GLOSSARY OF ABBREVIATIONS USED IN THIS REPORT

| | |
|---|---|
| A&E | Accident and Emergency department |
| AFE | Amniotic fluid embolism |
| APH | Antepartum haemorrhage |
| ARDS | Acute respiratory distress syndrome |
| ARM | Artificial rupture of membranes |
| βhCG | Beta human chorionic gonadotrophin |
| BMI | Body mass index |
| BP | Blood pressure |
| bpm | Beats per minute |
| CEMD | Confidential Enquiries into Maternal Death |
| CNORIS | Clinical Negligence and Other Risks Indemnity Scheme |
| CNST | Clinical Negligence Scheme for Trusts |
| CRAG | Clinical Resource and Audit Group |
| CS | Caesarean section |
| CSBS | Clinical Standards Board for Scotland |
| CTG | Cardiotocograph |
| CT | Computed tomography |
| CVP | Central venous pressure |
| D&C | Dilatation and curettage |
| DGH | District general hospital |
| DIC | Disseminated intravascular coagulation |
| DVT | Deep vein thrombosis |
| ECMO | Extra-corporeal membrane oxygenation |
| ECV | External cephalic version |
| FEV | Forced expiratory volume |
| GP | General practitioner |
| HAS | Human albumin solution |
| Hb | Haemoglobin concentration |
| Hb SC | Haemoglobin sickle cell |
| HDU | High-dependency unit |
| HELLP | Haemolysis, elevated liver enzymes, low platelets |
| HES | Hospital Episode Statistics |
| HIV | Human immunodeficiency syndrome |
| ICD9 | International Classification of Diseases, Injuries and Causes of Death, revision 9 |
| ICU | Intensive Care Unit |
| IVF | *in vitro* fertilisation |
| IV | Intravenous |
| JCVI | Joint Committee for Vaccination and Immunisation |
| MDR(UK)1 | Maternal Death Report Form for the United Kingdom (from October 1995) |
| MRI | Magnetic resonance imaging |
| NHS | National Health Service |
| NICE | National Institute for Clinical Excellence |
| OCD | Obsessive compulsive disorder |
| ONS | Office for National Statistics |
| PND | Postnatal depression |
| PPH | Postpartum haemorrhage |
| RCOG | Royal College of Obstetricians and Gynaecologists |
| SHO | Senior house officer |
| SIGN | Scottish Intercollegiate Guidelines Network |

| | |
|---|---|
| SLE | Systemic lupus erythematosus |
| SR | Specialist registrar |
| SUDEP | Sudden unexplained death in epilepsy |
| V/Q | Ventilation-perfusion |
| VTE | Venous thromboembolism |

# SUMMARY OF KEY RECOMMENDATIONS

## Reporting maternal deaths and assisting with the Enquiry

Any health professional who is aware of the death, from any cause, of a woman who is either pregnant or within one year following delivery, termination of pregnancy, ectopic pregnancy or miscarriage is required to report it to their director of public health or to the Enquiry direct.

All relevant hospital doctors and other health professionals are required to participate in the work of the Confidential Enquiry. Full case notes must be made available to the Enquiry Assessors and are treated in the strictest confidence. All professional staff who cared for the woman must provide information on request. Reports must be completed within nine months of the death.

## Auditable standards for maternity care

Each unit should identify a lead professional to develop and regularly update local multidisciplinary guidelines for the management of obstetric problems. This Report contains examples of such guidelines in a number of areas. As a minimum, guidelines should be provided for the following:

- follow-up procedures for women who regularly fail to attend for antenatal care
- the management of women who are at risk of a relapse or recurrence of a serious mental illness
- the management and local support strategies for women who disclose domestic violence
- the management of pre-eclampsia and eclampsia
- the management of obstetric haemorrhage
- the use of thromboprophylaxis
- the use of antibiotics for caesarean section
- the identification and management of ectopic pregnancy
- the identification of and support for women with higher-risk pregnancies and who appear unsuitable for midwifery-led care.

Clinical guidelines should be prominently placed in all antenatal and postnatal wards, the delivery suite and in accident and emergency (A&E) departments, and all guidelines should be given to all new members of staff.

The views of women who book late or fail to attend should be sought in helping to provide more appropriate services in future. The views of all women who use the services should also be sought on a regular basis.

The implementation of the guidelines should be subject to regular audit.

Each maternal death or case of severe morbidity should be discussed at multidisciplinary meetings and the report sent to the CEMD.

Units should organise regular drills for cases of massive haemorrhage so that when these emergencies occur all members of staff (including the blood bank) know exactly what to do to ensure that large quantities of crossmatched blood can be delivered to the delivery suite or theatre without delay.

## Health professionals

All staff should become familiar with the contents of this Report. Staff training, particularly in relation to audit and local guidelines, should be organised on a regular basis. The Report identified the need for further education and training in respect of signs of ectopic pregnancy, thromboembolism and the recognition and management of domestic violence and severe mental illness.

Continuing professional development should be accepted as the responsibility of the individual practitioner, as well as an employer, and knowledge and skills should be regularly updated using current research evidence.

Health professionals who work with disadvantaged clients need to be able to understand a woman's social and cultural background, act as an advocate for women with medical staff and colleagues and overcome their own personal and social prejudices and practice in a reflective manner.

All healthcare professionals should consider whether there are unrecognised but inherent racial prejudices within their own organisations, in terms of providing an equal service to all service users.

All health professionals should make themselves aware of the importance of domestic violence in their practice. They should adopt a non-judgemental and supportive response to women who have experienced physical, psychological or sexual abuse and must be able to give basic information to women about where to get help. They should provide or refer the woman to local sources of continuing support, whatever decision the woman makes made concerning her future.

Midwives should be prepared to decline to take responsibility for high-risk cases where the involvement of a consultant obstetrician is essential. The reasons for this should be explained to the woman and to the obstetrician.

## Commissioning for maternal health services

The importance of seeking antenatal care early in pregnancy should be part of health education and promotion materials prepared for different groups of society.

The planning and delivery of maternity services should focus on approaching each woman as an individual with different social, physical and emotional needs, as well as any specific clinical factors that may affect her pregnancy. Her pregnancy must not be viewed in isolation from other important factors that may influence her health or that of her developing baby.

Antenatal services should be flexible enough to meet the needs of all women, bearing in mind the needs of those from the most disadvantaged, vulnerable and less articulate groups in society are of equal if not more importance. Many women who died found it difficult to access or maintain access with the services and follow up mechanisms for those who failed to attend were poor. Women who regularly fail to attend clinics should be actively followed up.

When planning new methods of service provision, it is helpful to involve the women who might have difficulties in using the services in their design. Where this has been done, antenatal clinic attendances have significantly improved. Such flexibility may require imaginative solutions in terms of the timing and setting for antenatal clinics and the provision of outreach services.

Women at known higher risk of complications should not be delivered in maternity hospitals separate from acute hospital facilities. Clear and workable arrangements should be in place between all maternity units and their local intensive care unit to enable rapid transfer of any woman who suddenly requires intensive care.

The recent recommendations in the Department of Health of England's report *Comprehensive Critical Care*[1] should be considered in respect of the increased availability of intensive care and outreach services for pregnant or recently delivered women.

A perinatal mental health team which has the specialist knowledge, skills and experience to provide care for women at risk of, or suffering from serious postpartum mental illness should be available to every woman.

Women who require psychiatric admission following childbirth should ideally be admitted to a specialist mother and baby unit, together with their infant. Where this service is not available then a transfer should be considered.

Local trusts and community teams should develop guidelines for the identification of, and provision of support for women who suffer domestic violence, including developing multi-agency working to enable appropriate referrals or provision of information on sources of further help.

Information about local sources of help for domestic violence and emergency help lines, such as provided by Women's Aid, should be displayed in suitable places in antenatal clinic, for example in the women's toilets, and/or printed routinely at the bottom of the hand held maternity notes.

If at all possible partners, friends, family members and children should not be used to interpret for women unable to speak English. An interpreter should be provided.

In view the continuing evidence that doctors in both general and A&E medicine remain unaware of the recommendations made repeatedly in these Reports, it is again recommended that any pregnant woman sent to A&E must be seen by a senior obstetrician.

## At booking

At booking, a risk and needs assessment should take place to ensure that every woman will have a flexible care plan adapted to their own particular requirements for antenatal care. This should be reviewed regularly.

Clear and relevant information must be passed from the GP to the antenatal care team at booking concerning any past medical history including previous malignancies and abnormal cervical smears and any relevant family history. The GP booking letter should not be relied upon to provide all the information necessary to plan antenatal care.

All pregnant women should be given advice about the correct use of seat belts as soon as their pregnancy is confirmed.

All mothers should have their body mass index calculated at booking as part of the full risk assessment. Further, they should be offered advice about sensible weight reduction, including diet and exercise, and referral to a dietician where appropriate. A past history or family history of thromboembolism should be sought and if present, specialist advice should be obtained.

Enquiries about previous psychiatric history, its severity, care received and clinical presentation should be made routinely in a systematic and sensitive way at the antenatal booking clinic.

The term 'postnatal depression' or 'PND' should only be used to describe a nonpsychotic depressive illness of mild to moderate severity with its onset following delivery. It should not be used as a generic term to describe other mental illnesses.

The use of the term PND in the maternity records diminishes the severity of previous illness and the high risk of recurrence. Precise details of the type, onset and treatment for any previous illness should be sought and recorded. Women who have a past history of serious psychiatric disorder, postpartum or non-postpartum, should be referred to a psychiatrist and a management plan should be formulated in light of the high risk of recurrence.

All pregnant women should be routinely asked about domestic violence as part of their social history and should have the opportunity to discuss their pregnancy with a midwife, in privacy, without their partner present, at least once during the antenatal period.

Women with epilepsy should also be made aware of the dangers of bathing in pregnancy. They should be advised to bathe only in shallow water with someone else in the house or, alternatively, to shower.

All women should be encouraged to have HIV screening at booking.

## Continuing antenatal care

All providers of maternity services should ensure that there are clear protocols and routes of referral to primary or secondary care when rapid assessment, investigation and treatment are required. This will involve close collaboration with other professionals in both primary and secondary care.

When referring woman to general practitioners in primary care or to the obstetrician, midwives should make direct contact with the GP and not ask the woman or her family to do so on her behalf.

Midwives should have the ability to directly refer women they are concerned about to hospital services.

## Thromboembolism

Women with a past personal or family history of thromboembolism or other risk factors for deep vein thrombosis (DVT) – e.g. bed rest, pre-eclampsia, other medical disorders – should be carefully screened and consideration given to thromboprophylaxis.

All women undergoing caesarean section should receive prophylaxis against venous thromboembolism (VTE). Multiple risk factors are often present and the most effective method of prophylaxis, heparin at appropriate doses, should be used.

Wider use of thromboprophylaxis (not only after caesarean section) and better investigation of classic symptoms (particularly in high risk women) are urgently recommended.

Midwives, general practitioners and other medical staff should pay particular attention to women in the puerperium with chest or leg symptoms after either vaginal or operative delivery, in order to exclude the presence of DVT or potential pulmonary embolism.

If a pregnant woman displays chest or leg symptoms, Duplex ultrasound and/or ventilation/perfusion lung scanning should be used to exclude the presence of DVT or pulmonary embolism. Neither carries any significant risk to mother or fetus. Individual hospitals should have an agreed protocol for the objective diagnosis of suspected VTE during pregnancy.

These Reports have repeatedly stressed that chest X-ray is not contraindicated in pregnancy.

In clinically suspected DVT or pulmonary thrombembolism, treatment with unfractionated heparin or low-molecular-weight heparin should be given until the diagnosis is excluded by objective testing, unless treatment is strongly contraindicated. Subcutaneous unfractionated heparin is an effective alternative to intravenous unfractionated heparin for the initial management of DVT.

## Hypertensive diseases of pregnancy

Pregnant women with a headache of sufficient severity to seek medical advice or with new epigastric pain should have their blood pressure measured and urine tested for protein, as a minimum.

Clear, written, management protocols for severe pre-eclampsia should guide initial and continuing treatment in hospital.

Automated blood pressure recording systems can systematically underestimate blood pressure in pre-eclampsia, to a serious degree. Blood pressure values should be compared, at the beginning of treatment, with those obtained by conventional mercury sphygmomanometers.

Severe, life-threatening hypertension must be treated effectively.

Magnesium sulphate is the anticonvulsant drug of choice in the treatment of eclampsia.

There should be early engagement of intensive care specialists in the care of women with severe pre-eclampsia.

Women with moderate to severe pre-eclampsia require a level of clinical observation that may be incompatible with location in a single side room in hospital.

Women with multiple pregnancies are at increased risk of pre-eclampsia and their antenatal care should reflect that awareness.

## Haemorrhage

Every unit should have a protocol for the management of haemorrhage and this should be reviewed and rehearsed on a regular basis. It should also be included as part of life support training. All members of staff, including those in the blood bank, must know exactly what to do to ensure that large quantities of crossmatched blood can be delivered without delay.

It is recommended the guidelines for the management of women at known higher risk of haemorrhage (contained in Table 4.3 in Chapter 4) be followed.

The speed with which obstetric haemorrhage can become life threatening emphasises the need for women at known high risk of haemorrhage to be delivered in a hospital with a blood bank on site and appropriate laboratory facilities including haematological advice and therapy.

Placenta praevia, particularly in patients with a previous uterine scar, may be associated with uncontrollable uterine haemorrhage at delivery and caesarean hysterectomy may be necessary. A very experienced operator is essential and a consultant must be readily available.

On-call consultant obstetricians must consider all available interventions to stop haemorrhage, such as radical surgery or embolisation of uterine arteries, involving surgical or radiological colleagues as required.

It is essential that both obstetricians and anaesthetists be involved, at an early stage, in planning the elective management of very high-risk cases.

If haemorrhage occurs, experienced consultant obstetric and anaesthetic staff must attend.

## Amniotic fluid embolism register

A register of suspected cases of women who die or survive amniotic fluid embolism has been established. Such cases should be notified to Mr Derek Tuffnell, Consultant Obstetrician, Bradford Royal Infirmary, Duckworth Lane, Bradford, West Yorkshire BR9 6RJ.

## Ectopic pregnancy

All clinicians, and particularly those working in primary care and A&E

departments, need to be aware of atypical clinical presentations of ectopic pregnancy and especially the way it may mimic gastrointestinal disease. The possibility of atypical presentation should be taught to undergraduate medical and nursing students and highlighted in future textbooks.

Urinary dipstick testing for beta human chorionic gonadotrophin should be performed in any woman of reproductive age with unexplained abdominal pain. The test is now rapid, easy and sensitive.

Laparoscopic surgery for ectopic pregnancy has probable advantages over open surgery. However, it should only be undertaken by staff with training and experience meeting RCOG requirements.

Women with suspected ectopic pregnancies who have no signs of significant haemorrhage should not undergo surgery late at night if senior assistance is not immediately available.

Difficult surgical cases should not be delegated to unsupervised junior medical staff.

Cervical pregnancy may be associated with torrential haemorrhage. Care should be pre-planned carefully on a multidisciplinary basis.

## Genital tract sepsis

The onset of life-threatening sepsis at any stage of pregnancy can be insidious and all doctors and midwives must be aware of the symptoms and signs and be prepared to institute immediate treatment to avoid serious consequences.

A patient with prolonged rupture of the membranes who develops a fever and/or tachycardia should be carefully assessed by senior staff.

In patients with spontaneous rupture of the membranes not in labour, vaginal assessments should be avoided or kept to a minimum and undertaken with appropriately aseptic precautions.

There is clear evidence from controlled trials showing the benefits of prophylactic antibiotics for emergency caesarean section. This Report confirms that this policy is still not universally employed.

When infection develops and the patient is systematically ill, urgent and repeated bacteriological specimens including blood cultures must be obtained. Advice from a microbiologist must be sought at an early stage to assist with the use of appropriate antibiotic therapy.

There is some evidence in this Report of a failure to use the most appropriate antibiotics as recommended in hospital protocols.

In severe cases of sepsis doctors should be prepared, without delay, to give parenteral antibiotics before the diagnosis is confirmed.

## Medical problems in pregnancy

Prepregnancy counselling concerning the risks of pregnancy for women with potentially life-threatening conditions should not alienate the woman to such an extent that she does not come for antenatal care if she does become pregnant. These women need the best care that is available throughout pregnancy.

Previous Reports have repeatedly stressed, and this Report does so again, that pregnancy is not a contraindication for radiological investigations for women with severe and unremitting pain, including chest pain, particularly if the pain is so severe it requires management by major analgesia or epidural analgesia.

When any pregnant woman complains of episodes of vaginal bleeding in pregnancy, other than confirmed causes of haemorrhage, cervical cancer must be excluded by direct observation of the cervix and a cervical smear taken. This should be undertaken irrespective of her past medical history or reports of normal past cervical smears.

The importance of planned multidisciplinary care for women with cancer and other serious problems cannot be overstressed. Obstetricians, midwives, GPs, oncologists, surgeons, Macmillan nurses and palliative-care services may need to be involved, in conjunction with the woman and her partner, in planning a course of antenatal care that respects the wishes of the woman yet should optimise the outcome for the fetus.

Delivery for women with severe medical problems needs to be planned with care and, if possible, performed at an optimum time with consultants in attendance. A paediatrician should be involved antenatally, not only to optimise the care of the baby but also to discuss with the parents what may happen afterwards in regard to neonatal care. As the woman may require an elective caesarean section an anaesthetist should similarly be involved at an early stage in the pregnancy. A written and agreed care plan should be in her notes to pass this information on to colleagues who may have to attend for an emergency delivery.

Women with epilepsy need specific specialist advice in pregnancy. The ideal treatment for pregnant epileptic women, which has already been instigated in some centres, is a dedicated clinic to encompass prepregnancy counselling and attended by an obstetrician, a neurologist/obstetric physician and a specialist midwife or neurological nurse.

Pregnant women appear to be particularly susceptible to infectious diseases. Those who are not improving despite standard treatment should be admitted to hospital.

The risk to the fetus from poorly treated asthma is much greater than any possible risk to the fetus of steroid drugs. Steroid therapy can and should be continued in pregnancy without harm to the fetus.

Tertiary centres accepting the care of women with medical complications in pregnancy must be staffed at consultant level by physicians with relevant specialised medical experience and knowledge of obstetrics.

## Psychiatric disease

Enquiries about previous psychiatric history, its severity, care received and clinical presentation should be routinely made in a systematic and sensitive way at the antenatal booking clinic.

The use of the term postnatal depression or PND should not be used as a generic term for all types of psychiatric disorder. Details of previous illness should be sought and recorded in line with the recommendation above.

Women who have a past history of serious psychiatric disorder, postpartum or non-postpartum, should be assessed by a psychiatrist in the antenatal period and a management plan instituted with regard to the high risk of recurrence following delivery.

Women who have suffered from serious mental illness either following childbirth or at other times should be counselled about the possible recurrence of that illness following further pregnancies.

Protocols for the management of women who are at risk of a relapse or recurrence of a serious mental illness following delivery should be in place in every Trust providing maternity services.

A perinatal mental health team which has the specialist knowledge, skills and experience to provide care for women at risk of, or suffering from serious postpartum mental illness should be available to every woman.

Women who require psychiatric admission following childbirth should ideally be admitted to a specialist mother and baby unit, together with their infant. In areas where this service is not available then a transfer should be considered.

## Anaesthesia and intensive care

Early communication of anticipated problems and review of the patient by a critical care clinician would prevent delay in admission to intensive care in many cases. This applies particularly in cases identified to be at increased risk such as those with HELLP syndrome (haemolysis, elevated liver enzymes and low platelet count) which can deteriorate rapidly, as shown in this Report.

Dedicated obstetric anaesthesia services should be available in all consultant obstetric units. These services should be capable of taking responsibility for regional analgesia, anaesthesia, recovery from anaesthesia and the management and monitoring of intravenous fluid replacement therapy.

Adequate advance notice of elective caesarean sections in high-risk women must be given to the obstetric anaesthetic service. The notice must be sufficient to allow the consultation, investigation and assembly of resources needed for these cases to take place.

When presented with problem cases requiring special skills or investigations, obstetric anaesthetists should not hesitate to call on the assistance of anaesthetic colleagues in other sub-specialties as well as colleagues in other disciplines.

Invasive central venous and arterial pressure measurement can provide vital information about the cardiovascular system which can be life saving. Invasive monitoring via appropriate routes should be used particularly when the cardiovascular system is compromised by haemorrhage or disease.

Care of women at high risk of maternal haemorrhage must involve consultant obstetric anaesthetists at the earliest possible time.

Anaesthetists have a responsibility, as do all medical practitioners, to ensure that drugs are given in the correct dose, at the correct rate, by the correct route and by the most accurate means.

It seems not to be widely appreciated that oxytocin (Syntocinon®, Alliance) can cause profound, fatal hypotension, especially in the presence of cardiovascular compromise. Administration should follow the guidance in the *British National Formulary*, *Martindale* and other standard formularies. When given as an intravenous bolus the drug should be given slowly in a dose of not more than 5 iu.

## Reference

1.  Department of Health. *Comprehensive Critical Care*. London: Department of Health; 2000.

# CHAPTER 1

# Introduction and key findings

This Report, the first published in this millennium and the fifth covering the United Kingdom as a whole, continues the unbroken series of Confidential Enquiries into Maternal Deaths (CEMD) which started in 1952 for England and Wales, 1956 for Northern Ireland and 1965 for Scotland.

All CEMD reports are important, but this, covering maternal deaths occurring between 1997 and 1999, is possibly one of the most significant to have been published to date. The reasons for this include:

- For the first time, this Report has been able to evaluate more fully other factors that may have played a part in the woman's death. These findings are of great concern, showing that maternal mortality rates among the socially excluded, including women from lower socio-economic classes, very young girls and specific ethnic groups are higher than among the population as a whole. In summary:

  - ○ Women from the most disadvantaged groups of society were about 20 times more likely to die than women in the highest two social classes.

  - ○ Women from ethnic groups other than white were, on average, twice as likely to die than women in the white group. A large number of these women spoke little English.

  - ○ In a large number of cases, professionals used family members to interpret. There were several difficult cases where children were used inappropriately to interpret intimate personal or social details of the mother, and vital information was withheld.

  - ○ A disproportionate number of women from the traditional travelling community were likely to die.

  - ○ Twelve per cent of all the women whose deaths are included in this Report self-declared that they were subject to violence in the home.

  - ○ Access to care is also an issue for many of these groups of women. Twenty per cent of the women who died booked for maternity care after 24 weeks of gestation or had missed over four routine antenatal visits.

  - ○ Other factors were also associated with an increased risk of death; for example, young women under 18 years of age, increasing maternal age and increasing parity. Many women in this Enquiry were also obese. There also appeared to be over-representation of women with multiple pregnancies and those who had undergone *in vitro* fertilisation (IVF). Although some of these findings should be regarded with care because the very small numbers involved mean that they cannot necessarily be proven with statistical rigour, they nevertheless provide a unique indicator of the impact that social exclusion, inequality and other issues may have on a woman's reproductive health.

- The results show, sometimes in dramatic fashion, that the routine use of national guidelines can work. In this triennium, following the routine introduction and use of guidelines developed in part as a result of findings and recommendations from previous CEMD Reports, there have been significant decreases in deaths from pulmonary embolism and sepsis following caesarean section. In the very few cases where deaths occurred from these causes, guidelines do not appear to have been followed.

- Women are still dying of potentially treatable conditions where the use of simple diagnostic guidelines may help to identify conditions such as ectopic pregnancy, sepsis and pulmonary embolism. The diagnosis of many of these cases was missed in the primary care or accident and emergency (A&E) setting.

- For the first time the number of *Indirect* deaths, from medical conditions exacerbated by pregnancy, is greater than deaths from conditions that directly arise from pregnancy. *Indirect* deaths are of no less importance than *Direct* deaths and the recommendations in this Report for *Indirect* deaths must be regarded with equal importance to those that have been made for *Direct* deaths in previous Reports.

## The continuing importance of the Confidential Enquiries into Maternal Deaths and the value of this observational study

The findings of this Report demonstrate the contribution of such an observational study to both maternal and child health and the overall public health, and emphasise the need for it to continue in the future. This does not mean that further refinements to this Enquiry cannot be made and Chapter 21 discusses the possible future benefits of 'near miss' surveys of severe maternal morbidity.

Some people describe the Enquiry as a form of clinical audit, which could be used for performance monitoring. It is not. It is an observational and self-reflective study that identifies patterns of practice, service provision, and public health issues that may be causally related to maternal deaths.

Others question whether CEMD Reports are 'evidence based'. The highest level of evidence of clinical effectiveness comes from systematic reviews of randomised controlled trials. The most comprehensive and up-to-date systematic reviews of relevance to CEMD Reports are produced by the Cochrane Pregnancy and Childbirth Group, whose editorial structure is funded by the NHS Central Programme for Research and Development. The Co-ordinating Editor of the Group is a member of the CEMD Report writing panel.

Some Cochrane reviews are of direct relevance to topics highlighted by deaths described in recent Reports and have been cited to support recommendations. These include treatments for eclampsia and pre-eclampsia, and antibiotic prophylaxis before caesarean section. However, many problems tackled in successive Reports have not been addressed by randomised trials, including the prevention of thromboembolic disease and treatment of amniotic fluid embolism and of massive obstetric haemorrhage.

An important limitation of randomised trials is that, unless they are very large, they may provide little information about rare, but important, complications of treatments. Safety issues are, therefore, sometimes better illuminated by observational studies than by controlled trials.

Many causes of maternal death are very rare (e.g. cervical pregnancy) and treatment options for these may never be subjected to formal scientific study. Inevitably, recommendations for care to avoid such deaths in the future rely on lesser levels of evidence and frequently on 'expert opinion'. This does not mean that the Report is not evidence-based, merely that there is a lack of solid available evidence.

CEMD Reports could certainly be criticised legitimately if 'expert opinion' were given precedence over the findings of systematic reviews of randomised trials. The writing panel has gone to some effort to try to avoid any such error but would welcome feedback from readers if it is felt that, in any instance, it has failed in this objective.

## Results

The preceding section, Definitions of maternal mortality (page 7), gives a fuller explanation of the terminology used in this Report. Appendix 1 (page 329) gives details of the general trends in reproductive epidemiology. Details of the method of enquiry can be found in Appendix 2 (page 343).

## Overall maternal mortality rates

In the United Kingdom, maternal mortality rates can be calculated in two ways:

- through official death certification to the Registrars General (the Office for National Statistics, ONS, and its equivalents) or

- through deaths known to this Enquiry.

ONS data are based on death certificates where the cause of death is directly or secondarily coded for a pregnancy-related condition such as postpartum haemorrhage, eclampsia. Appendix 1 contains a summary table of ONS-derived maternal death rates.

The number of *Direct* and *Indirect* deaths identified by the Enquiry has always exceeded those officially reported. This is because a large proportion of women known to the Enquiry die of pre-existing medical conditions influenced by their pregnant state, for example cardiac disorders, epilepsy and some malignancies, but these are excluded from the official statistics. Also excluded are women who require long-term intensive care and whose final cause of death is registered as a non-pregnancy condition such as multiple organ failure even though the initiating cause was an obstetric event. Conversely, the maternal deaths known to the Registrars General may include *Late* deaths, as it is not possible to identify from the death certificate when the delivery or termination occurred.

Furthermore, in terms of international comparison, it is important to note two points:

1. The criteria used by the UK assessors for *Indirect* deaths are far more

inclusive than those used in other countries. For example, in this Enquiry all cases of cardiac disease, asthma and epilepsy are coded as *Indirect*, as are cases of suicide, unless obviously occurring in women with a longstanding previous psychiatric history.

2. Case ascertainment is lower in the vast majority of other countries because they do not undertake such comprehensive enquiries.

## Improved case ascertainment

The 1994–96 CEMD Report was the first to be produced using a new Office for National Statistics (ONS) computer program that helped to identify deaths that previously would have passed unrecognised. Before 1993, only the underlying cause of death was coded. For deaths occurring from 1993 onwards, computer programs have been used to code the cause of death automatically. As a result, all conditions given anywhere on the certificate are now coded and held on the computer record and the ONS has been able to undertake a more extensive search of death draft entry information to identify all conditions listed which suggest a maternal death. This has led to the identification of an extra 40 deaths in this triennium, compared with 67 deaths in 1994–96. Worryingly, 20 of these deaths were *Direct*. Eight had died in early pregnancy; five from ectopic pregnancy. Six unreported women died of thromboembolism, a further three had hypertensive disease of pregnancy, two died of sepsis and one from haemorrhage. There were also three *Late Direct* deaths. It may be more understandable why 17 *Indirect* deaths were also not notified to the CEMD, because the women died in the community and were out of touch with maternity or obstetric health professionals. Ten of these had cardiac disease.

The result of this improved case ascertainment has been to increase the numbers known to the Enquiry, and hence the overall and specific maternal mortality rates compared to data collected before 1993. This is reflected in the results as shown in Table 1.1 and Figure 1.1. It is not possible to know whether or not similar numbers remained undetected in previous triennia, but it is probable that such a degree of under-reporting existed in earlier years

**Table 1.1** Deaths notified to the Enquiry and rates per 100,000 maternities; United Kingdom 1985–99

| | 1985–87 | | 1988–90 | | 1991–93 | | 1994–96 | | 1997–99 | |
|---|---|---|---|---|---|---|---|---|---|---|
| | (*n*) | Rate | (*n*) | Rate | (*n*) | Rate | (*n*) | Rate | (*n*) | Rate |
| Type of death: | | | | | | | | | | |
| *Direct* | 139 | 6.1 | 145 | 6.1 | 129 | 5.6 | 134 | 6.1 | 106 | 5.0 |
| *Indirect* | 86 | 3.8 | 93 | 3.9 | 100 | 4.3 | 134 | 6.1 | 136 | 6.4 |
| *Direct* and *Indirect* | 223 | 9.9 | 238 | 10.1 | 228 | 9.9 | 268 | 12.1 | 242 | 11.4 |
| *Coincidental (fortuitous)* | 26 | 1.6 | 39 | 1.6 | 46 | 2.0 | 36 | 1.6 | 29 | 1.4 |
| *Late* | n/a | | 48 | 2.0 | 46 | 2.0 | 72 | 3.3 | 107 | 5.0 |
| **Total** | 249 | | 325 | 13.7 | 321 | 13.7 | 376 | 17.1 | 378 | 17.8 |
| **Total maternities (*n*)** | 2,268,766 | | 2,360,309 | | 2,315,204 | | 2,197,640 | | 2,123,614 | |

n/a = data not collected for this triennium

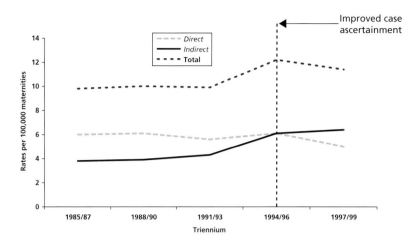

**Figure 1.1**    Direct and Indirect maternal death rates per 100,000 maternities;
United Kingdom 1985–99

### Office for National Statistics birth and maternal death linkage survey

In 2001, at the request of this Enquiry, the Office for National Statistics undertook a pilot study to test the feasibility and possible benefits of matching death records of women of fertile age with birth registrations up to one year previously. The aim was to identify all deaths in delivered women up to one year after birth and to see how many additional cases would be found. The results, which it is hoped to publish in a separate paper at a later date, can only be briefly summarised here. The methodology was successful and will be used to improve case ascertainment for future Reports.

It was gratifying to find that only three possible *Direct* deaths in women who had delivered had not been notified to the Enquiry. This gives a *Direct* case ascertainment rate of 97%.

Ten possible extra *Indirect* deaths, other than from mental illness, which occurred up to 42 completed days after delivery, were identified. This gives an ascertainment rate of 92%. These were probably deaths that occurred in the community after contact with maternity services had stopped.

By contrast with the reassuring findings for *Direct* and *Indirect* deaths, over 250 *Late* deaths that occurred three to twelve months after delivery were not notified. The greater the period of time between birth and the death of the mother the less likelihood there was of notification. None of these deaths was from *Direct* maternal causes and, apart from suicides, which are discussed in the next paragraph, there appeared to be only a few from *Indirect* causes. The vast majority were *Coincidental* and, of these, the leading cause of death was malignancy. Again, most of these deaths will not have been known to the maternity services. GPs, oncologists and cancer support teams are not used to reporting deaths to the CEMD.

### Deaths from mental illness

There has always been a large degree of under-ascertainment of deaths from mental illness or substance abuse by this Enquiry. Indeed, the CEMD only started to consider these deaths in detail in the last triennial Report. However, the ONS linkage study showed that the CEMD was unaware of over 40 extra deaths from suicide or deaths from violent causes, and another eight where the Coroner recorded an open verdict. In addition, 11 unreported women died from an accidental drug overdose. As it is not yet widespread practice for psychiatrists and community mental health or drug support teams to notify such deaths to this Enquiry, this degree of under-ascertainment is understandable. But, when all deaths up to one year from delivery are taken into account, the results of the study show that deaths from suicide are not only the leading cause of *Indirect* death but also the leading cause of maternal deaths overall.

In future, the investigation of deaths from mental illness will be more comprehensive through improved reporting from other professionals, closer ties to the Confidential Enquiry into Deaths from Suicide and Homicide and the adoption of the ONS record linkage pilot procedure as a routine part of case ascertainment.

## Summary of cases known to the Enquiry 1997–99

During this triennium, 378 deaths were reported to or identified by the Enquiry, a number remarkably similar to the 376 cases reported in 1994–96. There were very limited data for ten cases but it was still possible to code these deaths according to type.

Of the 378 deaths, 106 were classified as *Direct* and 136 as *Indirect* deaths, representing 28% and 36% of reported cases, respectively. Twenty-nine (8%) were classified as *Coincidental (Fortuitous)* and 107 (36%) as *Late*. The total number of *Direct* and *Indirect* maternal deaths reported to the Enquiry, 242, is lower than the 268 reported in the previous triennium. For the first time, however, the number of *Indirect* deaths exceeded the number of *Direct* deaths, as shown in Table 1.1 and Figure 1.1. Table 1.2 shows the actual deaths by cause and Table 1.3 the death rates per million maternities by cause of death for the last five triennia. For comparison, it is important to note that cases of sepsis in early pregnancy were counted as early pregnancy deaths until 1994 and some *Direct* causes of death were assigned to other specific chapters over the same period. Table 1.2 shows the cases as counted in the specific CEMD Reports for each triennium but, for purposes of comparison, Table 1.3 calculates the rates according to the classification used in this Report, i.e. all deaths from sepsis occurring at any point in pregnancy are included in the overall rate.

## Summary of overall findings 1997–99

In comparison with 1994–96, the first triennium in which the new system of case ascertainment was used, the overall findings for 1997–99 show:

- a small decrease in the combined overall maternal mortality rates (*Direct* and *Indirect* deaths) known both to the Registrars General and to this Enquiry. The maternal mortality rate for this triennium, derived from the CEMD data, is 11.4 deaths per 100,000 maternities.

**Table 1.2**  Maternal deaths reported to the Enquiry by cause; United Kingdom 1985–99

| Chapter in Report | Cause | 1985–87 (n) | 1988–90 (n) | 1991–93 (n) | 1994–96 (n) | 1997–99 (n) |
|---|---|---|---|---|---|---|
| *Direct*: | | | | | | |
| 2 | Thrombosis and thromboembolism | 32 | 33 | 35 | 48 | 35 |
| 3 | Hypertensive disease of pregnancy | 27 | 27 | 20 | 20 | 15 |
| 4 | Haemorrhage | 10 | 22 | 15 | 12 | 7 |
| 5 | Amniotic fluid embolism | 9 | 11 | 10 | 17 | 8 |
| 6 | Early pregnancy deaths: | | | | | |
| | Ectopic | 16 | 15 | 8 | 12 | 13 |
| | Spontaneous miscarriage | 5 | 6 | 3 | 2 | 2 |
| | Legal termination | 1 | 3 | 5 | 1 | 2 |
| | Other | – | – | 2 | – | – |
| | Total early pregnancy deaths | 22 | 24 | 18 | 15 | 17 |
| 7 | Genital tract sepsis | 6[a] | 7[a] | 9[a] | 16[b] | 14[b] |
| 8 | Other *Direct*: | | | | | |
| | Genital tract trauma | 6 | 3 | 4 | 5 | 2 |
| | Fatty liver | 6 | 5 | 2 | 2 | 4 |
| | Other | 9 | 9 | 8 | – | 1 |
| | Total other *Direct* | 27 | 17 | 14 | 7 | 7 |
| 9 | Anaesthetic | 6 | 4 | 8 | 1 | 3 |
| | Total *Direct* | 139 | 145 | 129 | 134 | 106 |
| *Indirect*: | | | | | | |
| 10 | Cardiac | 23 | 18 | 37 | 39 | 35 |
| 11 | Psychiatric | n/a | n/a | n/a | 9 | 15 |
| 12 | Other *Indirect* | 84 | 93 | 63 | 86 | 75 |
| 13 | *Indirect* malignancies | n/a | n/a | n/a | – | 11 |
| | Total *Indirect* | 107 | 111 | 110 | 134 | 136 |
| 14 | **Coincidental** | 26 | 39 | 46 | 36 | 29 |
| 15 | **Late** | | | | | |
| | Direct | n/a | 13 | 10 | 4 | 7 |
| | Indirect | n/a | 10 | 23 | 32 | 39 |
| | Coincidental | n/a | 25 | 13 | 36 | 61 |
| | Total *Late* | n/a | 48 | 46 | 72 | 107 |

N/A = Not available; [a] excluding early pregnancy deaths due to sepsis; [b] Including early pregnancy deaths from sepsis

- The *Direct* maternal mortality rate, 5.0 deaths per 100,000 maternities, is lower than in any of the other four preceding triennia for which UK data have been collected.

- The *Indirect* maternal mortality rate, 6.4 deaths per 100,000 maternities, is higher than in any of the preceding four triennia.

- For the first time, the number of *Indirect* maternal deaths is greater than *Direct* maternal deaths as shown in Figure 1.1.

### Deaths before delivery

Eighty-three women died of *Direct* or *Indirect* causes before delivery, 34 % of all such maternal deaths. In this group, the largest causes of *Direct* deaths were ectopic pregnancy and pulmonary thromboembolism. There was a variety of causes of *Indirect* deaths among undelivered women, with deaths from suicide, cardiac disease and malignancies among the largest groups.

**Table 1.3**    Death rates by major cause of death per million maternities; United Kingdom 1985–99

| Chapter in Report | Cause | 1985–87 Rate | 1988–90 Rate | 1991–93 Rate | 1994–96 Rate | 1997–99 Rate |
|---|---|---|---|---|---|---|
| 2 | Thrombosis and thromboembolism | 14.1 | 14.0 | 15.1 | 21.8 | 16.5 |
| 3 | Pregnancy-induced hypertension | 11.9 | 11.4 | 8.6 | 9.1 | 7.1 |
| 4 | Haemorrhage | 4.4 | 9.3 | 6.5 | 5.5 | 3.3 |
| 5 | Amniotic fluid embolism | 4.0 | 4.7 | 4.3 | 7.7 | 3.8 |
| 6 | Early pregnancy | 7.9[a] | 7.6[a] | 5.2[a] | 6.8 | 8.0 |
| 7 | Sepsis | 4.4 | 5.5 | 6.4 | 6.4[a] | 6.6[a] |
| 8 | Other *Direct*: | 11.9 | 7.2 | 6.0 | 3.2 | 3.3 |
|  | – uterine trauma | 2.6 | 1.3 | 1.7 | 2.3 | 1.0 |
|  | – other | 9.3 | 5.9 | 4.3 | 0.9 | 2.3 |
| 9 | Anaesthetic | 2.6 | 1.7 | 3.5 | 0.5 | 1.4 |
|  | *Indirect:* | | | | | |
| 10 | – cardiac | 10.1 | 7.6 | 15.9 | 17.7 | 16.5 |
| 11 | – psychiatric[b] | – | – | – | 4.1 | 7.1 |
| 12 | – other | 37.0 | 31.0 | 27.0 | 39.1 | 35.3 |
| 13 | – malignancies[c] | – | – | – | – | 5.1 |
|  | Total *Direct* and *Indirect* | 98.2 | 100.1 | 98.1 | 121.9 | 114.0 |
| 14 | *Coincidental (fortuitous)* | 11.3 | 16.5 | 19.9 | 16.4 | 10.8 |
| 15 | *Late* | – | 20.3 | 19.9 | 32.8 | 50.3 |

[a] Including sepsis in early pregnancy; [b] until 1993–96 counted as *Coincidental*; [c] until 1997–99 not classified separately

## Specific causes of death

Figure 1.2 shows the major causes of maternal deaths reported to the Enquiry by rate per million maternities.

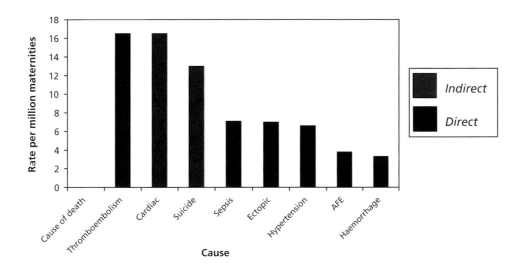

**Figure 1.2**    Major causes of maternal death, rates per million maternities; United Kingdom 1997–99

## *Direct* deaths

There has been a reduction in rates of death from several key causes of maternal death, while deaths from sepsis continue to slowly rise. This is shown in Figure 1.3.

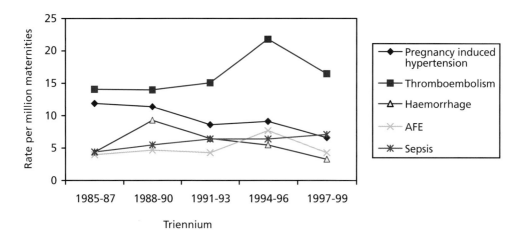

**Figure 1.3**  Major causes of *Direct* deaths; rates per million maternities; United Kingdom 1985–99

## Thrombosis and thromboembolism

Thrombosis and thromboembolism remain the major *Direct* cause of maternal death, although the rate, 16.5 per million maternities, has fallen from the all-time high of 21.8 per million maternities in last Report. They account for 33 % of all *Direct* maternal deaths. However, this overall death rate hides two key findings:

- The number of deaths from thromboembolism following caesarean section has fallen dramatically following the introduction and routine use of guidelines for thromboprophylaxis as shown in Figure 1.4.

- Conversely, there has been a significant rise in the number of deaths from thromboembolism in other women, in many of whom the diagnosis was missed in either general practice or A&E departments, or in women who, despite having known risk factors, were not offered appropriate thromboprophylaxis.

It is important to note that the rate of *Indirect* maternal deaths from cardiac disease is exactly the same as that for thromboembolism. It is thus the joint leading cause of death for reported cases overall.

## Hypertensive disease of pregnancy

Hypertensive disease of pregnancy remains the second leading cause of *Direct* deaths, as it was in the last triennium, although the rate has fallen to 7.1 per million maternities compared with 9.1 per million in the last Report. This may well again reflect the introduction of guidelines for the management of pre-eclampsia.

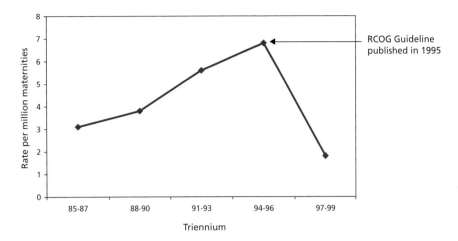

**Figure 1.4**    Deaths from thromboembolism following caesarean section, rates per million maternities; United Kingdom 1985–99

## Sepsis

Sepsis, including deaths in early pregnancy following miscarriage and ectopic pregnancy, is the third leading cause of *Direct* deaths. Unlike other leading causes of *Direct* deaths, the rate of maternal deaths from sepsis is slowly increasing. In this triennium the rate was 8.0 per million maternities, a rise from 6.8 per million maternities in the last Report.

## Deaths in early pregnancy

Although, when taken overall, deaths in early pregnancy are the second leading cause of *Direct* deaths, the deaths included in this category arise from a number of causes. The largest number are due to ectopic pregnancy, which comprises the fourth leading cause of *Direct* deaths. The 1997–99 rate for the occurrence of ectopic pregnancy is 11.1 per 1000 estimated pregnancies, of whom 0.4 per thousand died, compared with 11.5 per 1000 estimated pregnancies in 1994–96 with the same rate of death, 0.4 per thousand ectopic pregnancies. As with the last Report, most of the fatal cases were missed in the primary-care or A&E setting.

## Amniotic fluid embolism

Deaths from amniotic fluid embolism (AFE) have reduced by half compared with the last Report (a rate of 3.8 per million maternities compared with 7.7 per million). The reasons for this fall are not clear but some women are now surviving this previously fatal condition.

## Haemorrhage

Although the fall from 5.5 to 3.3 per million maternities in the rate of death attributable directly to haemorrhage is welcome, there are a number of other cases where haemorrhage played a significant part. Concern remains that care is not always as good as it should be, even in cases where problems could have been anticipated.

### Other *Direct* causes of death

There has been a slight decrease in deaths in this category, which mainly relates to uterine trauma and fatty liver. Deaths from uterine trauma have reduced to two compared with five in the last Report, while deaths from fatty liver of pregnancy have doubled to four. The combined rate of deaths in this category is 2.8 deaths per million maternities compared with 3.2 per million in the last Report.

### Anaesthesia

There were three deaths attributed to anaesthesia, an increase on the one case in the last Report, although still only accounting for 3% of *Direct* maternal deaths.

### Cardiac disease

Heart disease and thromboembolism are now the joint most common causes of maternal death reported to this Enquiry. Therefore, heart disease is still potentially dangerous in pregnancy even though disease patterns have changed. The most common causes are cardiomyopathy, including puerperal cardiomyopathy, dissecting aneurysm of the thoracic aorta and myocardial infarction.

Women with pulmonary vascular disease have a very high risk of dying in pregnancy. Typical estimates of mortality risk are 30% per pregnancy in Eisenmenger's syndrome and 30–50% in primary and secondary pulmonary hypertension.

### Other *Indirect* deaths

These deaths now outnumber those from *Direct* causes. The findings and recommendations made for the management of these women are of equal importance.

Nearly half the deaths in this category were from diseases of the central nervous system, including cerebral haemorrhage and epilepsy. Thirteen women died of infectious disease, five from asthma and four each from diabetes and blood disorders. There were also a number of deaths from other causes.

### Suicide

When the cases of suicide identified by the record linkage study are taken into account, deaths from suicide are the leading cause of maternal death. However, because only 28 such deaths were reported to the Enquiry this triennium, this is not evident in the figures given in this Report. In future, the adoption of the ONS record linkage methodology described earlier in this chapter will enable clearer conclusions to be drawn.

To date, it has not been routine practice to report all such deaths to the CEMD, especially after the woman has lost contact with the community midwives. Reporting mechanisms will be strengthened in future to improve case ascertainment and closer links with the Confidential Enquiry into Suicides and Homicides will also be developed with this aim in mind.

The assessors consider it illogical that the International Classification of Diseases should not count these deaths as having a maternal cause. As a consequence, the death certificate data are not always coded to a pregnancy-related suicide, thus increasing the possibility that many more of these cases remain unreported to the CEMD. It should be noted for statistical purposes that many of these deaths are counted as *Late* deaths, since they occurred later than 42 days post delivery.

## Substandard care

Box 1.1 gives the definitions of substandard care used in this Report.

| Box 1.1 | Definitions of substandard care used in this Report |
|---|---|
| Major | Contributed significantly to the death of the mother i.e. different management would reasonably have been expected to alter the outcome. |
| Minor | It was a relevant contributory factor. Different management might have made a difference but the mother's survival was unlikely in any case. |
| Incidental | Although lessons can be learned it did not affect the eventual outcome. |

Substandard care remained very difficult to evaluate in many of the cases in this Report due to the lack of key data from some records and case notes. While it is clear that many of the cases received less than optimum care, it has not always been possible to quantify these with certainty. Nevertheless, despite these limitations, the assessors classified 60·4% of *Direct* deaths as having some form of substandard care, as shown in Table 1.4. Fifty per cent of *Direct* deaths had major substandard care in which different treatment may have affected the outcome. Seventeen per cent of *Indirect* deaths and nine per cent of deaths from cardiac disease were associated with substandard care, as shown in Table 1.5. By contrast, only about 10% of both *Coincidental* and *Late* deaths had substandard care, with seven per cent in each category being classified as major. The major concerns about the care of these cases were failings in social services support for vulnerable young girls and in lack of multidisciplinary or coordinated care.

The specific cases and lessons to be learned are discussed in the relevant Chapters of this Report and lessons are highlighted and reflected in the recommendations.

Without direct access to case notes, it will never be possible adequately to establish the number of deaths due to substandard care, and it is for this reason **this Report recommends that the full case notes be made available to the CEMD Assessors in future.**

**Table 1.4**    *Direct* deaths assessed as having substandard care; United Kingdom 1997–99

| Cause of death | Major substandard care (n) | Minor substandard care (n) | Total cases of substandard care in Chapter (n) | Number of cases in chapter (n) | Overall substandard care (%) |
|---|---|---|---|---|---|
| 2 Thrombosis | 15 | 5 | 20 | 35 | 57 |
| 3 Hypertension | 12 | – | 12 | 15 | 80 |
| 4 Haemorrhage | 4 | 1 | 5 | 7 | 71 |
| 5 Amniotic fluid embolism | 2 | – | 2 | 8 | 25 |
| 6 Early pregnancy | 9 | 2 | 11 | 17 | 65 |
| 7 Sepsis | 6 | 1 | 7 | 14 | 50 |
| 8 Other Direct | 2 | 2 | 4 | 7 | 57 |
| 9 Anaesthetic | 3 | – | 3 | 3 | 100 |
| **Total** | 53 | 11 | 64 | 106 | 60·4 |

**Table 1.5**     *Indirect* deaths assessed as having substandard care; United Kingdom 1997–99

| Cause of death | Major substandard care | Minor substandard care | Total cases of substandard care in Chapter | Number of cases in chapter | Overall substandard care |
|---|---|---|---|---|---|
| | (n) | (n) | (n) | (n) | (%) |
| 10  Cardiac | 3 | – | 3 | 35 | 9 |
| 11  Psychiatric[a] | 9 | 8 | 17 | 43 | 39 |
| 12  Other Indirect | 11 | 2 | 13 | 75 | 17 |
| 13  Cancer | 3 | 10 | 13 | 52 | 25 |
| Total | 26 | 20 | 46 | 205 | 22 |

[a] until 1993–96 counted as *Coincidental*

The main causes of substandard care are given in Table 1.6. These can be summarised as:

- lack of communication and team work

- failure to appreciate the severity of the illness and suboptimal treatment

- wrong diagnoses

- failure of junior staff or general practitioners to diagnose or refer the case to a senior colleague or hospital

- failure of consultants to attend and inappropriate delegation of responsibility

- in some units, the continuing lack of a clear policy for the prevention or treatment of conditions such as pulmonary embolism, eclampsia or massive haemorrhage, and

- failure of the lead professional to identify diseases or conditions that do not commonly occur in their own specialty or to seek early advice.

**Table 1.6**     Major causes of substandard care, *Direct* and *Indirect* deaths

| Cause | Number | substandard care (% of all cases)[a] |
|---|---|---|
| Poor liaison between professionals | 32 | 42 |
| Failure to appreciate severity | 30 | 39 |
| Wrong diagnosis | 29 | 38 |
| Incorrect/suboptimal treatment | 29 | 38 |
| Failure of GP to refer to hospital | 16 | 21 |
| Senior doctor did not attend but gave advice by telephone | 10 | 13 |
| Intensive care unit full | 5 | 6 |
| Intensive care unit distant | 5 | 6 |
| Lack of blood products | 5 | 6 |

[a] More than one reason could apply in individual cases

## Delivery of care

### Antenatal care

Table 1.7 shows the type of antenatal care received by the women described in this Report. In most cases, care was shared between the GP, community or clinic midwife and the obstetricians – so-called traditional 'shared care'. In many of

**Table 1.7**     Maternal deaths by type of antenatal care; United Kingdom 1997–99

| Type of antenatal care | Classification of death | | | | Total |
| --- | --- | --- | --- | --- | --- |
| | *Direct* | *Indirect* | *Coincidental* | *Late* | |
| Consultant-led unit only | 15 | 27 | 1 | 13 | 56 |
| Traditional shared care | 35 | 67 | 19 | 69 | 190 |
| Midwife/GP[a] | 15 | 14 | 3 | 10 | 42 |
| Midwife only | 4 | – | 1 | 3 | 8 |
| Private clinic | – | 2 | – | 1 | 3 |
| Concealed pregnancy | – | 1 | 1 | 1 | 3 |
| No antenatal care | 2 | 2 | | 2 | 6 |
| Late booker/poor attender | 17 | 22 | 2 | 8 | 49 |
| Death before booking or after miscarriage or TOP | 18 | 1 | 2 | – | 21 |
| Total | 106 | 136 | 29 | 107 | 378 |

a see text; TOP = termination of pregnancy

these cases, the woman saw the obstetric staff only two or three times during the antenatal period. Fifty-six women, mainly perceived to have been at higher risk of complications (in most instances due to underlying or pre existing disease) had care provided by the obstetric unit, although they too were often seen at the hospital clinic by the midwife. Forty-one women had community-based shared care between midwives and/or GPs, going to the hospital only for scans and other tests. In eight cases, the woman received community-based midwifery-only care. Three women had private obstetric-led care.

Three of the women receiving midwife-led antenatal care were at higher risk and should have been supervised by an obstetrician. One of these women had a multiple pregnancy, another was a poorly controlled diabetic and the third was at very high risk of thromboembolism, being in a wheelchair due to an inherited disorder. For the other women, on the other hand, the midwifery-led care appeared excellent, with problems detected early and appropriate transfers made for specialist care. In one case, the midwife correctly diagnosed and referred a woman with postpartum thromboembolism, which had been missed by her GP. Three further women who had joint midwife/GP-led care were also at higher risk and should have been managed in an obstetric unit. These included a woman with a very poor past obstetric history due to severe pregnancy-induced hypertension in previous pregnancies, a woman with a very strong family history of primary pulmonary hypertension and another case of severe social exclusion and learning difficulties. Care for the other women appears to have been appropriate.

## Place of delivery

The place of delivery for the women who delivered is shown in Table 1.8. Most women were delivered in a consultant-led unit. Four women delivered in a midwife- or midwife/GP-led unit not adjacent to a consultant-led unit. Of the seven women who were classified as delivering at home, three were unexpectedly 'born before arrival' at hospital. Of the 'other' places for delivery, 15 caesarean sections were performed in A&E departments, being either 'postmortem' caesarean sections on women certified dead on arrival or 'perimortem' while the woman was still undergoing active cardiopulmonary resuscitation. One live birth and another early neonatal death were associated with the latter. Three unplanned emergency caesarean sections also took place in A&E with one live birth.

**Table 1.8**      Maternal deaths by place of delivery; United Kingdom 1997–99

| Type of death | Consultant unit | Stand-alone GP/ midwife unit | A&E | ICU | Hospital other | Home | Total |
|---|---|---|---|---|---|---|---|
| Direct | 60 | 0 | 5 | 1 | – | 1 | 67 |
| Indirect | 72 | 3 | 6 | 1 | 3 | 3 | 88 |
| Coincidental | 11 | – | 3 | 1 | 1 | – | 16 |
| Late | 98 | 1 | 1 | – | 4 | 3 | 107 |
| Total | 241 | 4 | 15 | 3 | 8 | 7 | 278 |

## Type of delivery

Table 1.9 shows the type of delivery, where known, for *Direct* and *Indirect* deaths occurring after 24 weeks of completed gestation.

**Table 1.9**      Cases by mode of delivery: *Direct* and *Indirect* deaths; United Kingdom 1997–99

| Type of delivery | Direct (n) | Indirect (n) | Total (n) |
|---|---|---|---|
| Spontaneous vaginal | 11 | 22 | 33 |
| Induced vaginal | 7 | 7 | 14 |
| Ventouse | 6 | 6 | 12 |
| Forceps | 3 | 2 | 5 |
| Vaginal breech | 1 | – | 1 |
| Caesarean section[a] | | | |
| – emergency | 14 | 9 | 23 |
| – urgent | 14 | 14 | 28 |
| – scheduled | 1 | 3 | 4 |
| – elective | 5 | 13 | 18 |
| – perimortem | 4 | 9 | 13 |
| – postmortem | 2 | 3 | 5 |
| – caesarean section total | 40 | 51 | 91 |
| Total delivered | 68 | 88 | 156 |
| Total undelivered more than 24 weeks of gestation | 5 | 19 | 24 |
| Total died before 24 weeks of gestation | 33 | 28 | 61 |
| Not known | – | 1 | 1 |
| Total | 106 | 136 | 242 |

[a] For RCOG definition see Chapter 20 Caesarean section

# Risk factors for maternal deaths

## Age

Maternal mortality is closely related to maternal age, as shown in Table 1.10 and Figure 1.5. For more robust analysis, the rates have been calculated for all maternal deaths by age between the years 1985 and 1999. A recent survey of severe maternal morbidity[1] also found a correlation between age and risk of severe maternal morbidity; women over 34 years of age were found to be at highest risk.

## Young mothers

Five school-age girls died aged 16 years or less and a total of 14 young women died aged 18 years or less. All but one were severely socially excluded. The characteristics of these deaths are shown in Table 1.11. Four of the five girls aged less than 16 years had been in the care of social services but three of these girls were homeless and living 'rough' at the time of their deaths. All but one of the deaths in women aged between 16 and 18 years were also characterised by social exclusion. Seven had suffered repeated episodes of domestic violence from within their own family and several of these also had suffered sexual abuse.

**Table 1.10** *Direct* and *Indirect* deaths by maternal age and rate per 100,000 maternities; United Kingdom 1985–99[a]

| Age | 1985–87 (n) | 1988–90 (n) | 1991–93 (n) | 1994–96 (n) | 1997–99 (n) | Overall (n) | 1985–99 (Rate) |
|---|---|---|---|---|---|---|---|
| < 20 | 15 | 17 | 7 | 15 | 19 | 71 | 8.2 |
| 20–24 | 47 | 38 | 30 | 40 | 35 | 190 | 7.2 |
| 25–29 | 53 | 74 | 87 | 71 | 61 | 346 | 9.0 |
| 30–34 | 60 | 57 | 61 | 70 | 66 | 314 | 11.5 |
| 35–39 | 35 | 31 | 36 | 53 | 50 | 205 | 20.7 |
| 40+ | 13 | 18 | 7 | 11 | 13 | 62 | 35.5 |
| Not stated | – | – | 1 | 8 | 4 | 9 | |
| Total | 223 | 238 | 229 | 268 | 242 | 1,200 | 12.1 |

[a] Denominator data supplied by ONS

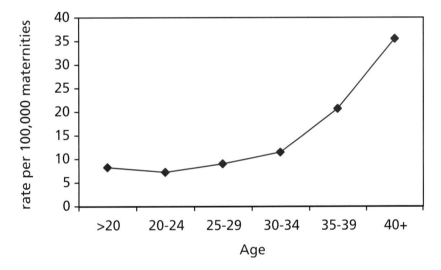

**Figure 1.5** Maternal mortality rate per 100,000 maternities, *Direct* and *Indirect* deaths by maternal age; United Kingdom 1985–99

**Table 1.11** Characteristics of maternal deaths in girls or young women aged 18 years or less

| Age (years) | (n) | Type of maternal death | | | Characteristics of social exclusion | | | | |
| | | Direct | Indirect | Coincidental | DV | Drug use | Homeless | Poor attender at clinic | Poor social circumstances |
|---|---|---|---|---|---|---|---|---|---|
| 16 or less | 5 | 3 | – | 2 | 3 | 3 | 3 | 3 | 5 |
| 17–18 | 9 | 2 | 4 | 3 | 4 | 3 | 1 | 4 | 8 |
| Total | 14 | 5 | 4 | 5 | 7 | 6 | 4 | 7 | 13 |

DV = domestic violence

## Parity

Maternal deaths are also more common in multiparous women, as shown in Table 1.12 and Figure 1.6. For more robust analysis, the rates have been calculated for all maternal deaths by age between the years 1991 and 1999. Due the large numbers of missing data for the triennia 1988–90 it has only been possible to calculate the overall rate from the data for the last three triennia.

**Table 1.12**  *Direct* and *Indirect* maternal deaths by parity and rate per 100,000 maternities; United Kingdom 1991–99

| Parity | 1991–93 (n) | 1991–93 Rate | 1994–96 (n) | 1994–96 Rate | 1997–99 (n) | 1997–99 Rate | Total 1991–99 (n) | Total 1991–99 Rate |
|---|---|---|---|---|---|---|---|---|
| 0 | 76 | 8.0 | 100 | 10.6 | 98 | 12.2 | 274 | 6.2 |
| 1 | 58 | 7.4 | 63 | 7.5 | 60 | 8.4 | 181 | 10.4 |
| 2 | 51 | 13.0 | 50 | 9.7 | 49 | 12.8 | 150 | 21.8 |
| 3 | 17 | 12.2 | 26 | 16.4 | 19 | 14.9 | 62 | 26.6 |
| 4+ | 18 | 25.6 | 13 | 10.8 | 16 | 37.7 | 47 | 35.0 |
| NS | 9 | – | 16 | – | – | – | 25 | – |
| Total | 229 | 9.8 | 268 | 12.0 | 242 | 11.4 | 739 | 11.3 |

NS = Not stated

Note: due to the large number of cases for the 1988–90 triennium, where parity was not stated, it is not possible to calculate meaningful overall rates before 1991

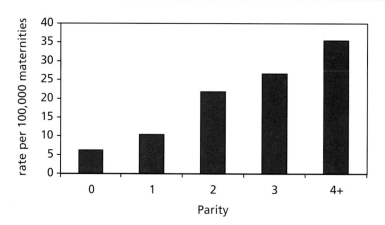

**Figure 1.6**  *Direct* and *Indirect* maternal deaths per 100,000 maternities by parity; United Kingdom 1997–99

## Multiple pregnancies

Eleven women had multiple pregnancies: nine sets of twins and two sets of triplets. These are shown in Table 1.13. Ten of these women delivered, nine by caesarean section. Six of these deaths were due to *Direct* causes, two were *Indirect* and three *Late*. Both sets of triplets were conceived by IVF. In all but one case an obstetrician supervised the antenatal care. The remaining case, in which the woman only received midwifery-led care until she developed severe complications, is discussed in Chapter 7.

Eight of these deaths were considered to be directly or indirectly associated with pregnancy. As shown in Table 1.14, this gives an overall maternal mortality rate

**Table 1.13**   Maternal deaths and multiple pregnancies; United Kingdom 1997–99

| Cause of death | Type of death | Twins (*n*) | Triplets (*n*) | Total (*n*) |
|---|---|---|---|---|
| Pregnancy-induced hypertension | *Direct* | 2 | 1 | 3 |
| Sepsis | *Direct* | 1 | 1 | 2 |
| Amniotic fluid embolism | *Direct* | 1 | – | 1 |
| Subarachnoid or berry aneurysm | *Indirect* or *Late Indirect* | 2 | – | 2 |
| Late coincidental | *Late* | 3 | – | 3 |
| Total | – | 9 | 2 | 11 |

**Table 1.14**   Maternal mortality rates for multiple pregnancies and rate per 100,000 maternities; United Kingdom 1997–99

| Type of pregnancy | *Direct & Indirect* deaths | Maternities | |
|---|---|---|---|
| | (*n*) | (*n*) | Rate |
| Singleton | 243 | 2093,965 | 11.2 |
| Twins | 6 | 29,628 | 20.3 |
| Triplets | 2 | 929 | 215.3 |
| Quads | – | 21 | – |
| Total | 242 | 2,123,614 | 11.4 |
| Data supplied by ONS | | | |

of 20.1 per 100,000 twin maternities and 21.5 per 100,000 triplet maternities compared with a maternal mortality rate of 11.2 for singleton pregnancies. These results should be interpreted with caution because of small numbers.

## Infertility

Ten women were known to have undergone IVF for infertility. Of these, there were two *Direct* deaths associated with the triplet pregnancies previously discussed. The other deaths related to singleton pregnancies, of which all eight were delivered. There were three *Direct* deaths in this group of eight, one each from pulmonary embolism, haemorrhage and ruptured ectopic pregnancy. There were three *Indirect* deaths and the remaining two were *Coincidental*. Thus, eight of the ten deaths were considered to be directly or indirectly associated with pregnancy. Figures from the Human Fertilisation and Fertilisation Authority, which are published on a financial-year basis, show that for the three financial years April 1997 to April 2000, there were 20,658 IVF maternities. Using these data as a proxy for January 1997 to December1999, the period of this Report, a maternal mortality rate of 48.4 per 100,000 IVF maternities can be estimated. As with multiple births, because of small numbers these results need to be interpreted with caution. In future, these Reports will continue to collect information on this group of women, with the aim of providing more a more robust data pool to enable more rigorous analysis.

## Ethnicity

As ONS data for the ethnic group of the mother were confined to country of birth, it is not possible to calculate directly maternal death rates by ethnic group, as many mothers will be second, third or more generation women born in the UK. Ethnic group information is now being collected as part of the Hospital Episode

Statistics (HES) system for England, but is not complete for the years covered by this Report. There was a 63% HES coverage of births by ethnic group for the period 1997–99.

Using the 1997–99 distribution by ethnic group as a best estimate for the period covered by this Report leads to the estimates of maternal death rates by ethnic group for *England*. Because specific coding was often incomplete, as with the last Report, the ONS codes for 'black African', 'black Caribbean', 'black Other' and 'black Mixed' have been grouped together, as have those from the Indian subcontinent.

As Table 1.15 shows, there is an increased risk of maternal mortality for all groups other than white. Women from India, Bangladesh and Pakistan appear to have a three-times higher risk for this triennium and black women (a composite of black African, black Caribbean, black Other and black Mixed) have a one-and-a-half times as great a risk. In the last Report, the findings for these two groups were reversed, with black women having a three times higher risk. The findings, averaged out for the last triennium and this one, show that, in general, women from ethnic groups other than white are at twice as much risk of a maternal death.

These findings also underline the care that needs to be taken in interpreting these results due to the small numbers and difficulty in coding involved.

**Table 1.15** Maternal deaths by ethnic group and rate per 100,000 maternities; England 1997–99

| Ethnic group | Direct & Indirect deaths[a] | Estimated maternities | |
|---|---|---|---|
| | (n) | (n) | Rate |
| White | 159 | 1,442,286 | 11.0 |
| Pakistani/Indian/Bangladeshi | 31 | 95,638 | 32.4 |
| Black African/Caribbean/Mixed/Other | 16 | 97,502 | 16.4 |
| Asian and Others | 7 | 50,409 | 13.9 |
| Total | 213 | 1,685,835 | 12.0 |

[a] English deaths only

There was no increase in any specific cause of maternal death by ethnic group, but there was a slight increase in the number of woman from ethnic minority groups other than white who were judged to have received major substandard care. The percentage for non-white women was 28% compared with 20% for white women.

In some cases, the care received by women from ethnic minority groups was of an exceptionally high standard. In other cases it was poor. Some of these women were recently arrived immigrants pregnant on arrival in the UK and many did not speak English. Several were late in booking and others were poor attenders at antenatal clinics. A number constantly moved address during their pregnancy making community follow up difficult.

Nearly half of the women who booked after 20 weeks in pregnancy or who were poor clinic attenders came from an ethnic minority group and half of these women did not speak English. Five women first arrived in the United Kingdom in advanced pregnancy but seem to have accessed the services relatively promptly. On the other hand, in a very few cases, some women from Asia were newly married to English men who did not appear to care about helping their wife to access antenatal care.

Chapter 10, on cardiac disease, highlights several cases where the desire to fulfil womanhood and their role in society meant that some women who knew they were at serious risk of dying from pre-existing cardiac disease minimised or ignored the seriousness of their symptoms.

Perhaps from concerns of stigmatisation, some families also refused help from the medical, midwifery and psychiatric services, preferring to care for women with severe postnatal mental illness themselves.

## Translation

In a number of cases in this Report, family members were used as interpreters for women who did not speak English. Several of these were the woman's own children, who may have been the only family members who could speak English, having learned it at school. The use of family members as translators causes concern because:

- the woman may be too shy to seek help for intimate concerns

- it is not clear how much correct information was conveyed to the woman, as the person who was interpreting did not have a good grasp of the language, or may have withheld information

- in some cases, the translator was a perpetrator of domestic violence against his partner, thus not enabling her to ask for advice or help

- in those cases where the woman's pre-existing medical condition meant that she was at significant risk of dying, it is not clear how much information was conveyed concerning the risks to her own health, and

- it is not appropriate for a child to translate intimate details about his or her mother and unfair on both the woman and child.

## Travellers

A striking finding was that six women who died in this triennium came from the travelling community. This community, to date, has not been included as a separate class by ONS when collecting ethnic group data. They are included in the 'white' category. It is therefore not possible to estimate the risk of maternal death in this group of women, despite attempts by ONS to identify suitable denominator data for this Report. Nevertheless, it is clear that this group is grossly over-represented when compared to the 'white' group of women as a whole, and quite possibly has the highest maternal death rate among all ethnic groups.

Three women died from *Direct* causes, all associated with major substandard care, and two were *Late* deaths also associated with substandard care. One woman had an *Indirect* death where the quality of care was difficult to judge. From the level of care taken over completing the report forms for this Enquiry and the tone of some of the comments contained within them, it appears that this community is at particular risk of substandard care from health service professionals.

The health of this community has already caused public health concern and Appendix 1 of this Report contains further information on this.

## Social class

For the first time, it has been possible to calculate the social class of women who had a maternal death. The highest scoring occupational code of either the woman or her partner, or the woman herself if she had no partner, was classified into one of the nine categories now used to describe social class. The UK maternities by social class used as the denominator data have been derived by using the 1999 data for 'England and Wales live births by social class' and applying the social-class proportions to the 1997–99 UK maternities (2,123,614).

**Table 1.16**  Social class of woman by type of death, estimated maternal mortality rate per 100,000 maternities and relative risk; United Kingdom 1997–99

| Social class | Direct (n) | Indirect (n) | Direct/Indirect combined (n) | Rate | 95% CI | Coincidental (n) | Late (n) | Total (n) | Rate | 95% CI |
|---|---|---|---|---|---|---|---|---|---|---|
| 1 | 3 | 2 | 5 | 2.94 | (0.96, 6.87) | 0 | 8 | 13 | 7.65 | (4.07, 13.08) |
| 2 | 9 | 16 | 25 | 4.19 | (2.71, 6.18) | 5 | 20 | 50 | 8.37 | (6.21, 11.04) |
| 3 | 13 | 18 | 31 | 15.21 | (10.33, 21.59) | 4 | 15 | 50 | 24.53 | (18.21, 32.34) |
| 4 | 9 | 24 | 33 | 5.32 | (3.66, 7.47) | 4 | 13 | 50 | 8.06 | (5.99, 10.63) |
| 5 | 14 | 12 | 26 | 8.31 | (5.43, 12.17) | 3 | 18 | 47 | 15.01 | (11.03, 19.96) |
| 6 | 8 | 4 | 12 | 11.35 | (5.87, 19.83) | 1 | 3 | 16 | 15.14 | (8.65, 24.58) |
| 7 | 0 | 7 | 7 | 23.81 | (9.57, 49.05) | 0 | 1 | 8 | 27.21 | (11.75, 53.61) |
| 8 | 1 | 4 | 5 | 38.96 | (12.65, 90.91) | 1 | 0 | 6 | 46.75 | (17.16,101.75) |
| 9 | 48 | 49 | 97 | 135.46 | (109.85, 165.25) | 11 | 29 | 137 | 191.33 | (159.32,223.33) |
| Not stated | 1 | 0 | 1 | | | 0 | 0 | 1 | | |
| Total | 106 | 136 | 242 | 11.40 | | 29 | 107 | 378 | 17.80 | |

**Key**

Social classes as defined by ONS:

Social class 1 = I Professional
Social class 2 = II Managerial
Social class 3 = IIIN Skilled occupations-non manual
Social class 4 = IIIM Skilled occupations-manual
Social class 5 = IV Partly skilled
Social class 6 = V Unskilled
Social class 7 = Armed forces
Social class 8 = Inadequately described occupations
Social class 9 = Housewife/husband, full-time carer, full-time student, permanently sick, independent means, no previous occupation, not stated

The results are shown in Table 1.16 and confirm what has long been suspected, that women in the lower social classes have a higher risk of maternal death. Women from the most deprived circumstances appear to have a twenty times greater risk of dying of *Direct* or *Indirect* causes than women from social classes 1 and 2.

**Table 1.17**  Characteristics of antenatal clinic attendance; United Kingdom 1997–99

| | Total deaths (n) | Late booker (>22 weeks) (n) | Late booker (<28 weeks) (n) | Poor attender at ANC[b] (n) | No antenatal care (n) | Total late or non-attenders (n) | Percentage of all deaths (%) |
|---|---|---|---|---|---|---|---|
| *Direct* | 89[a] | 3 | 4 | 10 | 2 | 19 | 21 |
| *Indirect* | 128[a] | 10 | 2 | 10 | 2 | 24 | 19 |
| *Coincidental* | 25[a] | | 1 | 2 | | 2 | 12 |
| *Late* | 71 | | 1 | 6 | 1 | 8 | 11 |
| Total | 313 | 13 | 8 | 28 | 5 | 53 | 17 |

[a] Excluding early deaths; [b] missed four or more appointments; ANC = antenatal clinic

The causes of death across all social classes will be the subject of a further study, to be published later but, in general, this disparity could be seen for all causes of maternal death apart from suicide, which showed little gradient.

## Access to care

For the first time, this Report has also been able to look in more depth at access to care. Table 1.17 shows that over one-fifth of the women who had a *Direct* death did not receive optimum antenatal care, in that they booked late or were described as poor attenders at the antenatal clinic. In the vast majority of cases these women were not actively followed up when they failed to attend the clinic.

## Women who booked late

Twenty per cent of the women who died from *Direct* and *Indirect* causes booked after 20 weeks of gestation. A disproportionate number of these women came from ethnic groups other than white.

HES data show that women from non-white ethnic groups are twice as likely to book later than 20 weeks of gestation. Late bookers constitute about 8% of the white pregnant population and 17% of the non-white pregnant population. Among the women who died from *Direct* or *Indirect* causes in this Report, 20% of those who booked late were from non-white ethnic groups compared with 12% of white women.

### *Further characteristics of women who booked late or who were poor attenders at clinic*

The predominant characteristics of these women are shown in Table 1.18. Poor attenders are defined as women who missed four or more antenatal visits. Sixteen per cent of deaths from *Direct* or *Indirect* causes were in women with obvious social exclusion. Strikingly, 38% of women who died from *Coincidental* (*Fortuitous*) causes also appeared to be socially excluded and lessons also need to be drawn from this group. By comparison, only 6% of women who died after 42 days after delivery

**Table 1.18**    Analysis of late bookers (> 20 weeks of gestation) or poor attenders by predominant characteristic

| Predominant characteristic[a] | Direct (n) | Indirect (n) | Coincidental (n) | Late (n) | Total (n) |
|---|---|---|---|---|---|
| Domestic violence (DV) | 4 | 3 | 1 | 2 | 10 |
| Little/no English | 5 | 3 | 1 | – | 9 |
| Substance misuse (3 with DV) | 1 | 2 | 2 | 1 | 6 |
| Extreme poverty | 1 | 5 | – | – | 6 |
| Just arrived in UK | 1 | 3 | 1 | – | 5 |
| Homeless/constant change of address | 1 | 3 | 2 | – | 6 |
| Grande multipara (2 had alcohol problems) | 1 | 1 | – | 2 | 4 |
| Under 16 years old | 1 | – | 2 | – | 3 |
| Always concealed pregnancies | – | – | 1 | 1 | 2 |
| Unaware pregnant | 1 | 1 | – | – | 2 |
| No reason obvious | 1 | 1 | 1 | – | 3 |
| Total late bookers | 17 | 22 | 11 | 6 | 56 |
| Total type | 106 | 136 | 29 | 107 | 377 |
| Total of maternal deaths by type (%) | 16% | 16% | 38% | 6% | 13% |

[a] Most had more than one characteristic

and reported to this Enquiry (*Late* deaths) had these features. Five women also had children on the at-risk register or who had been taken into care.

## Marital status

Thirty-three percent of the women who had a *Direct* or *Indirect* maternal death in 1997–99 were known to be married at the time of death and 45% were living in a stable relationship. Of the 22% of deaths that occurred in women who did not have a partner, more than half were in women who were alone and appeared to be unsupported by their families.

## Geographical distribution

There was no over- or under-representation among English regions, Scotland, Wales or Northern Ireland, or by individual hospital or community Trust, other than that which could have been expected by chance.

# Reference

1.  Waterstone M, Bewley S, Wolfe C. Incidence and predictors of severe obstetric morbidity: case–control study. *BMJ* 2001;322:1089–94.

# Key recommendations

1. The importance of seeking antenatal care early in pregnancy should be part of health education and promotion materials prepared for all groups in society.

2. The planning and delivery of maternity services should focus on approaching each woman as an individual with different social, physical and emotional needs, as well as specific clinical factors that may affect her pregnancy. Her pregnancy must not be viewed in isolation from other important factors that may influence her health or that of her developing baby.

3. Antenatal services should be flexible enough to meet the needs of all women. The needs of those from the most vulnerable and less articulate groups in society are of equal if not more importance. Many women in this Report found it difficult to access or maintain access with the services and follow-up for those who failed to attend was poor.

4. When planning new methods of service provision it is helpful to involve women who might have difficulties in using the services. Where this has been done, antenatal clinic attendances have significantly improved. Such flexibility may require imaginative solutions in terms of the timing and setting for antenatal clinics and the provision of outreach services.

5. At booking, a risk and needs assessment should take place to ensure every woman will have a flexible care plan adapted to her own particular requirements for antenatal care. This should be reviewed regularly.

6. Health professionals who work with disadvantaged clients need to be able to understand a woman's social and cultural background, act as an advocate for women, overcome their own personal and social prejudices and practise in a reflective manner.

7. All healthcare professionals should consider whether there are unrecognised but inherent racial prejudices within their own organisations, in terms of providing an equal service to all users.

8. Interpreters should be provided for women who do not speak English. The use of family members, including children as interpreters, should be avoided if at all possible.

# *Direct* deaths

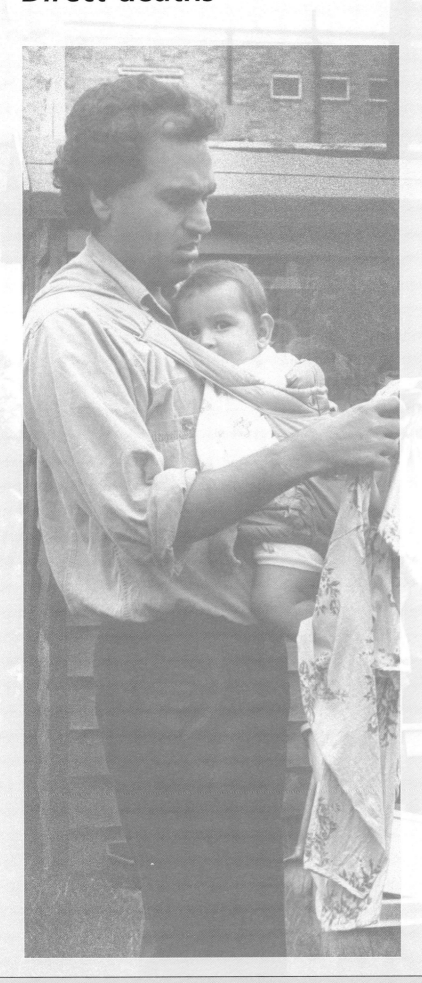

## CHAPTER 2

# Thrombosis and thromboembolism

JAMES DRIFE on behalf of the Editorial Board

## Thrombosis and thromboembolism: key recommendations

- At booking the body mass index (BMI) should be routinely calculated to identify women whose BMI is over 30 kg/m². A past history or family history of thromboembolism should be sought and, if present, specialist advice should be obtained.

- Women with other risk factors for deep vein thrombosis (DVT): e.g. bed rest, pre-eclampsia, other medical disorders, should be carefully screened and consideration given to thromboprophylaxis.

- All women undergoing caesarean section should receive prophylaxis against venous thromboembolism (VTE). Multiple risk factors are often present and the most effective method of prophylaxis, heparin at appropriate doses, should be used.

- Wider use of thromboprophylaxis (not only after caesarean section) and better investigation of classic symptoms (particularly in high-risk women) are urgently recommended.

- In view of the continuing evidence that doctors in general medicine and accident and emergency (A&E) medicine remain unaware of the recommendations made repeatedly in these Reports, we again recommend that any pregnant woman sent to A&E must be seen by a senior obstetrician.

- Midwives, general practitioners and other medical staff should pay particular attention to women in the puerperium with chest or leg symptoms after vaginal delivery in order to exclude the presence of DVT or potential pulmonary embolism.

- If a pregnant woman displays chest or leg symptoms, duplex ultrasound and/or ventilation/perfusion lung scanning should be used to exclude the presence of DVT or pulmonary embolism. Neither carries any significant risk to mother or fetus. Individual hospitals should have an agreed protocol for the objective diagnosis of suspected VTE during pregnancy.

- These Reports have repeatedly stressed that chest X-ray is not contraindicated in pregnancy.

- In clinically suspected DVT or pulmonary thromboembolism, treatment with unfractionated heparin or low-molecular-weight heparin should be given until the diagnosis is excluded by objective testing, unless treatment is strongly contraindicated.

- Subcutaneous unfractionated heparin is an effective alternative to intravenous unfractionated heparin for the initial management of DVT.

## Summary

There are 35 deaths from thrombosis and/or thromboembolism counted in this Chapter: 31 from pulmonary embolism and four from cerebral thrombosis. In addition, nine *Late* deaths from pulmonary embolism are counted in Chapter 15.

Of the deaths from pulmonary embolism, 13 were antepartum, eight being in the first trimester of pregnancy. One further death followed a miscarriage. Of the 17 postpartum deaths, ten followed vaginal delivery. The other seven postpartum deaths followed caesarean section but in three of these cases the operation had been performed in an attempt to save the baby after massive antepartum pulmonary embolism. Of the four other deaths, three women had received inadequate thromboprophylaxis and only one had received no thromboprophylaxis at all.

The total of 31 deaths from pulmonary embolism represents a substantial reduction from the 46 cases in 1994–96. This is mainly due to a dramatic fall in deaths after caesarean section, following the publication, in 1995, of Royal College of Obstetricians and Gynaecologists (RCOG) guidelines on thromboprophylaxis at caesarean section.[1] The fall was not due to delaying death from thromboembolism after operation; only one of the nine *Late* deaths followed caesarean section.

Risk factors for thromboembolism were present in 25 of the 31 cases. Thirteen women were overweight, five had had a period of bed rest, four had a family history, three had previous thromboembolism, two had undertaken long-haul flights during pregnancy and one had varicose veins. Some had multiple risk factors. In addition to these risk factors, 18 of the women were aged over 30 years.

Of the six women with no recorded risk factors, five died before 25 weeks of gestation. It is possible that thrombophilia may have been a factor in these deaths. A family history of thromboembolism should be carefully sought at booking.

Five of the nine *Late* deaths were associated with the oral contraceptive pill; all five women were overweight and in two their obesity should have contraindicated the combined oral contraceptive pill.

Substandard care was present in 57% of cases, usually in the form of failure to investigate classic symptoms in women with obvious risk factors. There is still an urgent need to educate GPs and casualty officers that the risk of thromboembolism is increased from early pregnancy until the late puerperium.

The gratifying reduction in deaths after caesarean section points the way to further improvements. More notice should be taken of other risk factors. The recommendation in the 1994–96 Report is repeated with added emphasis: 'Wider use of thromboprophylaxis *(not only after caesarean section)* and better investigation of classic symptoms (particularly in high-risk women) are urgently recommended'.

# Pulmonary embolism

Despite a fall in this triennium, pulmonary embolism (PE) is still the leading *Direct* cause of maternal death in the United Kingdom. The total of 31 deaths (excluding *Late* deaths) equates to a rate of 1.45 per 100,000 maternities. Table 2.1 shows the comparison with previous triennia.

**Table 2.1** Deaths from pulmonary embolism (excluding *Late* deaths) and rates per 100,000 maternities; United Kingdom 1985–99

| Triennium | Total (n) | After miscarriage/ ectopic (n) | Antepartum (n) | In labour (n) | After CS (n) | After vaginal delivery (n) | Rate[a] |
|---|---|---|---|---|---|---|---|
| 1985–87 | 30 | 1 | 16 | 0 | 7 | 6 | 1.3 |
| 1988–90 | 24 | 3 | 10 | 0 | 8 | 3 | 1.2 |
| 1991–93 | 30 | 0 | 12 | 1 | 13 | 4 | 1.3 |
| 1994–96 | 46 | 3 | 15 | 0 | 15 | 10 | 2.1 |
| 1997–99 | 31 | 1 | 13 | 0 | 4[a] | 10 | 1.4 |

Another 3 deaths followed caesarean section performed after antepartum collapse; CS = caesarean section

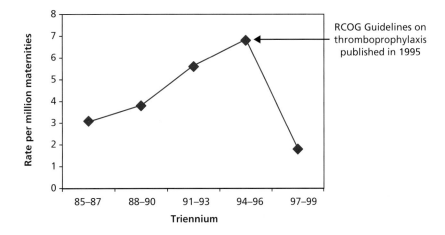

**Figure 2.1** Deaths from pulmonary embolism following caesarean section, rate per million maternities; United Kingdom 1985–99

Compared with 1994–96 there has been little change in most categories but a striking fall in deaths after caesarean section. The number of embolisms occurring after caesarean section fell from 15 to four. In another three cases death occurred after caesarean section, which had been undertaken in an attempt to save the baby after antepartum collapse. This fall, as shown in Figure 2.1, is all the more remarkable in view of the continuing rise in the caesarean section rate between 1994 and 1999.

### Cases counted in other Chapters

One case is counted in Chapter 8; Genital tract trauma:

A woman who had had a previous caesarean section developed a deep vein thrombosis (DVT) in the middle trimester of pregnancy. There was a family history of thrombophilia. Labour was induced with prostaglandins because of postmaturity and delivery was by vacuum extraction because of fetal distress. She developed primary postpartum haemorrhage and at laparotomy a scar dehiscence was repaired. Further severe bleeding occurred and she underwent hysterectomy. She was transferred to an intensive care unit (ICU) but developed multiorgan failure and died.

The cause of death was haemorrhage due to the dehiscence of the uterine scar. A history of anticoagulation may be relevant in cases of severe haemorrhage and it is not clear when the anticoagulants were stopped in this case.

## Risk factors

Risk factors for venous thromboembolism (VTE) were present in no fewer than 25 of the 31 women. Of the five who had no apparent risk factors, all died before 25 weeks of gestation. In one other case, details (including the woman's weight) were not recorded. It is possible that, in these six cases, risk factors such as a positive family history were present but unreported. All cases of VTE in the third trimester and after delivery were associated with one or more risk factors. In 13 of these 17 cases the woman was overweight (BMI greater than $30\text{kg/m}^2$).

### Age

Age has been identified in previous Reports as a risk factor for VTE. The age distribution of deaths from pulmonary embolism in 1997–99 is shown in Table 2.2.

Table 2.2    Age and pulmonary embolism: *Direct* and *Late* deaths; United Kingdom 1997–99

| Age (years) | *Direct* deaths (n) | *Late* deaths (n) | Total (n) | Rate per 100,000 maternities |
|---|---|---|---|---|
| < 20 | 1 | 1 | 2 | 1.2 |
| 20–24 | 4 | 3 | 7 | 1.6 |
| 25–29 | 6 | 1 | 7 | 1.1 |
| 30–34 | 11 | 3 | 14 | 2.2 |
| 35–39 | 8 | 1 | 9 | 3.5 |
| 40+ | 1 | | 1 | 2.2 |
| Total | 31 | 9 | 40 | 1.9 |

### Air travel

Two women died after long-haul flights in pregnancy. One died at 25 weeks of gestation and the other at 36 weeks. Annex D to this Chapter summarises the recent advice of the RCOG to help prevent thromboembolism in pregnant women who travel by air.

## Family history

Four women were known to have a strong family history of thromboembolism in a first-degree relative such as a mother or sister. In all four cases, embolism occurred before labour.

## Previous history

Three women had a previous thromboembolism. One of these women died before delivery and the other two died after vaginal delivery. Two were obese. In two cases the social circumstances were particularly poor.

## Immobility

In five cases embolism occurred after a period of bed rest. In four of these the embolism occurred before labour. In three, the woman's weight was also a risk factor.

## Maternal weight

Obesity is also well known to be a risk factor for thromboembolism but nowadays maternal weight is poorly recorded in maternity notes in the UK. Among the 31 deaths from pulmonary embolism, weight was recorded in only 21 cases, sometimes at autopsy rather than in the clinic. In three cases, there was no indication whatever of the weight or build of the woman. Of the remaining 28 cases, two women were described by the pathologist as 'well nourished'. The weights or descriptions of the other 26 are given in Table 2.3.

Of the nine *Late* deaths, the woman's weight was not recorded in one case. Of the remaining eight cases, one woman was described by the pathologist as 'heavily built'. The weights or description of the other seven are given in Table 2.3.

The table indicates that the risk of death from pulmonary embolism rises with increasing weight. This should be taken into account when thromboprophylaxis is considered.

Table 2.3     Weight and pulmonary embolism, *Direct* and *Late* deaths; United Kingdom 1997–99

| Clinical or pathological description | Maternal weight (kg) | *Direct* deaths (*n*) | *Late* deaths (*n*) |
|---|---|---|---|
| 'Thin' | | 2 | – |
| | 49–60 | 5 | 1 |
| | 61–70 | 2 | – |
| | 71–80 | 4 | 1 |
| | 81–90 | 4 | 1 |
| | 91–100 | – | 2 |
| | >100 | 6 | 1 |
| 'Obese'[a] | | 3 | 1 |
| Total | | 26 | 7 |

[a] Includes 'grossly obese' and 'morbid obesity'

## Oral contraception

Maternal weight is also important after delivery when contraception is discussed. Five of the nine *Late* deaths followed the prescription of combined oral contraceptives to overweight women. Two of these cases are described here:

> A primigravid woman aged over 30 years weighed over 110 kg at booking. She developed leg ulcers associated with swelling during pregnancy. A DVT was excluded in the puerperium and she was prescribed a low-dose combined oral contraceptive pill. Several months after delivery she developed a painful swollen leg and a few days later she collapsed and died. Autopsy showed DVT and massive pulmonary embolism.

This woman's BMI at booking was 41 kg/m$^2$. The combined contraceptive pill was therefore contraindicated. She did not seek medical advice for her leg swelling.

> A parous woman aged under 30 years had a normal pregnancy and delivery. She weighed over 90 kg at booking but lost weight during pregnancy and weighed about 85 kg at term. She was under five feet in height. About two months after delivery she started on the combined oral contraceptive pill and a few weeks later died of pulmonary embolism.

At booking, this woman's BMI was 39.5 kg/m$^2$, which would contraindicate the combined pill. At term, her BMI was 37.3 kg/m$^2$, which requires the pill to be used 'with caution'.

The importance of weight as a contraindication for the combined contraceptive pill seems insufficiently appreciated and is therefore summarised here. The *British National Formulary* (BNF) gives the advice shown in Box 2.1, in its section on the combined oral contraceptive pill.

---

**Box 2.1    BNF advice on combined oral contraceptive use and risk factors for venous thromboembolism**

Use with **caution** if any of following risk factors present but **avoid** if two or more factors present:

- *Family history of venous thromboembolism* in first degree relative aged under 45 years

- *Obesity* – BMI above 30 kg/m$^2$ (avoid if BMI above 39 kg/m$^2$)

- *Long term immobilisation*, e.g. in a wheelchair

- *Varicose veins* (avoid…where definite history of thrombosis).

---

Thus, the BNF advises that the combined pill should be 'used with caution' when the BMI is above 30 kg/m$^2$ and avoided altogether when the BMI is over 39 kg/m$^2$. Computer programs for GPs calculate the BMI automatically when the basic data are entered and simple plastic calculators are also available. Without such aids, the BMI is awkward to calculate: it is the woman's weight in kilograms divided by the square of her height in metres. Few people in the UK know their height in metres. As a guide, Box 2.2 gives examples of weights above which the combined oral contraceptive pill should be 'used with caution' or avoided altogether.

| Box 2.2 | Heights and weights when the combined oral contraceptive pill should be used with caution or avoided | |
|---|---|---|
| Height | BMI 30 kg/m² ('caution') | BMI 39 kg/m² ('avoid') |
| 5' (1.52 m) | 69 kg | 90 kg |
| 5' 3' (1.60 m) | 77 kg | 100 kg |
| 5' 6' (1.68 m) | 85 kg | 110 kg |

Among the five *Late* deaths associated with the combined pill in this triennium, the BMI of two women was probably above 39 kg/m² and was above 30 kg/m² in all five. It is therefore recommended that 'caution' in the puerperium should mean advising overweight women to delay starting the combined oral contraceptive pill until several months after delivery.

## Risk factors for thromboembolism: conclusions

More attention needs to be paid to risk factors for three reasons.

### Thromboprophylaxis

A combination of risk factors, or even a single factor, may indicate thromboprophylaxis during or after pregnancy. Caesarean section, formerly a major risk factor, has been made safer by the widespread use of appropriate thromboprophylaxis and this shows what could be achieved.

### Significance of symptoms

The presence of one or more risk factors should alert the clinician when a woman presents with symptoms suggestive of VTE. Several cases described below show substandard care in this regard.

### Contraception

Risk factors must be taken into account in discussing contraception after delivery.

## Antepartum deaths

A total of 13 patients died from pulmonary embolism during the antenatal period. The gestations were: up to 12 weeks (8); 13–24 weeks (3) and 24 weeks to term (2).

More than 50% of the antepartum deaths were in the first trimester. Even at this early stage, pregnancy carries a risk of thrombosis and additional risk factors such as bed rest, dehydration and hyperemesis should indicate thromboprophylaxis.

Both unfractionated heparin and low-molecular-weight heparins are safe in early pregnancy as they do not cross the placenta.

Many of these women were not under the direct care of an obstetrician at the time of their death, although several had seen their GP or a hospital specialist or had attended A&E. Details of the cases are summarised in Table 2.4.

### Failure of diagnosis

In three of the cases in Table 2.4 a GP failed to refer a woman for investigation of possible VTE after she complained of typical symptoms. In two of those cases, risk factors – obesity or family history – were also present:

> A primigravida with a very strong family history of thromboembolism complained of chest pain at eight weeks of pregnancy. A GP diagnosed intercostal muscle strain. The next day another GP found no evidence of DVT but diagnosed 'pulmonary embolism/infection'. On the third day, a further GP admitted her to hospital. She was treated with heparin but ten days later complained again of breathlessness and one day later she died.

The family history should have suggested testing for thrombophilia before pregnancy and should have alerted the doctors that pulmonary embolism was a likely diagnosis. The failure of heparin treatment in hospital suggests that the dosage may have been inadequate. This is discussed further below.

In other cases, hospital teams failed to carry out appropriate investigations:

> A woman aged over 30 years was referred by her GP at eight weeks of gestation to A&E with a three-week history of dyspnoea at rest and slight cyanosis of the lips on exertion. A junior doctor noted mild tachycardia, diminished air entry at the right base and a palpable liver edge, and wrote that pulmonary embolism should be excluded. Her respiratory rate was 24 bpm and the D dimer was positive. A medical registrar wrote that chest X-ray was contraindicated in pregnancy. The case was discussed with an obstetric registrar and the woman was discharged without treatment. She died at home next day of massive pulmonary embolism.

Although pulmonary embolism can be elusive, in this case it is difficult to know what other diagnosis could have explained this constellation of signs and symptoms. **These Reports have repeatedly stressed that chest X-ray is not contraindicated in pregnancy.**

> An overweight woman aged over 30 years and with a strong family history of thromboembolic disease developed thrombophlebitis and was admitted to A&E at eight weeks of gestation with chest pain. The GP had suggested a diagnosis of PE but a medical registrar again believed that chest X-ray or anticoagulation were contraindicated by pregnancy and the woman was allowed home with diagnosis of 'musculoskeletal pain'. Three days later she saw the GP who thought that PE had been excluded. Two days later, she attended hospital with classic symptoms including haemoptysis. She was transferred to major

**Table 2.4**      Antepartum deaths from pulmonary embolism (PE); United Kingdom 1997–99

| Gestation (weeks) | Risk factors | Features |
|---|---|---|
| 8 | Bed rest | Age < 31 years<br>3-week history of hyperemesis<br>Admitted for rehydration, collapsed next day |
| 8 | Bed rest<br>Age > 35 years | Complained of leg pain – calves symmetrical |
| 8 | Family history<br>Previous PE<br>Gross obesity<br>Age > 35 years | Admitted with PE at 8 weeks<br>Anticoagulated with low-molecular-weight heparin<br>No account taken of her weight in calculating the dose |
| 8 | Family history | Complained of chest pain to three GPs:<br>– one diagnosed muscle strain<br>– one diagnosed infection<br>– third diagnosed pulmonary embolism<br>Inadequately heparinised in hospital |
| 8 | None apparent | Referred to A&E with 3-week history of dyspnoea and slight cyanosis on exertion<br>Diminished air entry at right base<br>Respiratory rate 24/min<br>D dimer positive<br>Discharged without treatment<br>Died next day |
| 8 | Family history<br>Overweight<br>Thrombophlebitis | Admitted with chest pain<br>'No chest X-ray due to pregnancy'<br>Diagnosis: musculoskeletal pain<br>GP thought PE had been excluded by hospital<br>Seen at hospital with pain and haemoptysis<br>Transferred to major centre: 'not typical' of PE<br>Waited 24 hours for a ventilation/perfusion scan: died while waiting |
| 8 | High parity<br>'Well nourished' | 4 days after pregnancy confirmed, complained of shortness of breath and chest pains<br>Collapsed and died at home |
| 10 | None apparent | Age < 31 years<br>Collapsed twice in early pregnancy: no diagnosis made<br>Remained in coma until middle trimester |
| 21 | Age > 35 years | Dyspnoea at 16 weeks<br>PE looked for but not found<br>Collapsed and died five weeks later |
| 23 | None apparent | Age < 25 years<br>Sudden death at home |
| 24 | Long flight | Age < 25 years<br>Very long flights at 15 and 19 weeks<br>At 24 weeks, walked into A&E with 1 day history of dizziness and dyspnoea<br>Collapsed within five minutes |
| 25 | None apparent | Consulted GP with breathing disturbance and tingling fingers<br>Diagnosis: hyperventilation due to panic attacks<br>Collapsed and died a few days later |
| 34 | Obese | Phoned GP with breathlessness and pain on inspiration<br>Routine visit arranged<br>Died before she was seen |

centre where the clinical picture was considered 'not typical' of PE. A V/Q scan was arranged for the following day but she died in the meantime.

In this case, the family history was ignored, the GP's clinical diagnosis was overridden for erroneous reasons, there was failure of communication between hospital and GP and there was delay in arranging a ventilation/perfusion scan.

**In view of the continuing evidence that doctors in general medicine and A&E remain unaware of the recommendations made repeatedly in these Reports, we again recommend that any pregnant woman sent to A&E must be seen by a senior obstetrician.**

### Failure of treatment

One case of failure of heparin treatment has already been described. Another treatment failure can be attributed to failure to recognise the importance of maternal weight:

> A woman aged over 35 years with a strong family history of PE and a past history of PE in the puerperium was admitted with a DVT and PE in the first trimester of pregnancy. She weighed over 140 kg. She was treated with twice-daily dalteparin injections and allowed home on this regimen. She died two weeks later of massive PE.

This woman probably had hereditary thrombophilia in addition to her gross obesity. The therapeutic dose of dalteparin is 200 units/kg/24 hours, which in this patient would be 29,600 units/day. According to the manufacturer's data sheet, the maximum daily dose is 18,000 units. This woman received no more than 10,000 units daily. No account seems to have been taken of the fact that the therapeutic dose of dalteparin is weight-dependent.

A recent RCOG Guideline, *Thromboembolic Disease in Pregnancy and the Puerperium: Acute Management*,[2] gives detailed advice on the initial therapeutic dosage of low-molecular-weight heparin and this is reproduced in Box 2.3.

| Box 2.3 Therapeutic dosage for low molecular weight heparin | |
| --- | --- |
| **Early pregnancy weight** | **Initial dose of enoxaparin** |
| < 50 kg | 40 mg twice daily |
| 50–69 kg | 60 mg twice daily |
| 70–89 kg | 80 mg twice daily |
| > 90 kg | 100 mg twice daily |

## Deaths after caesarean section

Caesarean section, like other major surgical procedures, is a risk factor for VTE. After the introduction of RCOG guidelines on thromboprophylaxis,[3] the number of cases of postoperative embolism has been reduced from 15 in 1994–96 to four in the present triennium. Three other deaths occurred after antepartum embolism followed by caesarean section, performed in an attempt to save the baby after maternal collapse. These cases are described in Table 2.5.

In the last triennium, 1994–96, most deaths after caesarean section occurred 15–42 days after delivery, and there was concern that thromboprophylaxis might be delaying but not fully preventing the formation of thrombus. This is not supported by the 1997–99 figures, which show a completely different pattern. In the present triennium, all the *Direct* deaths occurred within the first week after operation. One *Late* death occurred eight weeks after operation.

Of the seven women in Table 2.5, four were socially disadvantaged. In one such case the woman had limited English and this may have made her reluctant to seek medical help:

> A woman who had limited English booked at hospital and had midwifery care at home. After being seen at 25 weeks, she undertook a long-haul flight and returned several weeks later. At 35 weeks, she developed intermittent breathlessness but was reluctant to call her GP. The midwife visited her at home. Three days later she collapsed. Cardiopulmonary resuscitation was unsuccessful and she underwent postmortem caesarean section in the A&E department.

Midwives should not have to take responsibility for excluding general disease during pregnancy but should know that pregnancy increases the risk of pulmonary embolism, which presents with breathlessness. In this case, there were communication difficulties due to the woman's limited English. The midwifery assessor commented that the midwife should have contacted the GP herself and requested a visit, based on the fact that the patient had been abroad and was unwell.

Three of the women in Table 2.5 were overweight and another two were obese:

> A young primigravida who had suffered childhood asthma developed pre-eclampsia at 34 weeks, when her weight was over 150 kg. After failed induction of labour she underwent caesarean section. She wore anti-embolism stockings during the operation and received heparin (5000 units twice daily) for three days after operation. She mobilised early and was discharged on day six. On day 28, she complained of pain in the leg and buttock. On day 35, she complained of breathlessness and the GP diagnosed asthma. Later that day, she was readmitted to hospital, where pulmonary embolism was diagnosed. She was treated with heparin but died within two hours of admission. Autopsy confirmed DVT and pulmonary embolism.

In view of her high-risk status, anticoagulation might have been started during pregnancy and continued for longer than three days. Heparin levels may not have been adequate in view of her weight. The significance of her leg and chest symptoms was not appreciated soon enough.

> An obese primigravida had a breech presentation diagnosed at 34 weeks. At 36+ weeks she was admitted with ruptured membranes and underwent caesarean section. She went home on day 4 with a

**Table 2.5** Deaths from pulmonary embolism (PE) following caesarean section; United Kingdom 1997–99

| PE (days after delivery) | Risk factors | Features |
|---|---|---|
| Before delivery | Overweight<br>Bed rest | Age < 25 years<br>Disadvantaged background<br>Admitted at 30 weeks with diarrhoea, vomiting and pyrexia<br>? chest infection<br>Breathing problems required oxygen, intubation and ventilation<br>CS<br>Died after 7 days in ICU<br>Autopsy showed multiple thrombi/emboli of several days' duration |
| Before delivery | Long flight | Limited English<br>Intermittent breathlessness at 36 weeks after long-haul flight<br>Reluctant to involve GP<br>Visited by midwife<br>Collapsed at home 3 days later<br>Arrested<br>Postmortem CS in A&E |
| Before delivery | Family history<br>Bed rest | IVF pregnancy<br>Polyhydramnios<br>Admitted for rest at 32 weeks<br>DVT confirmed by venogram at 34 weeks<br>Collapsed 1 week later<br>Perimortem CS and thoracotomy |
| 1 | Overweight | Failed induction at 38 weeks<br>CS<br>Collapsed on day 1 and died on day 11<br>Thromboprophylaxis probably inadequate |
| 2 | Overweight<br>Bed rest | SROM at 34 weeks<br>Thromboprophylaxis started after CS<br>Leg swelling noted on day 2<br>Died later that day |
| 6 | Obese | CS and discharged on day 4<br>Breathlessness on day 5<br>GP visited<br>Collapsed on day 6<br>Died on day 21 |
| 35 | Obese<br>Bed rest | Age < 25 years<br>Diabetic, weight > 150 kg<br>Pre-eclampsia<br>4 weeks in hospital<br>Failed induction at 34 weeks<br>CS<br>Anti-embolism stockings and boots<br>Heparin 5000 units bd for 3 days after delivery<br>Complained of breathlessness, died soon after admission to ICU |

CS = caesarean section; DVT = deep vein thrombosis; ICU = intensive care unit; IVF = *in vitro* fertilisation; SROM = spontaneous rupture of membranes haemoglobin of 8.4 gm%. The next day the midwife noted that she was breathless and had pain in upper back. The GP visited her at home. On day 6 she collapsed at home, and despite intensive treatment she died two weeks later.

External cephalic version (ECV) might have avoided the need for caesarean section but was not offered. She received no thromboprophylaxis despite her obesity. Her weight was not recorded. The midwife was concerned about pulmonary embolism but, as in the previous case above, the GP did not investigate her symptoms despite her high-risk status.

The most striking feature of Table 2.5, however, is that it includes many fewer cases than in the last Report and three of the four women who dies after caesarean section did receive some form of thromboprophylaxis, although it was inadequate. This attests to the importance of the major recommendation in the last Report, which is repeated here. **All women undergoing caesarean section should receive prophylaxis against VTE. Multiple risk factors are often present and the most effective method of prophylaxis, heparin at appropriate doses, should be used.**

## Deaths after vaginal delivery

There were ten deaths from thromboembolism after vaginal delivery, the same number as in 1994–96. The details of these ten cases are summarised in Table 2.6. In contrast to the pattern following caesarean section, only one of these deaths occurred in the first 12 days after vaginal delivery. Only one of these cases involved instrumental delivery. The other nine deaths followed normal deliveries.

### Inadequate thromboprophylaxis

Risk factors were present in at least nine cases. Seven of the ten women were overweight and in one other case the weight was not recorded. Of the three women who were not known to be overweight, all were aged over 35 years, one had a history of previous thromboembolism and one had had previous varicose vein surgery. All the women aged under 35 years were overweight and four of them had another risk factor. The recommendation in the previous Report is repeated here. **Women with risk factors for DVT (e.g. bed rest, pre-eclampsia, other medical disorders, family history) should be carefully screened and consideration given to thromboprophylaxis.**

There is a clear need for the development of national guidelines on thromboprophylaxis after normal delivery. The 1995 RCOG Guideline[1] focuses largely on caesarean section. Many maternity units have now drawn up their own guidelines for vaginal delivery, whereby women, such as those over 35 years and the obese, receive thromboprophylaxis. One such guideline, developed in the Glasgow Royal Maternity Hospital, is reproduced at the end of this Chapter (Annex A).

### Failure of diagnosis

In two cases, the woman was seen by her GP but the diagnosis was missed. In another case, the diagnosis was missed by both the GP and the A&E department:

> An overweight primigravida had a normal delivery at term and went home on day two. On day 12, she developed back pain due to a 'disc lesion' and was immobilised for two weeks. She developed chest pain, which the GP diagnosed as 'musculoskeletal'. That evening she called the midwife because she was clammy and was losing consciousness. She had a tachycardia. She was sent to A&E where slight vaginal bleeding was noted. This was diagnosed as 'postpartum haemorrhage' and she was transferred to an obstetric unit on another site. She died en route.

Obesity and immobility are risk factors for DVT, particularly in the puerperium. Prophylactic heparin should have been considered. Chest pain after two weeks of immobilisation should not be dismissed as 'musculoskeletal', particularly in an overweight patient. It is of particular concern that the A&E department missed the diagnosis when the woman was mortally ill.

**Midwives, GPs and other medical staff should pay particular attention to women in the puerperium with chest or leg symptoms after vaginal delivery in order to exclude the presence of DVT or potential pulmonary embolism.**

### Failure of heparin treatment

In three cases, the social circumstances were poor and, in two of those cases, disadvantaged women who had a previous history of VTE were discharged soon after delivery with a supply of heparin for self administration. One of those women had concealed her pregnancy and the other had a history of poor attendance at the anticoagulant clinic. The combination of early discharge and self-administered injections may not be appropriate in such cases.

In another case of failure of treatment, a woman had a pulmonary embolism diagnosed and was treated with low-molecular-weight heparin in hospital. When she deteriorated, streptokinase was administered but she deteriorated further and died.

### Drug adverse effects

An adverse effect of antipsychotic medication has been reported very recently:

> A woman aged over 30 years with a previous history of postnatal mental illness had a normal delivery at term and went home on day two. On day six, she was admitted to a psychiatric hospital with puerperal psychosis. She was treated with risperidone and fluoxetine and discharged after two weeks. Two weeks later, she collapsed at home and died.

The pathologist confirmed a massive pulmonary embolism and reported that she was moderately obese. There is no other record of her weight. A recent study in the *Lancet*[3] reports an increased risk of thromboembolism among patients taking antipsychotic drugs. The overall odds ratio is 7 but the risk is lower for 'high-potency' drugs than 'low-potency' drugs. Risperidone appears to be a 'high-potency' antipsychotic drug. Fluoxetine is an antidepressant (selective serotonin reuptake inhibitor) and was not implicated in the *Lancet* report.

**Table 2.6** Deaths from pulmonary embolism after vaginal delivery; United Kingdom 1997–99

| Days after delivery | Risk factors | Features |
|---|---|---|
| 7 | Phlebitis | Age > 35 years<br>Multipara<br>Previous varicose vein surgery<br>Varicose veins and phlebitis in pregnancy<br>Short labour<br>Early mobilisation<br>Complained of difficulty breathing and dizziness<br>Died soon after admission to hospital |
| 13 | Obese | Primigravida<br>Stillbirth in last trimester<br>Collapsed at day 13 |
| 13 | Obese | Intrauterine death at 29 weeks<br>Vaginal delivery, home the next day<br>Chest pain on day 6<br>On day 8 GP diagnosed PE<br>Hospital started heparin but V/Q scan showed 'abnormalities not diagnostic of PE'<br>Heparin stopped, patient discharged<br>Died several days later |
| 20 | Overweight | Age < 25 years<br>Normal delivery at term<br>Admitted at day 20 with PE<br>Rx low molecular weight heparin<br>Deteriorated<br>Rx streptokinase<br>Further deterioration: surgery arranged but died that night |
| 20 | Obese<br>Previous emboli | Grande multipara<br>Anaemic<br>Poor attender at anticoagulant clinic<br>On heparin: ? compliance<br>Normal delivery: retained placenta and neonatal death<br>Home on heparin<br>Admitted on day 20 with PE<br>Collapsed and died next day |
| 25 | Overweight<br>Bed rest | Normal delivery at term<br>Disc lesion at day 12, immobilised for 2 weeks<br>Called GP on day 25, chest pain: diagnosis 'musculoskeletal'<br>Called midwife because losing consciousness<br>Sent to A&E: diagnosis 'PPH', transferred to obstetric unit<br>Arrested en route |
| 28 | None apparent | Age > 35 years<br>Learning difficulties<br>Weight not recorded<br>Normal delivery<br>Breathless and slight tachycardia at day 21<br>GP visited<br>Died one week later |
| 34 | Obese<br>Medication | Normal delivery at term<br>Home on day 2<br>Admitted to psychiatric hospital on day 6 with psychosis<br>Rx risperidone and fluoxetine<br>Discharged at day 19<br>Died at day 34 |
| 35 | Past history of VTE | Age > 35 years<br>Poor social circumstances and concealed pregnancy<br>Delivered at home<br>Hospital transfer, discharged with 7 day supply of heparin |
| 40 | Overweight<br>On pill | Age < 25 years<br>Vacuum delivery at term<br>Commenced combined contraceptive pill on day 21<br>Died on day 40 |

PE = pulmonary embolism; PPH = postpartum haemorrhage

## *Late* deaths

Nine *Late* deaths related directly to pulmonary embolism are recorded in this triennium and are counted in Chapter 15. Only two such deaths were recorded in the previous triennium. It is uncertain whether there has been a real increase or whether case ascertainment has improved. Eight of the *Late* deaths followed vaginal delivery and only one followed caesarean section (Table 2.7).

Five of the nine women were overweight (four weighing over 80 kg). Another was described by the pathologist as 'heavily built' and another was 'grossly obese'. At least five of these overweight women had taken the combined oral contraceptive pill after delivery. Two cases were described early in this chapter and the other two are described here:

**Table 2.7**    Interval between delivery and pulmonary embolism: *Direct* and *Late* deaths; United Kingdom 1997–99

| Delivery | Days postpartum | | | | | Total |
|---|---|---|---|---|---|---|
| | 0–7 | 8–14 | 15–28 | 29–42 | 42–365 | |
| Vaginal | 1 | 2 | 4 | 3 | 8 | 18 |
| Caesarean section[a] | 3 | – | – | 1 | 1 | 4 |
| Total | 4 | 2 | 4 | 4 | 9 | 23 |

[a] Another 3 deaths followed caesarean section performed after antepartum collapse

> A young primigravid woman weighing 85 kg had a vaginal delivery at term and started the combined pill one month later. Five months after delivery, she complained of shortness of breath, chest pain and dyspnoea on exertion. Her GP prescribed amoxycillin. The next day she was admitted to a medical ward where pulmonary embolism was diagnosed but she was inadequately heparinised. She was transferred to the ICU where, despite treatment with streptokinase, she died.

The diagnosis of pulmonary embolism is always easy in retrospect but this case illustrates the importance of taking risk factors into account. She was overweight (with a BMI of 31 kg/m²), she was taking the combined contraceptive pill, which she had started a month after delivery, and she presented with shortness of breath, chest pain and dyspnoea on exertion: classic symptoms of pulmonary embolism, not chest infection. In hospital, she was inadequately heparinised.

> A 'grossly obese' parous woman aged over 30 years was admitted in spontaneous labour at the end of the second trimester. She smoked ten cigarettes a day and had not attended for antenatal care. She delivered a macerated stillbirth and went home the same day. She later received the combined oral contraceptive pill from her GP. She collapsed and died almost a year after the delivery and autopsy showed pulmonary embolism.

Although this woman's weight was not recorded, the comment that she was 'grossly obese' suggests a BMI of over 39, which contraindicates the combined oral contraceptive.

Of the other two overweight women, few details are available about one, who died three months after a normal delivery at term and was noted to be of 'heavy build'. The other is briefly described here:

> A parous woman weighing 98 kg was admitted to hospital at the end of the first trimester with a DVT, which was treated with low-molecular-weight heparin. She also developed insulin-dependent diabetes. In the second trimester she was readmitted as an emergency with pre-eclampsia. A long intravenous line was inserted. She suffered an intrauterine death and after medical induction of labour delivered a macerated stillbirth. She remained in hospital for two months and collapsed and died seven months after delivery. Autopsy showed pulmonary embolism due to atrial mural thrombosis.

The adequacy of the thromboprophylaxis has been queried in this case and was substandard in another *Late* death:

> A primigravida aged over 35 years had 'cold auto-agglutinin' in the serum at booking. Early in the third trimester she was admitted with eclampsia and delivered by caesarean section, in a different maternity unit from where she had booked. The baby survived. Thromboprophylaxis was with TED stockings but not heparin. The woman was transferred to an ICU on another site and was discharged on day eight. On day 18 she was admitted to another district general hospital with a chest complaint. Her leg veins were checked by Doppler and a diagnosis of chest infection was made. No ventilation/perfusion scan was done. She was discharged after five days. A week later she attended her GP with chest pain and was given analgesia. A month later, she collapsed and died. Autopsy showed pelvic vein thrombosis, multiple emboli and old infarction.

According to RCOG guidelines she should have been considered for subcutaneous heparin as well as TED stockings as she had two risk factors – age over 35 years and emergency caesarean section. There was a failure to investigate symptoms suggestive of pulmonary embolism. Multiple-site care may have caused poor communication between carers.

In one other *Late* death there was also failure to carry out a ventilation/perfusion scan:

> A parous woman of normal build had a normal delivery at term. Six weeks later she attempted suicide and was admitted to a psychiatric ward. She complained of haemoptysis and chest pain, and felt she had a fishbone stuck in her throat. Her C-reactive protein was markedly raised and her pulse rate was 110 bpm. Two chest X-rays were normal. A junior trainee in general medicine examined her and noted 'clinically no evidence of pulmonary embolism'. Two weeks after admission she collapsed and died of pulmonary embolism.

The diagnosis of pulmonary embolism was considered and excluded by the help of two chest X-rays. Nevertheless the 'gold standard' test is a ventilation/perfusion scan and this test needs to be performed if there is reasonable suspicion of this difficult diagnosis.

## Cerebral thrombosis

There were four cases of cerebral thrombosis in this triennium:

> A young parous woman was admitted in the third trimester with a history of ten days of diarrhoea and three days of vomiting. She had abdominal pain, which settled, but she then developed neurological symptoms that progressed to hemiparesis and coma. A computed tomography (CT) scan showed infarction with secondary haemorrhage and sagittal sinus thrombosis. She was transferred to tertiary neurological centre and treated with streptokinase directly into the sagittal sinus via burr holes and cannulae. Fetal distress developed and an emergency caesarean section was carried out. The baby survived but the woman died in ICU a few days later.

The care seems to have been good at all stages. Three days of vomiting had led to dehydration, which can predispose to thrombosis.

> An older primigravida with a BMI of 30 kg/m$^2$ and a long history of infertility became pregnant by IVF. Severe growth restriction occurred, followed by placental abruption. Caesarean section was carried out and a stillborn infant was delivered. One week later she was admitted with unsteadiness and headache. A CT scan showed small infarcts. She was discharged after a week but readmitted with drowsiness and right sided weakness. Another CT scan showed sagittal sinus thrombosis. Despite anticoagulation and thrombolytic therapy she deteriorated and died.

No thromboprophylaxis was given at the time of the caesarean section, possibly because the indication was placental abruption. The decision to undertake caesarean section is debatable, as the baby was premature, growth restricted and possibly already compromised by the abruption.

> A primigravid woman, whose mother had died of pulmonary embolism and whose father had had two strokes, booked late in pregnancy. She attended regularly and had a normal delivery at term. Eight days after delivery she developed a severe headache and became drowsy. She was admitted unconscious with a dense hemiplegia. A CT scan showed an intracerebral haematoma and thrombotic occlusion of the left transverse and sigmoid sinuses. Despite thrombolytic therapy she deteriorated and died.

Despite the family history, a thrombophilia screen was negative after her admission with cerebral thrombosis. It is not clear whether the family history had been noted at the booking clinic: a thrombophilia screen at that time might have been more useful.

> A parous woman who had been born with an occipital encephalocoele underwent caesarean section at 38 weeks for fetal distress. Although she received antibiotic prophylaxis she developed a wound infection. More than two weeks after delivery she collapsed. Brain stem infarction was confirmed and she died ten days later. Autopsy confirmed vertebral vein and dural sinus thrombosis, with congenital hydrocephalus.

Heparin thromboprophylaxis might have prevented the fatal thrombosis but she was not at high risk of thromboembolism according to RCOG guidelines.

## Substandard care

Care was judged to be substandard in 20 cases, 57% of all such deaths. As in the previous triennium, the main reasons were failure to appreciate risk factors and provide adequate thromboprophylaxis, and failure to arrange adequate investigation of patients with symptoms.

## Comments

After a sharp rise in 1994–96, the number of deaths from thromboembolism in 1997–99 has fallen back to a level similar to that in earlier triennia. The fall is due to a welcome reduction in deaths after caesarean section, despite a continuing rise in the national caesarean section rate.

Nevertheless, pulmonary embolism remains the major cause of *Direct* maternal deaths in the UK. The number of deaths can and must be further reduced. Obvious risk factors were present in at least 25 of the 31 cases in this triennium. Combinations of factors, such as age and operative delivery, can lead to an increase in risk greater than the additive effect of the two factors.[4] The key to reducing the death rate lies in identifying risk factors and taking appropriate action.

### Identification of risk factors at booking

The most common risk factor is being overweight. It is recommended that the BMI should be routinely calculated at booking to identify women whose BMI is over 30 kg/m$^2$.

A **past history** of pulmonary embolism and/or DVT is a high risk factor for recurrence in pregnancy. Many of these women, particularly those with a family history, will have underlying thrombophilia, which can be found in around 50% of patients with VTE in pregnancy. Knowledge of this condition is rapidly evolving and patients with thrombophilia should be seen by specialists with particular expertise in this area.

A **family history** of thromboembolism should also be sought at booking. When this is positive, specialist guidance should be sought from a haematologist with regard to thrombophilia screening.

### During pregnancy

Awareness of the risk of VTE in early pregnancy needs to be increased among all doctors, not just obstetricians and gynaecologists. In this triennium, as in previous ones, several women presented to general practitioners or A&E departments with symptoms of chest pain and shortness of breath but were discharged home. More complete investigation might have led to treatment that could have prevented the fatal pulmonary embolism. In most cases, diagnosis can be made using Duplex ultrasound scanning, which is now available in virtually all major hospitals. Its use is recommended in any case where there is suspicion, as clinical diagnosis is notoriously unreliable. Women and indeed doctors need to be reassured that nowadays very low radiation doses are required for ventilation perfusion scanning, chest X-ray and even X-ray venography.

**If a pregnant woman displays chest or leg symptoms Duplex ultrasound and/or ventilation/perfusion lung scanning should be used to exclude the presence of DVT or pulmonary embolism, both of which carry no significant risk to mother or fetus.**

Bed rest and immobilisation in women who are pregnant should be recognised as risk factors for the development of DVT and prophylaxis is advised.

The thromboprophylactic method chosen will depend on the patient but heparin is the most effective technique presently available. Low-molecular-weight heparins have not yet been proven to be more effective than unfractionated heparin in pregnancy but they have fewer adverse effects and only have to be given once a day.

### At surgery

Thromboprophylaxis for caesarean section is now routine and this must be maintained if the number of deaths from this cause is to be kept low. Previous Reports have also included deaths after other forms of surgery in pregnancy, including treatment of ectopic pregnancy.

The 1995 RCOG Guidelines[1] included a risk assessment chart (given at the end of this chapter as at Annex B) that highlights the need for more effective prophylaxis when multiple risk factors are present, as they were in many of the deaths in this triennium. Such women need subcutaneous heparin as the preferred option at appropriate doses and for appropriate duration.

Annex C at the end of this chapter provides an example of a suggested guideline for epidural anaesthesia in women receiving heparin thromboprophylaxis.

### After delivery

In this triennium, as in the last, there were failures to appreciate the risk of thromboembolism after vaginal delivery in patients with multiple risk factors. Prolonged thromboprophylaxis may be advisable in patients with continuing risk factors. Specific notice must be taken of any symptoms of breathlessness, chest or leg pain, which might well herald the development of VTE.

## Guideline development

As recommended in the last Report, each unit should develop its own guideline based on existing national guidelines which can be applied within the requirements of their own unit. **Implementation of such guidelines in local health care contracts, care and audit plans have the potential to reduce significantly deaths from pulmonary embolism in the next triennium.**

## Management of thromboembolic disease

The recent RCOG Guideline on the acute management of thromboembolic disease in pregnancy and the puerperium[2] makes five key recommendations and these are reproduced in Box 2.4.

---

**Box 2.4    Key recommendations from RCOG guidelines on the management of thromboembolic disease in pregnancy**

- Any woman with signs and symptoms suggestive of VTE should have objective testing performed expeditiously to avoid the risks, inconvenience and costs of inappropriate anticoagulation. Individual hospitals should have an agreed protocol for the objective diagnosis of suspected venous thromboembolism during pregnancy.

- In clinically suspected DVT or pulmonary thromboembolism, treatment with unfractionated heparin or low-molecular-weight heparin should be given until the diagnosis is excluded by objective testing, unless treatment is strongly contraindicated.

- Subcutaneous unfractionated heparin is an effective alternative to intravenous unfractionated heparin for the initial management of DVT.

- Low-molecular-weight heparins are more effective than unfractionated heparin with lower mortality and fewer haemorrhagic complications in the initial treatment of DVT in nonpregnant subjects. Low-molecular-weight heparins are as effective as unfractionated heparin for treatment of pulmonary thromboembolism.

- During pregnancy, adjusted-dose subcutaneous, unfractionated heparin or subcutaneous low-molecular-weight heparin are effective alternatives to oral anticoagulants in maintenance treatment of VTE.

All the above recommendations except the first are classed as 'Grade A' (requiring at least one randomised controlled trial as part of a body of literature of overall good quality and consistency). The first recommendation is classed as Grade B (requiring well controlled studies).

---

This Chapter has been seen by and discussed with Professor Ian Greer MD MRCP FRCOG, Glasgow Royal Infirmary.

## References

1. Royal College of Obstetricians and Gynaecologists. *Report of a Working Party on Prophylaxis against Thromboembolism in Gynaecology and Obstetrics.* London: RCOG; 1995.
2. Royal College of Obstetricians and Gynaecologists. *Thromboembolic Disease in Pregnancy and the Puerperium: Acute Management. Guideline No 28.* London: RCOG; 2001.
3. Zornberg GL, Jick H. Antipsychotic drug use and risk of first-time idiopathic venous thromboembolism: a case-control study. *Lancet* 2000;356:1219–23.
4. Greer I, editor. Thrombo-embolic disease in obstetrics and gynaecology. *Bailliere's Clin Obstet Gynaecol* 1997;11:403–615.

## ANNEX A
## Guidelines for thromboprophylaxis in vaginal deliveries

### Low risk

Assessment | Uncomplicated pregnancy
Therapy | Early mobilisation and avoidance of dehydration

### Moderate risk

Assessment | Any two of these factors:
– age over 35 years
– obesity (greater than 80 kg at booking)
– parity four or more
– labour 12 hours or more
– gross varicose veins
– current infection
– pre-eclampsia
– immobility prior to labour for four or more days
– mid-cavity or rotational forceps delivery
– major current medical illness

Therapy | Subcutaneous enoxaparin 40 mg once daily
Where heparin is contraindicated, use elasticated compression stockings immediately (contact physiotherapist)

Commence | Within six hours (allow three hours between removal of the epidural cannula and first administration)

Duration | Should continue until discharge
– if discharged prior to day five, discontinue therapy
– if hospital stay continues beyond day five, review by medical staff

### High risk

Assessment | **Any vaginal delivery with any one of these factors:**
– patient with four or more moderate risk factors
– extended major pelvic or abdominal surgery
– patient with family history of DVT/pulmonary embolism or thrombophilia
– paralysis of lower limbs
– patient with antiphospholipid antibody or lupus anticoagulant

Therapy | Subcutaneous enoxaparin 40 mg plus graduated elastic compression stockings

| | |
|---|---|
| Commence | Within six hours (allow three hours between removal of the epidural cannula and first administration) |
| Duration | Should continue until discharge |
| | Patients with a past history of venous thromboembolism or underlying thrombotic problem, should continue for a minimum of six weeks |
| | Specialist advice should be sought for those with a family history of thrombophilia |

**Heparin and warfarin are not contraindicated in breastfeeding**

## ANNEX B
## Prophylaxis against thromboembolism in caesarean section

The following recommendations, taken from the RCOG Working Party report on prophylaxis against thromboembolism,[1] are of relevance to patients requiring caesarean section.

A risk assessment of all patients undergoing elective or emergency caesarean section should be performed and prophylaxis instituted as appropriate. See box below.

---

**RCOG Risk assessment profile for thromboembolism in caesarean section**

**Low risk: early mobilisation and hydration**

- Elective caesarean section – uncomplicated pregnancy and no other risk factors.

**Moderate risk: consider one of a variety of prophylactic measures:**

- Age over 35 years
- Obesity (80 kg or greater)
- Parity four or more
- Labour 12 hours or more
- Gross varicose veins
- Current infection
- Pre-eclampsia
- Immobility prior to surgery (four days or more)
- Major current illness; e.g. heart or lung disease, cancer, inflammatory bowel disease, nephrotic syndrome
- Emergency caesarean section in labour.

**High risk: heparin prophylaxis with or without leg stockings**

- A patient with three or more moderate risk factors from above
- Extended major pelvic or abdominal surgery; e.g. caesarean hysterectomy
- Patients with personal or family history of DVT, pulmonary embolism or thrombophilia, paralysis of lower limbs
- Patients with antiphospholipid antibody (cardiolipin antibody or lupus anticoagulant).

## Management of different risk groups

### *Low-risk patients*

Patients undergoing elective caesarean section with uncomplicated pregnancy and no other risk factors require only early mobilisation and attention to hydration.

### *Moderate-risk patients*

Patients assessed as of moderate risk should receive subcutaneous heparin (doses are higher during pregnancy) or mechanical methods. Dextran 70 is not recommended until after the delivery of the fetus and is probably best avoided in pregnant women.

### *High-risk patients*

Patients assessed as high risk should receive heparin prophylaxis and, in addition, leg stockings would be beneficial.

Prophylaxis until the fifth postoperative day is advised (or until fully mobilised if longer).

The use of subcutaneous heparin as prophylaxis in patients with an epidural or spinal block remains contentious. Evidence from general and orthopaedic surgery does not point to an increased risk of spinal haematoma.

## Prophylaxis against thromboembolism in pregnancy

The RCOG Working Party also made recommendations for prophylaxis against thromboembolism in pregnancy, which are summarised in the box below.

---

**RCOG guidelines for prophylaxis against thromboembolism in pregnancy**

Patients with a previous history of thromboembolism in pregnancy or the puerperium and no other thrombotic risk factor should receive thromboprophylaxis for up to six weeks postpartum (subcutaneous heparin and then oral warfarin if desired).

Patients at higher risk, e.g. those having had multiple episodes of thromboembolism, may require heparin throughout the pregnancy.

---

## ANNEX C
## Suggested guidelines for epidural anaesthesia in women receiving heparin thromboprophylaxis*

**Heparin** (subcutaneous low-dose heparin)

- Wait four hours after giving dose before siting block or removing catheter

- Next dose no less than two hours after giving block.

**Low-molecular-weight heparin (LMWH)**

- Wait 10–12 hours after dose before inserting block or removing catheter

- Next dose no less than six hours later

- All LMWH prescribed at 18.00 daily

- Beware other anticoagulants/nonsteroidal anti-inflammatory drugs may increase risk.

In all patients, extreme vigilance is required to detect new numbness, weakness or bladder or bowel dysfunction.

Any neurological problem must be investigated as an emergency.

*Adapted from departmental guidelines, Bristol Royal Infirmary

## ANNEX D
## Summary of advice on preventing deep vein thrombosis for pregnant women travelling by air[1]

There are no direct evidence-based data to guide thromboprophylactic advice for pregnant air travellers. However, it seems prudent that precautionary conservative measures advised for all travellers should also be recommended in pregnancy. These include isometric calf exercise (as increasingly advised in flight by major airlines), walking around the cabin where possible, avoiding dehydration by drinking plenty of water/juices/soft drinks and by minimising alcohol and caffeine intake.

Pregnant women are recommended to wear properly fitting elastic compression stockings for long-haul flights or for all flights if they have additional risk factors.

For women at increased risk of thromboembolism undertaking long-haul flights pharmacological thromboprophlyaxis is recommended. Although low molecular weight heparin is to be preferred, there are pragmatic difficulties in arranging for women to receive or self-administer injections, not only before an outbound flight but also before the return flight from another country. Low-dose aspirin is an acceptable alternative, which should be considered in those women with additional risk factors in whom heparin is contraindicated or impractical to administer.

---

**Summary table of RCOG Scientific Advisory Committee Advice on preventing thromboembolism in pregnant women travelling by air**

| Any gestation and up to six weeks post-partum | Short haul flight (up to four hours) | Long haul flight (four hours or more) |
|---|---|---|
| No additional risk factors | Calf exercise; move around cabin; avoid dehydration; minimise alcohol and coffee consumption. | Calf exercise; move around cabin; avoid dehydration; minimise alcohol and coffee consumption; well-fitting elastic below-knee compression stockings. |
| Additional risk factors[a] Weight ≥ 100 kg or BMI at booking ≥ 30+ Multiple pregnancy Thrombophilia Past personal or strong family history Medical disorders with increase risk of DVT | Calf exercise; move around cabin; avoid dehydration; minimise alcohol and coffee consumption; well-fitting elastic below-knee compression stockings. | Calf exercise; move around cabin; avoid dehydration; minimise alcohol and coffee consumption; well-fitting elastic below-knee compression stockings; low molecular weight heparin[b] on day of travel (pre-flight) and day after.[c] |

[a]   Women with additional risk factors may need to seek appropriate medical advice; some, for instance will already be on thromboprophylatic medication
[b]   thromboprophylactic doses are 5000 units dalteparin or 40 mg enoxaparin
[c]   Low-dose aspirin (75 mg per day for three days before travel and on day of travel) is an acceptable alternative in those unable to take low-molecular-weight heparin

---

### Reference

1.   Royal College of Obstetricians and Gynaecologists. Advice on *Preventing Deep Vein Thrombosis for Pregnant Women Travelling by Air*. Scientific Advisory Committee Opinion Paper 1. London: RCOG Press; 2001.

## CHAPTER 3

# Hypertensive diseases of pregnancy

JAMES P NEILSON on behalf of the Editorial Board

### Pre-eclampsia and eclampsia: key summary points

- The largest single cause of death among women with pre-eclampsia and eclampsia was intracranial haemorrhage – reflecting a failure of effective antihypertensive treatment.

- Five deaths were associated with HELLP syndrome, a variant form of pre-eclampsia that can be characterised by rapid clinical decline before delivery and further deterioration after delivery.

- Four deaths occurred after sudden clinical deterioration between the decision to deliver and the actual act of delivery.

### Pre-eclampsia and eclampsia: key recommendations

- Pregnant women with a headache of sufficient severity to seek medical advice or with new epigastric pain should have their blood pressure measured and urine tested for protein, as a minimum.

- Clear, written, management protocols for severe pre-eclampsia should guide initial and continuing treatment in hospital.

- Automated blood pressure recording systems can systematically underestimate blood pressure in pre-eclampsia, to a serious degree. Blood pressure values should be compared, at the beginning of treatment, with those obtained by conventional mercury sphygmomanometers.

- Severe, life threatening, hypertension must be treated effectively.

- Magnesium sulphate is the anticonvulsant drug of choice in the treatment of eclampsia.

- There should be early engagement of intensive care specialists in the care of women with severe pre-eclampsia.

- Women with moderate to severe pre-eclampsia require a level of clinical observation that may be incompatible with location in a single side room in hospital.

- Women with multiple pregnancies are at increased risk of pre-eclampsia and their antenatal care should reflect that awareness.

## Summary

There were 15 confirmed deaths from eclampsia or pre-eclampsia counted in this Chapter. This represents a reduction from the 20 deaths counted in the last Report. The rate has declined to 7.5 per million maternities from 9.0 per million in the last Report, as is shown in Table 3.1. Figure 3.1 shows the decline in rates over the last 30 years. The age-specific rates are shown in Table 3.2, which shows that mortality rates from hypertensive disorders in pregnancy rise with age but are also higher than average in women under the age of 25 years.

**Table 3.1** Maternal deaths from hypertensive disorders of pregnancy and rates per million maternities; United Kingdom 1985–99

| Triennium | Pre-eclampsia | | Eclampsia | | Total | |
|---|---|---|---|---|---|---|
| | (n) | Rate | (n) | Rate | (n) | Rate |
| 1985–87 | 15 | 6.7 | 12 | 5.4 | 27 | 12.1 |
| 1988–90 | 12 | 5.1 | 14 | 5.9 | 27 | 11.0 |
| 1991–93 | 12 | 5.3 | 8 | 3.4 | 20 | 9.0 |
| 1994–96 | 12ª | 5.4 | 8 | 3.6 | 20 | 9.0 |
| 1997–99 | 10 | 5.2 | 5 | 2.4 | 15 | 7.1 |

ª In three of these deaths only death certificate information is available and there is no record of eclampsia

**Table 3.2** Maternal deaths from hypertensive disorders by age band and rates per million maternities; United Kingdom 1985–99

| Age (years) | 1985–87 (n) | Rate | 1988–90 (n) | Rate | 1991–93 (n) | Rate | 1994–96 (n) | Rate | 1997–99 (n) | Rate | 1985–99 (n) | Rate |
|---|---|---|---|---|---|---|---|---|---|---|---|---|
| Under 25 | 10 | 11.9 | 8 | 9.6 | 3 | 4.4 | 11 | 18.6 | 3 | 5.5 | 35 | 13.0 |
| 25–29 | 5 | 6.4 | 5 | 5.6 | 11 | 13.4 | 2 | 2.7 | 3 | 4.6 | 26 | 8.5 |
| 30–34 | 7 | 16.0 | 8 | 16.0 | 4 | 7.2 | 4 | 6.5 | 4 | 6.4 | 27 | 11.7 |
| 35–39 | 3 | 19.7 | 4 | 23.8 | 2 | 10.6 | 2 | 9.1 | 5 | 19.2 | 16 | 19.1 |
| 40+ | 2 | 75.1 | 2 | 63.5 | – | – | – | – | 1 | 22.3 | 5 | 31.3 |
| NS | – | – | – | – | – | – | 1 | – | – | – | – | – |
| All ages | 27 | 12.1 | 27 | 11.4 | 20 | 8.6 | 20 | 9.1 | 15 | 7.1 | 108 | 9.6 |

NS = not stated

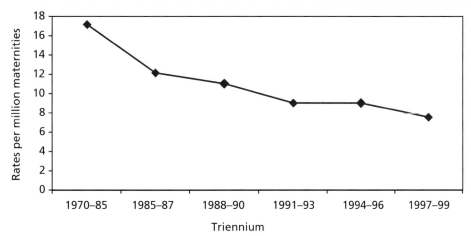

**Figure 3.1** Maternal mortality rates per million maternities for deaths from hypertensive diseases of pregnancy, 1970–99 (England and Wales rates used until 1985; from 1985, rates for the United Kingdom are shown)

Of the cases counted in this Chapter, seven were from intracranial haemorrhage, three from intra-abdominal haemorrhage, one from eclampsia, one from acute respiratory distress syndrome (ARDS), two from multi-organ failure that included ARDS and one from septicaemia while undergoing intensive care. The broad classes of death are compared with figures from recent triennia in Table 3.3. Although there has been a steady trend towards fewer deaths, 12 of the 15 (80%) showed clear features of substandard care and there were, undoubtedly, avoidable deaths. Intracranial haemorrhage, as the single largest cause of death, indicates a failure of effective antihypertensive therapy.

**Table 3.3**     Causes of death due to eclampsia and pre-eclampsia; United Kingdom 1985–99

| Cause of death | 1985–87 (n) | 1988–90 (n) | 1991–93 (n) | 1994–96 (n) | 1997–99 (n) |
|---|---|---|---|---|---|
| *Cerebral* | | | | | |
| Intracranial haemorrhage | 11 | 10 | 5 | 3 | 7 |
| Subarachnoid | – | 2 | 0 | 1 | 0 |
| Infarct | – | 2 | 0 | 0 | 0 |
| Oedema | – | 0 | 0 | 3 | 0 |
| Total cerebral | 11 | 14 | 5 | 7 | 7 |
| | | | | | |
| *Pulmonary* | | | | | |
| ARDS | 9 | 9 | 8 | 6 | 1 |
| Oedema | 2 | 1 | 3 | 2 | 0 |
| Total pulmonary | 11 | 10 | 11 | 8 | 1 |
| | | | | | |
| *Hepatic* | | | | | |
| Rupture | 0 | 0 | 0 | 2 | 2 |
| Failure/necrosis | 1 | 1 | 0 | 1 | 0 |
| Total hepatic | 1 | 1 | 0 | 3 | 2 |
| | | | | | |
| Other | 3 | 2 | 4 | 2 | 5 |
| **Overall Total** | **27** | **27** | **20** | **20** | **16** |

Although most substandard care was seen in the hospital sector, there were examples in primary care of general practitioners failing to appreciate the possible significance of headache and epigastric pain as symptoms of pre-eclampsia, or at least failing to make the appropriate response by measuring blood pressure and testing urine for proteinuria.

Nine women were primigravid and six were parous. Two women had chronic hypertension, with superimposed pre-eclampsia. Three women (19%) had multiple pregnancies.

All deaths that are recorded in this Chapter occurred in hospital. In two cases, the woman was found dead in a single room in the antenatal ward.

In two cases, the first indication of clinical concern was the observation of fetal growth restriction, predating signs of pre-eclampsia.

## Cases counted in other Chapters

Women with pre-eclampsia whose deaths are discussed in other Chapters and are not counted in this one, include two cases in Chapter 12; *Indirect* deaths. These were a woman who died of basilar artery thrombosis three weeks after termination of pregnancy and a woman who was found unexpectedly to have acute purulent meningitis at autopsy. A woman who died from haemorrhage after caesarean section for placenta praevia is discussed in Chapter 4; Haemorrhage.

Cases are listed in this Chapter on a thematic basis, rather than by the pathological complication that ultimately caused death.

## Eclampsia

The last Report described eight women who died after eclamptic seizures, while in this triennium, five women died after definite or probable eclamptic fits. All five women had eclamptic seizures following admission to hospital, in contrast with the previous triennium, when six of the eight women first fitted outside hospital.

Magnesium sulphate has been shown to be the anticonvulsant of choice in eclampsia[1,2] and it is now used widely in pre-eclampsia in the UK when a need is seen for anticonvulsant prophylaxis. The precise role of magnesium sulphate in the treatment of pre-eclampsia has yet to be established with clarity[3] and British obstetricians have traditionally had a high threshold for the use of anticonvulsants. The multinational Magpie trial is assessing the benefits and risks of magnesium sulphate for women with pre-eclampsia and their babies, and should report its findings early in 2003.[4]

In the following case of eclampsia, the seizure was potentially preventable, as there had been inadequate assessment of the woman in a primary care setting and there was delay in initiating treatment once she reached hospital. The delay in implementing effective antihypertensive treatment was more important than the delay in starting anticonvulsant therapy:

> The woman had a blood pressure of 100/60 mmHg at booking. She developed vomiting and diarrhoea in mid third trimester and was referred to the maternity unit, as a case of gastroenteritis, by her GP who did not, apparently, check her blood pressure. On arrival in hospital, she was found to have a blood pressure of 210/120 mmHg with proteinuria ++++. Difficulty was encountered in contacting the on-call consultant and, one hour after admission and before any treatment was given, she had an eclamptic fit. She was treated with magnesium sulphate and labetalol and delivered by caesarean section. Continuing management was discussed with the consultant in charge of the local intensive care unit (ICU), which was on another site, and the decision was made to continue her care in the high dependency unit in the maternity unit. Despite further treatment with labetalol and hydralazine, the patient remained hypertensive and she had a cardiac arrest four hours after delivery. She was resuscitated and transferred to the ICU but a computed tomography (CT) scan revealed a massive intracranial haemorrhage, and she died some hours later.

Clear, written, management protocols for severe pre-eclampsia should determine initial treatment, even when the on-call consultant is not immediately available.

As an example, a management protocol in use in all maternity units in the Mersey

Region is attached as Annex A to this Chapter. This was developed through multidisciplinary discussion and consensus, identification of good evidence where that existed and study of other management guidelines in the UK, notably from Newcastle, Leeds, Birmingham and Oxford.

Another important point to note from this case is the potential for misleading blood pressure measurements from automated recording systems, which can systematically underestimate both systolic and diastolic blood pressures in pre-eclampsia to an alarming degree.[5] These systems are useful to monitor trends during treatment but the values should be compared, at the beginning, with those obtained by conventional sphygmomanometers. It is critically important in ensuring that life-threatening, severe hypertension is treated effectively, that the blood pressure is measured accurately. The degree of hypertension in this case may have been underestimated. The recognised hypertension certainly was not treated effectively. In a woman with such severe disease there may have been merit in the insertion of an arterial line to measure blood pressure. The absence of a resident anaesthetist in this stand-alone small maternity hospital may have contributed to the outcome.

In the following case, antenatal care was substandard through a failure to appreciate the significance of the past obstetric history and to plan care accordingly. Whether this would have averted the fatal outcome is less clear:

> This woman's previous pregnancies had been complicated by pre-eclampsia and fetal growth restriction and had ended in caesarean sections before term. Despite these unequivocally high-risk features, the booking visit and subsequent antenatal clinic visits up to the beginning of the third trimester were performed exclusively by a community midwife without the involvement of a consultant obstetrician. The only risk features noted in the maternity records were 'previous preterm deliveries'. However, when seen by a consultant early in the third trimester, the woman's blood pressure was normal and fetal size, clinically and ultrasonically, was also satisfactory. There was a trace of proteinuria, also detected when the woman was seen again by the midwife two weeks later. Four days after that, the woman was admitted to hospital with symptomatic pre-eclampsia. The fetus was found to be dead and it was assumed that she had suffered a placental abruption. Soon after admission, she had an eclamptic seizure, which was treated with intravenous diazepam and magnesium sulphate. She was in labour and was transferred to the ICU, where she delivered vaginally. The extent of the accompanying disseminated intravascular coagulation was not, initially, fully appreciated because of an ambiguous report from the laboratory that clotting factors were not obtainable, which meant, in fact, that no clotting factors were identified in the patient's blood, rather than there being technical problems in performing the test. The patient had a massive postpartum haemorrhage after delivery, requiring hysterectomy after the usual uterotonic treatments. Following this, she entered a state of coma and was found to have a large intracerebral haemorrhage, which was, ultimately, the cause of her death.

This case illustrates the importance of multidisciplinary teamwork and while there was early engagement of intensive-care specialists the death might have been preventable had there been proactive involvement by a haematologist after the grossly abnormal, but ambiguously reported, clotting screen.

> A woman was admitted to hospital with what appeared to be mild pre-eclampsia and planned induction of labour was delayed because the delivery suite was busy. In the meantime, she developed fulminating pre-eclampsia accompanied by epigastric pain and unusual patterns of behaviour and she received treatment with hydralazine but no anticonvulsant. Two hours later, she had an eclamptic fit, which was treated with intravenous diazepam and phenytoin infusion. Some hours after delivery by caesarean section, she became drowsy and developed focal neurological signs. She had suffered an intracranial haemorrhage and was transferred to a regional neurosurgical unit where she underwent three craniotomies, but to no avail. A previously undiagnosed arteriovenous malformation was found at the site of haemorrhage.

Use of the anticonvulsant regimen in this case represents substandard care. The management protocol has now been changed in this unit to include the use of magnesium sulphate. The delay in performing induction of labour may be seen as a system failure.

In the following case, there were concerns about possibly over-hasty discharge from the ICU:

> A parous woman presented first for antenatal care in mid-pregnancy and was found to have a blood pressure of 90/50 mmHg. Subsequent attendance for antenatal care was sporadic and communication between the maternity team and the patient was mediated through a series of relatives because of the woman's limited knowledge of English. When seen at the clinic close to term, she was found to have a blood pressure of 170/100 mmHg and proteinuria ++. She was admitted directly from the clinic to the hospital for induction of labour but, within minutes of a prostaglandin pessary being inserted into the vagina, she had an eclamptic fit. A second seizure occurred shortly after the start of magnesium sulphate treatment but there were no further fits. A caesarean section was performed at this time because of a fetal bradycardia. Further management was based on a well-structured, written, clinical protocol and involved anaesthetists and obstetricians. The patient was admitted to the ICU two days after delivery because of increasing respiratory difficulty, which was attributed to pulmonary oedema and which improved after diuretic treatment. She was discharged from the ICU the same day but had a cardiac arrest on the postnatal ward four days later. Resuscitation proved difficult and, although successful eventually, the patient had severe hypoxic cerebral damage. Histology of the brain at autopsy showed features compatible with pre-eclampsia/eclampsia; there was also evidence of acute respiratory distress syndrome (ARDS).

There were several aspects of substandard care in the following case:

A woman was detected as having a small-for-dates fetus early in the third trimester. While waiting to be seen at the specialist antenatal clinic one week later, she consulted her general practice because of headaches and was told to take paracetamol. At the clinic, she was found to have a blood pressure of 180/100 mmHg (booking blood pressure 100/70 mmHg) and +++ proteinuria, and was admitted to a side-room in the antenatal ward and treated with labetalol and, subsequently, nifedipine. Ultrasound confirmed the clinical diagnosis of fetal growth restriction and a decision was made to deliver by caesarean section after a two-day course of corticosteroids. She had ++++ proteinuria with a normal platelet count, an elevated urea and modest elevation of serum urate. Later the same day, the patient was found dead on the floor of the side-room. She was resuscitated and was transferred to the ICU of another hospital, where fetal death was diagnosed and labour was induced. Ventilation was discontinued after diagnosis of brain-stem death. There was no evidence of cerebral haemorrhage at autopsy.

Whether or not this woman died as result of an eclamptic seizure must remain a matter of speculation, but it seems probable. Certainly, the standard of care was substandard in that staff failed to ensure that she was in a location within the hospital in which she could receive the level of observation that the severity of her pre-eclampsia merited. The standard of resuscitation is also a matter of concern, since the cardiac arrest team did not arrive until 13 minutes after the initial call. The GP was also at fault in advising paracetamol over the telephone to a pregnant woman with severe headache. It is essential to check the blood pressure, at a minimum, in such circumstances.

A case in which a woman had puffy fingers and subsequently collapsed and died at home is described in Chapter 14; *Coincidental* deaths, as there is insufficient evidence to classify this as an eclamptic death. Cases where the cause of death cannot be finally determined are also traditionally counted in this Chapter. Briefly, her blood pressure was normal and she had no proteinuria two weeks before death. She reportedly 'fitted' at home and was found to be in asystole by the attending paramedics. A postmortem caesarean section was performed but the baby was stillborn. The autopsy was grossly inadequate and provides little insight into the cause of death.

## HELLP syndrome

Five deaths were associated with HELLP syndrome (haemolysis, elevated liver enzymes, low platelets), which can represent a particularly aggressive form of pre-eclampsia with a rapidity of clinical deterioration that may leave effective therapy lagging. These cases require direct input by clinicians with special expertise in the management of pre-eclampsia, including regional obstetric experts, obstetric anaesthetists, haematologists and the early engagement of ICU consultants, especially if the maternity unit is 'off-site'.

Although some have argued that acute fatty liver may have a similar pathophysiological basis, deaths from acute fatty liver are, as is traditional in the Reports, discussed in Chapter 8 as 'Other *Direct*' deaths.

In HELLP syndrome, there may be serious initial clinical deterioration, rather than improvement, after delivery, as illustrated by the following case, which did not reveal evidence of substandard care:

> A woman who had suffered an eclamptic fit during her first labour had an uncomplicated second pregnancy and her third, index, pregnancy was also uncomplicated until she had a small antepartum haemorrhage in mid third trimester. She was delivered by caesarean section because of some evidence of fetal compromise. She had been normotensive throughout and there was no retroplacental clot at caesarean section. On the first day after delivery, she was found to be drowsy and there was biochemical evidence of deteriorating renal and hepatic function, together with haematological signs of thrombocytopenia, disseminated intravascular coagulation and haemolysis. Despite prompt transfer to the ICU after the diagnosis of HELLP syndrome, her clinical condition progressively declined and she died of multi-organ failure five days later.

The following case was also characterised by rapid clinical deterioration:

> A woman was admitted to hospital in late pregnancy with what appeared to be mild pre-eclampsia. Her blood pressure was modestly elevated at 150/90 mmHg, there was proteinuria +++ and her uric acid levels and platelet counts were normal. Induction of labour was started but she complained of severe abdominal pain and became markedly hypertensive. She was treated with labetalol and magnesium sulphate and delivered by caesarean section. It was apparent that she had HELLP syndrome, with dropping haemoglobin concentration and platelet counts and rapidly rising liver function test results. There was also deteriorating renal function. A decision was made to transfer the patient to an ICU (the maternity unit was isolated) after she became drowsy some six hours after delivery. On arrival at the ICU, she was found to have pulmonary oedema. She did not have a central line. Also, there was evidence of intracranial haemorrhage, which, ultimately, was responsible for her death. Autopsy revealed subdural blood and a large intracerebral haematoma, as well as liver necrosis.

Where the time course of disease is as explosive as this, it is prudent to anticipate the need for intensive care and make preparations especially if working 'off-site'. A central line is essential despite accompanying coagulopathy in such severe disease. Coagulation factor support can provide cover for the placement of the line.

> A very young woman was admitted to hospital early in the third trimester because her fetus was small for gestational age and there had been reduced fetal movement. Ultrasound examination confirmed the presence of fetal growth restriction and steroids were given in anticipation of early delivery. The maternal blood pressure was normal on admission; biochemistry was also normal except for a marginally raised uric acid level. Three days later, the woman complained of visual disturbance and abdominal pain and, the next day, was noted to have elevated blood pressure, proteinuria, hyper-

reflexia and grossly disordered biochemical and haematological results, compatible with HELLP syndrome. Delivery was effected by caesarean section but the fulminating pattern of disease continued, requiring treatment with magnesium sulphate (subsequently stopped because of oliguria), haematological input, and transfer to the ICU, some 16 hours after delivery. There, ventilation was commenced but the woman remained gravely ill and she died four days later. Autopsy confirmed the presence of multi-organ damage including ARDS, acute tubular necrosis, liver changes typical of severe pre-eclampsia/HELLP syndrome, pituitary infarction and hypoxic changes in the brain.

It was impossible to judge whether facets of the care of this young woman could, or should, have been better, because of thin documentation. The delay in transfer to the ICU clearly merits scrutiny. However, the best account of events available to this Enquiry was the clinical summary on the autopsy report. Such a lack of documentation provided by the clinicians caring for this woman for this Enquiry is manifestly and deeply unsatisfactory and is incompatible with the Chief Medical Officer for England's vision of the NHS as an 'organisation with a memory'.[6]

In the following case, the obstetricians concerned have also failed, despite repeated requests, to provide the Enquiry with anything more than minimal information. The following account summarises the helpful report by one of the midwives:

> A parous woman with no previous obstetric problems booked with a blood pressure of 80/60 mmHg. She remained normotensive during the remainder of her pregnancy including labour, which occurred at term. Within hours of delivery, she complained of epigastric pain and her blood pressure rose to 185/110 mmHg. After some delay, she was treated with a single sublingual dose of nifedipine, with some subsequent and transient lowering of her blood pressure before it again rose, to 195/110 mmHg. There was further delay before laboratory results became available, showing elevated uric acid levels and grossly elevated liver enzymes. The haemoglobin value and platelet count have not been made available to the Enquiry but the patient was bleeding spontaneously from her gums and she had gross haematuria when eventually catheterised. It seems clear that she had HELLP syndrome. During this time, she complained of severe headache and was found to be hyper-reflexic. Some hours later, transfer to an ICU in another hospital was arranged by the on-call anaesthetist. There is no record of a consultant obstetrician having seen the patient or even having been consulted during a phase of progressive deterioration over a period of several hours. On arrival at the ICU she was still hypertensive, but had also become comatose. A CT scan revealed a frontal-lobe haematoma. After attempts to correct her coagulopathy, the haematoma was evacuated through a burr hole, but she never recovered and died the following day.

The care of this patient was seriously substandard in many respects: failure to recognise the serious nature of her condition, slow and ineffective treatment, inadequate monitoring and absence of senior obstetric input. It is difficult to believe that this unit had a written protocol for the management of severe pre-eclampsia.

> A woman with a multiple pregnancy was delivered by caesarean section because of upper abdominal pain, thought to be suggestive of placental abruption, two weeks before the date of a planned caesarean section. The woman was noted to be yellow prior to delivery and she became frankly jaundiced afterwards. There was no evidence of abruption at caesarean section. It became obvious after delivery that she was developing HELLP syndrome and she was transferred to an ICU, from where she required open surgical drainage of a retroperitoneal haematoma. After a week in the ICU, she was showing some signs of improvement when there was a rapid decline suggestive of septicaemia. Autopsy revealed an undiagnosed candida septicaemia.

There was delay in making the diagnosis of HELLP syndrome in this case. Relevant blood results were not available until after delivery. Earlier diagnosis might have prompted earlier referral to the ICU. It is accepted that candida septicaemia is notoriously difficult to diagnose.

In a further case of HELLP syndrome, clinical management was prompt and effective and involved care in the ICU. The condition occurred unusually early in pregnancy, well before fetal viability, and was accompanied by fetal growth restriction. The patient recovered after termination of the pregnancy and went home, but was readmitted three weeks later, unconscious. Investigations revealed basilar artery thrombosis. She died within a few days of admission. It seems possible that she might have had antiphospholipid syndrome to account for both pathological processes. This case is counted in Chapter 12 *Indirect* deaths.

## Intra-abdominal haemorrhage

Three women died after intra-abdominal haemorrhage, in two cases after hepatic rupture:

> A woman was admitted to hospital, close to term, with severe pre-eclampsia, superimposed on essential hypertension. Her hypertension was treated with a cocktail of hydralazine, labetalol and nifedipine. Attempted induction of labour was unsuccessful because of the occurrence of fetal distress after a second dose of vaginal prostaglandin. An emergency caesarean section was performed under general anaesthesia. At induction of anaesthesia, the woman's blood pressure was 250/160 mmHg. She was transferred to the recovery area one hour and 40 minutes after the delivery of her baby, with a note estimating intraoperative blood loss at 1.5–2 litres. There were no explanations in the papers available to the Enquiry for the unusual timescale or the unusual amount of blood loss. Ten minutes after arrival in the recovery room, the patient's blood pressure was 48/23 mmHg with other signs of hypovolaemic shock. Blood was taken for crossmatching and two units of O negative blood were transfused. The patient was receiving her fourth unit of blood when she had a cardiac

arrest, some two hours after reaching the recovery room. She remained profoundly hypotensive (given her pre-existing hypertension) throughout this time and a haemoglobin estimate gave a result of less than 6 g/dl. Attempts at resuscitation proved futile. The quality of the autopsy report is deeply unsatisfactory and is discussed in Chapter 18.

This woman died of haemorrhagic shock and the standard of her care is unsatisfactory in many respects. The on-call anaesthetist had not been made aware of the presence on the delivery ward of a woman with such severe pre-eclampsia that she required no less than three antihypertensive drugs. There appears to have been an inappropriate persistence in trying to achieve vaginal delivery, which eventually led to a 'crash' caesarean section, with its attendant hazards. Whatever happened in the operating theatre to cause such severe blood loss is not documented in the papers available to the Enquiry. There was serious delay before blood was taken for crossmatching. There was inadequate appreciation of the state of hypovolaemia after the caesarean section. In this patient with severe pre-eclampsia and major blood loss, there was an obvious need for a central line to guide blood replacement. There was no senior involvement for many hours before death. Even after death, the patient received substandard attention, in the form of an inadequate autopsy.

In contrast, in the next case, there was no evidence of substandard care:

A woman was admitted to hospital at 36 weeks with pre-eclampsia. Proteinuria was generally + during her in-patient stay. Induction of labour was initiated but caesarean section was required for fetal distress. After delivery, the mother's blood pressure rose and she required treatment with hydralazine and nifedipine. There was sudden clinical deterioration two days after delivery accompanied by falling levels of haemoglobin and platelets, disordered liver function tests, dropping oxygen saturation and a metabolic acidosis. Provisional diagnoses of possible HELLP syndrome or intra-abdominal haemorrhage were made, and the patient was transferred to the ICU. Ultrasound examination revealed a large subcapsular haematoma in the liver. There was some speculation that the haemorrhage might have occurred into a pre-existing liver adenoma, rather than de novo, but the basis for this suggestion is unclear. Hepatic artery embolisation was performed by an interventional radiologist but the patient's condition remained unstable. She was transferred to a regional centre where she underwent two liver transplants but, despite intensive care of high quality, she subsequently died.

In a further case of death following hepatic rupture, care was substandard because the woman was discharged home despite persisting proteinuria. Whether her transient absence from hospital materially contributed to the fatal outcome is not certain:

A parous woman with pre-eclampsia was admitted to hospital. Her blood pressure was modestly elevated and there was persistent proteinuria +. She was allowed home but returned later the same day after the GP was called and found her blood pressure to be 220/120 mmHg. In hospital, the blood pressure was 160/120 mmHg and the woman complained of epigastric pain. She had proteinuria +++, haematuria, thrombocytopenia and brisk reflexes. Urgent delivery by caesarean section was planned but was delayed somewhat because of another acute problem in the hospital. In the meantime, the patient became shocked and the fetal heart stopped. At caesarean section, a major haemoperitoneum was found, arising from a ruptured subcapsular haematoma of the liver. There was also a major postpartum uterine haemorrhage requiring hysterectomy after the usual methods of medical treatment. The patient was transferred to a regional centre of excellence where she underwent partial hepatectomy and was considered for liver transplantation but, although a liver did become available, her poor clinical state by then made this option non-viable.

Another woman, whose case is counted in Chapter 4; Haemorrhage, had her delivery precipitated by hypertension but died from intra-abdominal haemorrhage. Briefly, a morbidly adherent placenta praevia was encountered at a planned caesarean section and the patient died in the operating theatre. The timing of planned delivery seems appropriate. Other aspects of care were unsatisfactory and these are discussed in Chapter 4.

## Delay in delivery

Two cases have already been discussed in which there was delay in performing a planned delivery because the hospital concerned was busy. There were two further cases in which delay was associated with fatal outcomes. In the first, delay was triggered by excessive concern for hospital routines and compounded by a failure of recognition of the severity of the patient's condition because of problems of processing a blood specimen. In the second, a considered decision to delay delivery was made by a consultant, for legitimate clinical reasons, and the standard of care was not seen as wanting:

> A woman with a high multiple pregnancy following assisted conception, underwent apparently standard antenatal care at a community clinic. Proteinuria was noted over a four-week period during the early third trimester. When seen by a senior obstetrician at 34 weeks, the patient's blood pressure had risen to 130/80 mmHg from a booking level of 90/55 mmHg and she had proteinuria ++. No laboratory investigations were performed and the patient was asked to return in two weeks to be seen by a midwife. The patient was, in fact, admitted to hospital ten days later with severe epigastric pain and was found to have severe pre-eclampsia with hypertension, proteinuria and hyper-reflexia. She was treated with magnesium sulphate and the decision was made to deliver by caesarean section. It was decided, possibly because of the multiple pregnancy, to wait several hours before delivery so that this would happen during the normal working day. The blood specimen that was taken for laboratory studies haemolysed and was unsuitable for analysis. Unfortunately, during the

wait for delivery, the patient had an intracranial haemorrhage, which ultimately led to her death. She developed a severe headache and become unrousable. Prior to caesarean section, a low platelet count (less than 40,000) was detected. Subsequent autopsy did not identify the vessel responsible for the haemorrhage. There was accompanying cerebral oedema.

High multiple pregnancies are *par excellence* high-risk pregnancies and antenatal care should not be devolved primarily to midwifery staff based in community clinics. There is a well-recognised association of multiple pregnancy with pre-eclampsia and, in this case, there were several indications of evolving disease, long before the acute crisis occurred. Investigation of the patient's proteinuria at the antenatal clinic was inadequate, as were arrangements for follow-up. There was an opportunity to retrieve the situation when the patient herself sought emergency admission to hospital with symptoms of what proved to be severe pre-eclampsia. Unfortunately, delivery was delayed for many hours to suit hospital routines and the patient had what was to be a fatal intracranial haemorrhage in the meantime, perhaps associated with unrecognised thrombocytopenia as well as hypertension.

An unusual case of possible sleep apnoea is counted and also discussed in Chapter 12; *Indirect* deaths, but this occurred in a woman who was an inpatient for treatment of pre-eclampsia:

> A very overweight and highly parous woman who had diabetes and chronic hypertension, developed superimposed pre-eclampsia and was admitted to hospital and monitored carefully with substantial consultant input. A considered decision was made to delay delivery to try to avoid caesarean section as the fetal head was very high at that time and there seemed no immediate threat to the mother. The woman's obesity was an important factor in this decision. She was found dead, one night, in her room in hospital at 35 weeks of gestation. The immediate cause of death is unclear but she had complained of breathlessness during the preceding days and had been reviewed twice by a consultant physician. The breathlessness was attributed to asthma and seemed to respond to standard asthma therapy. There was no trauma to the tongue to suggest an eclamptic fit. Autopsy showed features in the kidneys compatible with pre-eclampsia but no evidence of seizures that might have occurred with eclampsia. The woman had received thromboprophylaxis and there were no signs of thromboembolic disease. There were signs in the lungs suggesting the possibility of an acute viral infection but no definitive cause of death, other then sleep apnoea, could be reached.

## Care after delivery

The need for vigilant monitoring after delivery of women with pre-eclampsia is illustrated by the following case:

> A woman with a multiple pregnancy had a blood pressure at booking of 90/60 mmHg. She was admitted to hospital during the pregnancy

with pre-eclampsia and was subsequently delivered by caesarean section. Immediately prior to delivery, her blood pressure was 140/80 mmHg and she had proteinuria +++. There was inadequate monitoring of the patient's blood pressure after delivery but the pressure was found to be 260/140 mmHg some eight hours after the birth. The patient developed neurological symptoms and was transferred to the ICU, where it became obvious that she had suffered a cerebral haemorrhage. Autopsy revealed a pontine haemorrhage.

In this case, postoperative monitoring of blood pressure was substandard, as was the failure to treat, promptly and effectively, a rise of blood pressure greatly in excess of baseline levels.

This Chapter has been seen and discussed with Steven Robson MD FRCOG, Professor of Obstetrics at the University of Newcastle, and Professor Michael Greaves MD MRCPath FRCP, Professor of Haematology and Head of Department of Medicine and Therapeutics, University of Aberdeen. We are also grateful to Dr G Edwards, Mersey Perinatal Epidemiology Unit, for the regional guidelines.

# References

1. Duley L, Henderson-Smart DJ. Magnesium sulphate versus diazepam for eclampsia. *Cochrane Database Syst Rev* 2001; Issue 2.
2. Duley L, Henderson-Smart DJ. Magnesium sulphate versus phenytoin for eclampsia. *Cochrane Database Syst Rev* 2001; Issue 2.
3. Duley L, Gulmezoglu AM, Henderson-Smart DJ. Anticonvulsants for women with pre-eclampsia. *Cochrane Database Syst Rev* 2001; Issue 2.
4. www.magpietrial.org.uk
5. Natarajan P, Shennan AH, Penny J, Halligan AW, de Swiet M, Anthony J. Comparison of auscultatory and oscillometric automated blood pressure monitors in the setting of pre-eclampsia. *Am J Obstet Gynecol* 1999;181:1203–10.
6. Department of Health. *An Organisation with a Memory*. London: Department of Health; 2000.

## ANNEX A
## Guidelines for the management of severe pre-eclampsia

### Introduction

Eclampsia and pre-eclampsia continue to be a leading cause of maternal mortality and morbidity.[1] Eclampsia is a rare occurrence, with a UK incidence of 4.9/10,000 maternities. Almost half of the seizures (44%) occur in the postnatal period, with over one-third (38%) occurring antenatally and 18% occurring in the intrapartum period.[2] The incidence of pre-eclampsia is unknown. The Collaborative Eclampsia Trial (1995)[3] established that magnesium sulphate is more effective in preventing recurrent seizures following eclampsia than either phenytoin or diazepam. An earlier audit of current practice within Merseyside and Cheshire highlighted variations in the standard of guidelines currently being used.[4]

These guidelines have been formulated following collaboration between obstetricians, midwives and anaesthetists from all the obstetric units within the former Mersey Region. The guidelines represent the consensus agreement of an evidenced based approach to the management of severe pre-eclampsia.[5] The aim of the guidelines is to increase the safety and stability of the woman although, if the fetus is still *in utero*, constant monitoring of fetal wellbeing should be an integral part of management protocol.

### Criteria for inclusion

Any woman with severe proteinuric hypertension where the decision has been made to deliver and with one of the following criteria (either 1, 2 or 3).

1.  Hypertension ( ≥ 140/90 mmHg) with proteinuria (≥ 0.3 g/day or ≥ 2+)

    **and at least one of the following:**

    i)   Headache, visual disturbance, epigastric pain
    ii)  Clonus (≥ 3 beats)
    iii) Platelet count less than $100 \times 10^9$, ALT (alanine aminotransferase) > 50 iu/l
    iv)  Creatinine greater than 100 or creatinine clearance less than 80.

2.  Severe hypertension (systolic ≥ 160 mmHg or diastolic ≥ 110 mmHg) with proteinuria (≥ 0.5 g/day or ≥ 2+)

3.  Eclampsia

4.  Clinical discretion should be used to include women who present with atypical symptoms.

### Key personnel to be contacted

- obstetric registrar on call

- anaesthetic registrar on call

- senior labour-ward midwife

- consultant obstetrician on call

- consultant anaesthetist on call.

### Maternal observations and investigations

- All maternal observations should be recorded on a specialised pregnancy-induced hypertension chart or an ICU chart.

- Oxygen saturation should be continuously monitored.

- Blood-pressure recordings should be made every 15–20 minutes.

- Maternal temperature should be recorded hourly.

- A Foley catheter should be *in situ* and hourly urinary output measured.

- Routine blood samples should be taken every 12–24 hours, including full blood count, urea and electrolytes, creatinine and liver function tests.

### Fetal observations

Minimum assessment of fetal wellbeing should include the following:

- growth assessment scan

- liquor volume assessment

- continuous external fetal monitoring

- umbilical cord Doppler if the woman's condition allows.

### Management of seizures

- All women with eclampsia should be treated with magnesium sulphate as the first-line drug of choice. The intravenous (IV) route is preferable.

- A loading dose of 4 g magnesium sulphate should be given over 5–10 minutes, followed by a maintenance infusion of 1–2g/hour IV at the discretion of the consultant in charge, continued for at least 24 hours after the last seizure. Recurrent seizures should be treated by a further bolus of 2 g magnesium sulphate.

- Diazepam may be administered if fits continue, at the discretion of the consultant in charge.

- Magnesium levels should be monitored when repeat fitting occurs or renal compromise is evident (therapeutic range 2–4 mmol/litre).

- Deep tendon reflexes should be monitored hourly when magnesium therapy is commenced. If reflexes are absent, or respirations are less than

14 per minute, or $SaO_2$ less than 95%, magnesium therapy should be stopped.

- If the fits continue, it is important to exclude other causes of fits and a CT scan should be considered.

## Management of hypertension

Severe hypertension is defined as greater than 160/110 mmHg or mean arterial pressure (MAP) greater than 125 mmHg.

- Hydralazine is the first-line drug of choice for management of severe hypertension titrated against blood pressure, except in the presence of tachycardia (greater than120 bpm). The agreed dose is 5 mg IV repeated every 20 minutes, to a maximum cumulative dose of 20 mg.

- Labetalol should be used as a second choice, given 20 mg IV followed at ten-minute intervals by 40 mg, 80 mg and 80 mg, up to a cumulative dose of 300 mg.

- Prophylactic $H_2$ antagonists should be given until the woman is transferred to normal postnatal care.

## Fluid balance management

- Fluid intake should be restricted to 85 ml/hour.

- Urinary output should be measured hourly.

- 500 ml human albumin solution (HAS) should be considered:
  - prior to hydralazine therapy
  - prior to caesarean section
  - if oliguria is evident (defined as urinary output less than 100 ml in a consecutive four-hour period)
  - prior to the administration of regional anaesthesia.

- If HAS has previously been administered, the insertion of a central venous pressure (CVP) line should be considered. If further complications occur, especially oliguria, after the administration of HAS, a line is recommended. Although the success rate of the subclavian-vein route is greater than the antecubital-fossa route, clinicians should use the route with which they are more familiar.

- If the central venous pressure value is greater than 10 mmHg, 20 mg frusemide should be considered.

- If the central venous pressure value is less than 10 mmHg, HAS 500 ml should be considered.

- A further dose of 20–40 mg frusemide should be considered if there is persistent oliguria.

## Informing ICU personnel

There should be locally agreed criteria regarding the physical transfer of women to the adult ICU.

- ICU is not a place, it is a service.

- Effective communications are of the utmost importance.

- The labour ward may be the most appropriate place to care for pregnant women.

- Non pregnancy-related problems such as cerebral vascular accident and pulmonary oedema need to be considered.

## References

1. Department of Health. *Report on Confidential Enquiry into Maternal Deaths 1991–1993*. London: HMSO; 1996.
2. Douglas KA, Redmond CWG. Eclampsia in the United Kingdom. *BMJ* 1994;309:1395–400.
3. Eclampsia Trial Collaborative Group. Which anticonvulsant for women with eclampsia? Evidence from the Collaborative Eclampsia Trial. *Lancet* 1995;345:1455–63.
4. Unit of Perinatal and Paediatric Epidemiology, University of Liverpool. *Regional Audit of the Management of Severe Pre eclampsia and Eclampsia. Mersey Perinatal Annual Report*. Liverpool: University of Liverpool; 1996.
5. Royal College of Obstetricians and Gynaecologists. *Management of Eclampsia. Guideline No. 10*. London: RCOG; 1996.

## CHAPTER 4

# Haemorrhage

MARION H HALL on behalf of the Editorial Board

## Obstetric haemorrhage: key recommendations

- Every unit should have a protocol for the management of haemorrhage and this should be reviewed and rehearsed on a regular basis. It should also be included as part of life support training. All members of staff, including those in the blood bank, must know exactly what to do to ensure that large quantities of crossmatched blood can be delivered without delay.

- The speed with which obstetric haemorrhage can become life threatening emphasises the need for women at known high risk of haemorrhage to be delivered in a hospital with a blood bank on site and appropriate laboratory facilities, including haematological advice and therapy.

- Placenta praevia, particularly in patients with a previous uterine scar, may be associated with uncontrollable uterine haemorrhage at delivery and caesarean hysterectomy may be necessary. A very experienced operator is essential and a consultant must be readily available.

- On-call consultant obstetricians must consider all available interventions to stop haemorrhage such as radical surgery or embolisation of uterine arteries, involving surgical or radiological colleagues as required.

- It is essential that both obstetricians and anaesthetists be involved, at an early stage, in planning the elective management of very-high-risk cases.

- If haemorrhage occurs, experienced consultant obstetric and anaesthetic staff must attend.

- It is recommended the guidelines for the management of women at known higher risk of haemorrhage, contained in Table 4.3 of this Chapter, be followed.

## Summary

Of the seven deaths directly due to antepartum and postpartum haemorrhage counted in this Chapter, three were due to placenta praevia, three to abruption of the placenta and one to postpartum haemorrhage (PPH). There were seven other deaths in which haemorrhage played a significant part and these are discussed here as well as being counted and discussed in other Chapters. In 11 of the 14 cases discussed in this Chapter care was substandard but this did not necessarily lead directly to death. Intrapartum and acute care was very poor in some cases and some hospitals were inadequately equipped to offer care to women with serious problems arising as an emergency. Even elective surgery was, on occasion, undertaken by staff without appropriate training and experience. Although the number of *Direct* deaths from haemorrhage continues to show a welcome decline, as shown in Figure 4.1 and Table 4.1, lessons can still be learned from the cases discussed in this Chapter.

**Table 4.1**   Deaths from haemorrhage by cause and rate per million maternities; United Kingdom, 1985–99

| Triennium | Placental abruption (n) | Placenta praevia (n) | Postpartum haemorrhage (n) | Total (n) | Rate per million maternities |
|---|---|---|---|---|---|
| 1985–87 | 44 | 0 | 6 | 10 | 4.5 |
| 1988–90 | 6 | 5 | 11 | 22 | 9.2 |
| 1991–93 | 3 | 4 | 8 | 15 | 6.4 |
| 1994–96 | 4 | 3 | 5 | 12 | 5.5 |
| 1997–99 | 3 | 3 | 1 | 7 | 3.3 |

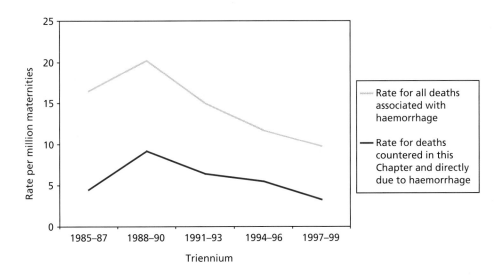

**Figure 4.1**   Death rates per million maternities from haemorrhage by cases counted in Chapter 4 and by total number of cases associated with haemorrhage; United Kingdom 1985–99

## Abruption

Abruption of the placenta presents without warning and a successful outcome requires good arrangements for emergency investigation and treatment. In this triennium, there were three deaths directly related to abruption, which are counted in this Chapter. These three deaths may not have been preventable, for various reasons, but do illustrate that there is a very short window of opportunity for intervention to promote a successful outcome:

> A woman with a known history of domestic violence and drug abuse
> lived in poor social circumstances. She had been diagnosed late in the

second trimester as having pulmonary hypertension secondary to possible subacute bacterial endocarditis. Appropriate plans were made for her delivery but she was admitted in hypovolaemic shock several weeks later, with clear evidence of abruption of the placenta and of right heart failure. There were also signs of bruises on her abdomen and arms. As there was fetal distress a rapid caesarean section was performed for the benefit of both the baby and mother. The baby survived but the mother could not be resuscitated from cardiogenic shock, in spite of the presence of three consultant anaesthetists, one of whom had previously assessed the patient.

The clinical care in this case was excellent. The total blood loss was estimated as 1200 ml, but she had prior severe anaemia, and pallor had been noted before admission. The abruption was unlikely to have been fatal without the concurrent pulmonary hypertension. Domestic violence was also considered to be a possible contributory factor in the aetiology of the abruption and the case is also discussed in Chapter 16.

After recurrent minor haemorrhage, a woman with orthopaedic problems was admitted in late second trimester with further bleeding and abruption of the placenta with an intrauterine death diagnosed by a consultant obstetrician. Because the laboratory and blood bank were several miles away, treatment for disseminated intravascular coagulation (DIC) was not started until five hours later and, even when it was provided, was inadequate. Blood loss at delivery was estimated as one litre. She was also anuric. A massive cerebral haemorrhage then occurred but her transfer to a neurosurgical unit did not occur until after her pupils were fixed and dilated and brain-stem death was diagnosed. It is not clear whether hypertension was a contributory factor to the cerebral haemorrhage as well as the DIC.

The main problem with this case was that the coagulopathy appears not to have been managed aggressively enough and was compounded by the fact that the unit for which she was booked was unable to provide prompt blood transfusion and therapy for DIC. There also seems to have been little anaesthetic involvement in planning or monitoring her care.

A woman with a previous PPH was admitted just prior to term with spontaneous rupture of her membranes. She was diagnosed by the admitting midwife as having had abruption of the placenta and an intrauterine death. She was promptly investigated with consultant obstetric and haematological advice and DIC was diagnosed. However, no transfusion of blood or blood products had been commenced by the time she delivered about three hours after admission. She collapsed shortly after delivery, having passed a massive blood clot, and there was uncontrollable haemorrhage. She died shortly afterwards despite the administration of blood, blood products and oxytocics, and with consultant obstetric and anaesthetic staff in attendance. Attempts at resuscitation by the cardiac arrest team were, as expected, unsuccessful for another hour. Her autopsy showed amniotic fluid embolism.

The care of this woman was satisfactory, except that earlier blood transfusion and therapy for DIC may have given a better chance of success to the treatment given after catastrophic haemorrhage began, although it is probable that she may have died anyway. The autopsy showed amniotic fluid embolism as well as abruption, but this was probably secondary. This case is also mentioned in Chapter 5.

## Placenta praevia

There were four deaths due to placenta praevia, three of which are counted in this Chapter. The fourth case is counted in Chapter 9 as an anaesthetic death. Previous reports have repeatedly emphasised the importance of having senior and experienced staff available at the time of caesarean section for placenta praevia and, when the surgery is elective, there should be no difficulty in providing this in any unit. It is therefore disappointing that three deaths from placenta praevia in this triennium illustrate again the problems that can arise when provision falls short of this.

The following is the case is counted in Chapter 9; Anaesthetic deaths:

> An elective caesarean section was performed by a registrar on a woman with known placenta praevia, fibroids and a history of previous uterine surgery. At operation, the immediate blood loss was 1200 ml but bleeding continued and, at an early repeat laparotomy when a hysterectomy was performed by a consultant obstetrician, a further five-litre blood loss was recorded. The bleeding continued and the woman proceeded to a splenectomy, where a further five-litre loss occurred. Two further general anaesthetics were required and the woman finally died of acute respiratory distress syndrome (ARDS) after she had aspirated her gastric contents.

Here, the initial surgery was likely to have presented problems for even the most experienced consultant but should certainly have been performed by a consultant. The role that anaesthesia may have contributed to her death is discussed in Chapter 9.

In two other cases of placenta praevia, there were also anaesthetic and surgical problems:

> In the first case, a consultant obstetrician performed an elective caesarean section for placenta praevia in a woman who had also had two previous caesarean sections. However, the general anaesthetic was given by an inexperienced registrar and no special precautions (such as extra cannulae or central venous pressure line) were taken. The estimated blood loss (attributed to the presence of placenta accreta) was 6.5 litres and her abdomen had to be re-opened, with a view to hysterectomy, within 30 minutes of closure. The woman died before the operation was completed.

It would seem that the abdomen was closed prematurely. The registrar anaesthetist was unable to cope with this serious emergency and should have had consultant help throughout.

In the second case, a woman who had suffered a previous PPH after a vaginal delivery was admitted in the third trimester of pregnancy with pre-eclampsia and a decision to deliver her early, by caesarean section, was taken. Although there was known to be an anterior placenta praevia and pre-operative anaemia, the operation was undertaken by a registrar with a registrar anaesthetist. The placenta was found to be morbidly adherent and there was excessive bleeding. The consultant obstetrician, consultant anaesthetist and the haematologist were then called. The abdomen was closed but re-opened because bleeding persisted. The woman died of hypovolaemic shock during the subsequent hysterectomy.

In this case, the report form was so inadequately completed, especially on the obstetric side, that it is difficult to know what really happened, but it is unacceptable for registrar staff to be operating alone on such a case. Placenta accreta is often not able to be diagnosed antenatally but placenta praevia is and was.

In contrast, exemplary care was provided for one woman:

A multiparous woman with a number of previous caesarean sections (the first for strong fetal indications, the following elective) was diagnosed as having placenta praevia on ultrasound scan at about 20 weeks of gestation. She had recurrent episodes of bleeding from then on and was managed as an inpatient from 25 weeks of gestation onwards. The risk of placenta accreta and major haemorrhage was repeatedly discussed with the woman and among all relevant staff, and detailed multidisciplinary plans were made for a planned caesarean section at 36 weeks and for an emergency section should bleeding or labour occur before this. Heavy bleeding, in the early hours of the morning, did occur just before the planned section and the prepared plan was immediately put into action. Surgery, including caesarean section, a hysterectomy and cross-clamping of the aorta was performed by three consultant obstetricians and a consultant vascular surgeon. The consultant anaesthetist was fully supported by staff from the intensive care unit (ICU) and extra experienced midwifery and theatre staff were on duty. Sixty units of blood were given in the first two hours and 200 units in all. After a few hours the situation appeared to be temporarily stable and she was transferred to ICU. Unfortunately, further bleeding occurred and she eventually died a few weeks later without recovering consciousness.

Although the eventual outcome was fatal, this case illustrates the value of having foreseen major problems and having a massive haemorrhage protocol, which was obviously well rehearsed and put into place very efficiently.

## Postpartum haemorrhage

There were six deaths in which postpartum haemorrhage (PPH) played a significant role, of which only one is counted in this Chapter. Five are counted in other Chapters (two in Chapter 3; Hypertension and one each in Chapter 7; Genital tract sepsis, Chapter 8; Other *Direct* (vaginal trauma) and Chapter 9; Anaesthesia. Again, because delivery can occur at any time during the day or night, a good outcome depends on adequate emergency care. If there are known risk factors some precautions can be taken but if the predisposing problem is a very serious one, the prognosis is worse:

> A woman who had suffered a retained placenta with postpartum haemorrhage in her previous deliveries (the first occasion being recorded as placenta accreta) had an induced delivery. Labour was induced over a weekend and, when the placenta was retained, there was midwifery delay in calling the registrar. When haemorrhage became profuse there was then a further delay before the registrar called the consultant and more delay in proceeding to hysterectomy under general anaesthesia. This was compounded by further delays in obtaining crossmatched blood from a hospital several miles away. Uncrossmatched O negative blood was appropriately given but, by then, the situation was out of control and cardiac arrest occurred. Ergometrine had been given at delivery but was not repeated.

It was inappropriate for this very-high-risk woman to be booked for confinement in a hospital without an on-site blood bank. There was no overwhelming reason for induction, which increases the risk of third-stage complications, and certainly not at a weekend.

> In a case counted in Chapter 9, a grand multiparous woman of very short stature was a heavy smoker and had a very regular alcohol intake. She also had had previous third-stage complications and was known to have irregular antibodies. After an uneventful vaginal delivery she sustained a significant postpartum haemorrhage estimated to be about three to four litres of blood. Haemostasis was achieved after examination under general anaesthesia but, due to difficulty in obtaining crossmatched blood, she may have been over-infused with other fluids and bronchospasm and pulmonary oedema occurred. She then developed ARDS and renal failure and eventually died after airway problems.

The intensive care of this woman was excellent. The only respect in which her care may have been substandard was in over-infusing her during the initial PPH. It is not clear whether coagulopathy was considered in the resuscitation, but there was clear evidence of consumptive coagulopathy from the platelet count of $26 \times 10^9/l$ when she was transferred to ICU. The carboprost, which was given as an oxytocic, and her heavy smoking may have contributed to the bronchospasm and insufficient attention may have been given to her very small size.

The following two cases are counted and also discussed in Chapter 3; Hypertensive disease of pregnancy:

> A woman with a multiple pregnancy was admitted as an emergency near term with pre-eclampsia and severe abdominal pain, which was diagnosed by a consultant obstetrician as a possible abruption. A decision was made to undertake an urgent caesarean section. The

anaesthetist noted jaundice but this was not investigated preoperatively. At operation, abruption was not confirmed and there was average blood loss. Over the next few hours she rapidly developed florid HELLP syndrome and was admitted to ICU. A wound haematoma developed, as did a massive retroperitoneal haematoma which was drained at a repeat laparotomy, but this recurred subsequently and was drained again. She eventually died of cerebral oedema and *monilial* septicaemia.

The decision to undertake the caesarean section was not unreasonable but it exposed the mother to the risk of surgical haemorrhage, as well as haemolysis, as there was clear evidence that hepatic pain and jaundice were present on admission. Her coagulopathy was profound. In the light of this, the failure to diagnose HELLP earlier is a source of concern. The management of the coagulopathy appears not to have been sufficiently aggressive and this would have contributed to the haemorrhage.

A multiparous woman in her late thirties was admitted with pre-eclampsia superimposed upon essential hypertension a few weeks from term. Induction of labour by dinoprostone gel was begun and antihypertensive treatment with nifedipine, hydralazine and labetalol given. After the second (larger) dose of dinoprostone was given, uterine hypertonus and fetal distress occurred and immediate caesarean section was performed by a registrar with general anaesthetic given by a registrar anaesthetist. During the procedure, massive blood loss occurred (her haemoglobin fell from 13.2 to 5.5 g/l) and within a short time she became grossly hypotensive. Blood and replacement fluid therapy were totally inadequate and she died of hypovolaemic shock after two hours. The only consultant involvement in her care was that the consultant obstetrician on call concurred in the decision to induce her but did not see her and was not called at all until after she had died, neither was there any no consultant anaesthetic involvement. The key medical staff were absent at the time of her death from cardiac arrest, although they were aware of her condition.

The ready availability of a cardiac arrest team contrasts with the poor recovery care provided for this woman. The very poor standard of care received suggests a lack of leadership, teamworking and protocols. It is to be noted that hypotension may be more difficult to treat after anti-hypertensive therapy.

A woman with septicaemic shock and an intrauterine death developed DIC secondary to sepsis from group-A haemolytic streptococcus. The seriousness of her condition was not recognised until several hours after admission when she was in extremis. Resuscitation was then undertaken, but the treatment of the DIC was delayed as the laboratory was not on site and platelets had to come from 60 miles away. A few hours after admission, because delivery was not imminent, a caesarean section was performed in case the sepsis was intrauterine, although this proved not to be the case. After the operation, the DIC and vaginal bleeding persisted and she was transferred to an ICU where she received in all 56 units of blood, 36 units of fresh frozen plasma, 13 units of platelets and 14 units of cryoprecipitate. Her condition did not improve and her uterine arteries were embolised the next day, but this did not provide any long-term benefit. Antibiotic treatment was inhibited by a history of penicillin allergy.

The key problem in this case was the failure of the midwifery and obstetric staff to recognise the seriousness of her condition on admission, when immediate treatment may have given her a chance of survival. DIC is usually self-limiting but persisted here because of her profound septic shock. This case is counted in Chapter 7.

> Labour was induced in a woman with a previous caesarean section because of a malformation in the fetus. Intravenous oxytocin was given in the second stage. After a ventouse delivery there was a massive PPH, the bleeding being at least partly due to multiple vaginal tears. Eighteen units of blood were transfused and a laparotomy showed the caesarean section scar to be intact, but internal iliac ligation and hysterectomy were required. The haemorrhage was then well controlled but a vesicovaginal fistula occurred and death occurred after repair ten months later.

Administration of oxytocin in the second stage of labour was considered to be substandard care in a woman with a previous caesarean section, and the ventouse delivery was very traumatic. The abdominal surgery was successful in controlling the bleeding but should not have resulted in a fistula. This is classified as a *Late Direct* maternal death and counted in Chapter 15.

A woman who ultimately died of severe respiratory infection is counted in Chapter 12; *Indirect* deaths, but is also discussed here:

> A multipara with prior normal deliveries and a very poor social history was admitted with ruptured memranes at 36 weeks of gestation. After two days, oxytocin was given but after a short time it was suspected that there was malposition of the head, and a caesarean section was performed. Inferolateral extension of the incision caused massive haemorrhage (four litres). The spinal anaesthetic was appropriately converted to a general. The consultant obstetrician, anaesthetist and haematologist were called and the situation was controlled using oxytocics, blood, fresh frozen plasma and other fluids. Postoperative heparin prophylaxis was given. She recovered and went home but was readmitted with a severe respiratory infection and died, in spite of intensive care.

The haemorrhage was primarily due to surgical trauma, although sepsis may have exacerbated the coagulopathy. Her obstetric care was good but it is not clear whether the caesarean section was essential. There is no criticism of her anaesthetic care but the prolonged anaesthetic associated with her massive PPH may have contributed to her respiratory infection, although there were other factors, such as heavy smoking.

## Comment

Although it is gratifying that there has been a reduction in the number of cases of haemorrhage ascribed to this Chapter, there were six other cases in which haemorrhage played a significant part. The recent survey of severe maternal morbidity[1] suggests that severe, possibly life-threatening, haemorrhage may occur in 6.7 per 1000 deliveries, which means there could be around 1400 cases of severe haemorrhage in the United Kingdom every year. Therefore, despite the continuing reduction in deaths from haemorrhage, important lessons remain to be learned from the cases described in this Report.

Obstetric haemorrhage is a life-threatening condition and can occur extremely rapidly. Therefore the following recommendations are made:

**A multidisciplinary massive haemorrhage protocol should be available in all units and updated and rehearsed regularly in conjunction with the blood bank. It should also be included in life-support training.**

**Women at known higher risk of haemorrhage should be delivered in a consultant unit with an on-site blood bank. The CEMD suggested guidelines for the management of such women are summarised in Table 4.3.**

**Table 4.3**    Recommendations for the management of women at known risk of haemorrhage

> Where a delivery is known to be one with a higher risk of major bleeding, for example placenta praevia, especially with previous caesarean section, myomectomy scars, uterine fibroids, placental abruption or previous third-stage complications, the following steps are essential.
>
> - Possible prepartum anaemia should be checked and corrected in the antenatal period if possible.
>
> - All elective or emergency surgery should be performed by a consultant.
>
> - Any anaesthetic should be given by a consultant.
>
> - Adequate intravenous access (two large-bore cannulae) should be in place before surgery starts.
>
> - At least four units of blood should be crossmatched and immediately available.
>
> - A central venous pressure line should be in place, either pre-operatively or whenever it is apparent that bleeding is excessive.
>
> - If bleeding is excessive, the obstetrician should consider either embolisation of uterine arteries by an interventional radiologist or further surgical procedures, such as internal iliac ligation, hysterectomy, B-Lynch suture or Billings suture. Any obstetrician who does not feel competent to perform any of the above should immediately call a colleague to assist or, if necessary, a vascular surgeon.
>
> - The advice of a consultant haematologist should be sought to assist in the management of coagulopathy, for example due to disseminated intravascular coagulation or massive transfusion. The most appropriate blood product replacement is dependent on the result of coagulation tests and full blood count and may involve cryoprecipitate, fresh frozen plasma and platelets.

This Chapter has been seen and discussed with Michael Greaves MD MRCPath FRCOG, Professor of Haematology and Head of Department of Medicine and Therapeutics, University of Aberdeen.

## Reference

1. Waterstone M, Bewley S, Wolfe C. Incidence and predictors of severe obstetric morbidity: case control study. *BMJ* 2001;**322**:1089–93.

# CHAPTER 5

# Amniotic fluid embolism

JAMES DRIFE on behalf of the Editorial Board

## Summary

There were eight deaths due to amniotic fluid embolism in the United Kingdom in 1997–99, less than half the number in the last triennium. All but one of the women were aged over 25 years. Three were nulliparous and none had had more than four previous deliveries. Five of the women had had induction or augmentation of labour but one woman collapsed during normal labour of spontaneous onset and two collapsed before labour, one dying undelivered. Four were delivered by caesarean section and three by forceps, the indication for intervention being maternal collapse in four cases and acute fetal distress in three cases. In six cases, the interval between collapse and death was four hours or less and in two cases the interval was greater than six hours.

Eight *Direct* deaths were attributed to amniotic fluid embolism (AFE) and classified under the International Classification of Diseases code ICD 673.1. Although the Reports now accept a clinical diagnosis, in this triennium the diagnosis was confirmed in all cases by the finding of squames or hair in the lungs on histological examination. A brief summary of these cases is given in Table 5.1.

## Cases counted in other Chapters

Three cases are mentioned here but counted in other Chapters:

> A woman aged under 25 years underwent vaginal termination of pregnancy by suction at 14+ weeks of gestation. The procedure was straightforward but after its completion she was found to have reduced oxygen saturation and bradycardia. Resuscitation was started but she developed disseminated intravascular coagulation (DIC). She was transferred to an intensive care unit but died six days later of multiple organ failure.

This case is counted in Chapter 6; Early pregnancy deaths but the clinical picture of collapse and DIC is characteristic of AFE. The diagnosis was not confirmed at autopsy but confirmation is difficult when death occurs several days after delivery. AFE has not previously been described in the first half of pregnancy, although the last Report included a case at 22 weeks of gestation.

> An obese woman aged over 30 years experienced shortness of breath at 18 weeks of gestation. She was treated with heparin and then warfarin for suspected pulmonary embolism. Two weeks later she was admitted with vaginal bleeding and was found to have an international normalised ratio (INR) of 8.3, which was treated with

vitamin K. She miscarried. A few hours later she complained of chest pain and breathlessness. Next day she became drowsy and suffered cardiac arrest shortly after transfer to a medical unit. At autopsy there was bilateral pulmonary oedema and pleural effusions. Histological examination of the lungs showed multiple platelet emboli and possible fetal squames.

This case is counted in Chapter 10; Cardiac disease. Despite the suspicion of 'fetal squamous debris' in the lungs, the clinical presentation is atypical of AFE. On her first admission, a ventilation/perfusion scan was not performed to confirm the diagnosis of pulmonary embolism and her breathlessness may have been due to anxiety. It is thought that she died from congestive cardiac failure caused by platelet thrombi in the coronary arteries, associated with heparin-induced thrombocytopenia.

**Table 5.1**  Clinical features of amniotic fluid embolism cases; United Kingdom 1997–99

| Complications before labour | Induction or augmentation of labour | Collapse | Complications during labour | Fetal outcome |
|---|---|---|---|---|
| Fibroid | Augmentation (ARM+oxytocin) | Sudden ICU[a] (7 h to death) | Pyrexia, felt unwell Sudden fetal distress CS, adherent placenta | LB |
| Previous SB Pyelonephritis Para 4 | Induction (prostaglandin) | Sudden ICU (4h to death) | Cardiac arrest Kielland's forceps | LB |
| Previous CS | No | Sudden No ICU (<1h to death) | Bloodstained discharge Sudden pain, coughing Collapse CS (no anaesthetic) Adherent placenta | LB |
| Late booking IUGR | Augmentation (ARM in labour) | Slow ICU[a] (62 h to death) | CS for fetal distress PPH, collapse | LB |
| Previous retained placenta | Induction (ARM + prostaglandin) | Sudden No ICU (4+h to death) | Fetal distress Ventouse Retained placenta, PPH Hysterectomy | NND |
| Headaches ? SROM | Undelivered | Sudden (Immediate death) | Postmortem CS | SB |
| APH Para 3 + 1 | Induction (ARM + oxytocin) | Sudden ICU (? 4h to death) | Collapse Forceps delivery PPH | LB |
| Twin pregnancy Collapsed at home | No | Sudden | Undelivered | |

APH = antepartum haemorrhage; ARM = artificial rupture of the membranes; CS = caesarean section; ICU = intensive care unit; LB = live birth; NND = neonatal death; PPH = postpartum haemorrhage; SB = stillbirth

[a] elements of substandard anaesthetic care identified

A parous woman aged over 30 years was admitted at term with classical features of placental abruption and had a vaginal delivery of a stillborn baby. Soon after delivery she developed postpartum haemorrhage and DIC. Despite major transfusion she died in the delivery suite. Autopsy showed AFE in addition to placental abruption.

This case is counted and described in Chapter 4 Haemorrhage. Both placental abruption and AFE cause DIC but, in this case, the abruption was thought to be the primary pathology because she had classic features of abruption for some hours before developing DIC.

**Table 5.2**     Maternal deaths and the rates per million maternities from amniotic fluid embolism by age; United Kingdom 1988–99

| Age | 1988–90 (n) | Rate | 1991–93 (n) | Rate | 1994–96 (n) | Rate | 1997–99 (n) | Rate | Total (n) | Rate |
|---|---|---|---|---|---|---|---|---|---|---|
| < 25 | 0 | 0.0 | 0 | 0.0 | 1 | 1.6 | 1 | 1.8 | 2 | 0.7 |
| 25–29 | 6 | 7.2 | 4 | 4.9 | 3 | 4.0 | 2 | 3.1 | 15 | 4.9 |
| 30–34 | 4 | 8.0 | 4 | 7.2 | 6 | 9.8 | 3 | 4.7 | 17 | 7.3 |
| 35–39 | 0 | 0.0 | 2 | 10.6 | 4 | 18.1 | 2 | 7.6 | 8 | 9.5 |
| 40+ | 2 | 63.3 | 0 | 0.0 | 3 | 79.3 | 0 | 0.0 | 5 | 31.2 |
| **Total** | **12** | **4.7** | **10** | **4.3** | **17** | **7.7** | **8** | **3.7** | **47** | **5.1** |

## Age

Of the eight deaths counted in this Chapter, only one of the women was aged under 25 years. Table 5.2 and Figure 5.1 show how the risk of the condition increases with age.

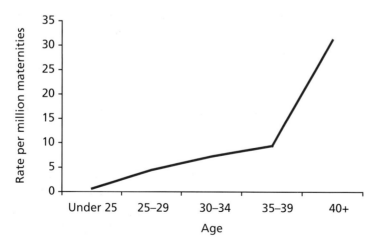

**Figure 5.1.** Amniotic fluid embolism; rates of death by maternal age per million maternities; United Kingdom 1997–99

## Parity

There was no association with parity. Three women were primigravid and two had one previous delivery. The other three women had two, three and four previous deliveries, respectively.

## Ethnic origin

Five women were white and two were Asian. Information was not available about one woman.

## Antenatal complications

Antenatal complications were present in four cases. One woman had fibroids, one had a twin pregnancy, one had a pregnancy complicated by intrauterine growth restriction and another had suffered antepartum haemorrhage. Among the other four women, the past obstetric history was possibly relevant in three cases: one woman had a previous caesarean section, one had a previous retained placenta and one had a previous stillbirth.

## Induction or augmentation of labour

Three women had labour induced: one received prostaglandin pessaries and two underwent artificial rupture of the membranes (together with prostaglandins in one case and intravenous oxytocin in the other). Two women had labour augmented: one received intravenous oxytocin and the other underwent amniotomy in labour. Of the other two women, one collapsed during normal labour of spontaneous onset and the other collapsed before labour began.

## Mode of delivery

None of the women had a normal delivery. In all cases, obstetric intervention was indicated by maternal collapse or fetal distress. One woman died undelivered. Four women were delivered by caesarean section. In one case, postmortem caesarean section resulted in the delivery of a stillborn baby. In another case, caesarean section was carried out without anaesthesia after maternal collapse. The baby survived, possibly with brain damage. The other two caesarean sections were performed because of sudden fetal distress. In two cases, the placenta was found to be abnormally adherent at caesarean section. In one case, caesarean section was followed by hysterectomy.

Two women were delivered by forceps and one by vacuum extraction. One forceps delivery was carried out after maternal cardiac arrest and the baby survived. The other forceps delivery was carried out after maternal collapse and the baby also survived. The vacuum extraction was indicated by acute fetal distress and was followed by a neonatal death.

Five of the eight babies were born alive but one of these may have brain damage.

## Speed of collapse

In three cases, the interval between collapse and death was about four hours. Two of these women reached an intensive care unit (ICU) but one died on the operating table after hysterectomy for postpartum haemorrhage. In one case, the interval between collapse and death was less than one hour and the woman did not reach ICU. In two cases the woman collapsed at home: one was dead on arrival at hospital and the other died very soon after admission.

In one case, the interval between death and collapse was seven hours and in another case the woman died on the third day after delivery. Both these cases were treated in ICU and in both cases care was considered to be substandard.

## Pathology

These cases are discussed in Chapter 18; Pathology.

## Substandard care

There were no cases of substandard obstetric care but in two cases the anaesthetic care was judged to be substandard:

> A primigravid woman aged over 30 years went into spontaneous labour at term. Progress was slow despite intravenous oxytocin. Pyrexia and maternal tachycardia were noted and the woman felt unwell and began shivering. Caesarean section was carried out under general anaesthesia for acute fetal distress. The placenta was abnormally adherent. After the operation the patient remained hypotensive and acidotic with a tachycardia of 150 bpm. She was transferred to the ICU but developed DIC. Some hours after delivery there was sudden deterioration. She was reintubated and a central venous line was inserted but she died within a few hours.

The clinical picture is consistent with overwhelming infection but the autopsy confirmed AFE. The anaesthetic care was felt to be substandard as the patient was extubated after operation, although she still had a marked tachycardia and hypotension.

> A primigravid woman aged under 25 years of age was seen late in pregnancy soon after she arrived in the UK. Intrauterine growth restriction was diagnosed. Labour was complicated by fetal distress and caesarean section was carried out. Within two hours she developed a tachycardia of 140 bpm and excessive oozing from the wound, which was re-explored. DIC was diagnosed. After further deterioration she was re-intubated and transferred to the ICU, where a central venous pressure line was inserted. Vaginal bleeding became torrential, despite a well-contracted uterus, and subtotal hysterectomy was performed. A further laparotomy was carried out because of renewed bleeding. She developed renal failure and was transferred to a tertiary centre for dialysis but quickly deteriorated further and died.

Autopsy did not at first confirm AFE but review of the histology showed possible foci of squames and lanugo hair in spite of the three-day interval between delivery and death, and this was accepted as confirming AFE.

The obstetric care was satisfactory but the anaesthetic care was felt to be substandard as a CVP line should have been inserted earlier, before admission to ICU.

## Comment

The number of deaths from amniotic fluid embolism rose from 10 in 1991–93 to 17 in 1994–96 and but now has fallen again to eight. The present Report and the previous two have accepted that cases can be diagnosed on clinical grounds. In 1991–93 there were two such cases, in 1994–96 there were four (and three cases in which information was inadequate) but in the present triennium there were none. The number of histologically confirmed deaths has varied little over the last five Reports – from eight in 1997–99 to ten in 1994–96.

The Reports have shown consistently that age is a risk factor for AFE. In the present triennium, as in 1994–96, only one woman was aged under 25 years. Of the other seven, five were aged 30 years or over. Although the average age of childbearing in the UK continues to rise, it is gratifying that, despite this trend, the number of deaths from AFE has remained fairly constant.

The use of oxytocic drugs has been thought to be a risk factor for AFE. Four of the eight women in this triennium received either prostaglandin or oxytocin and one had labour augmented by amniotomy. Nevertheless, three of the eight women received no intervention to induce or augment labour.

As in 1994–96, no single obstetric intervention was identified as a risk factor for AFE. In two cases, the condition complicated an entirely straightforward pregnancy but one of these women had a previous caesarean section. Antenatal complications included antepartum haemorrhage, fibroids, multiple pregnancy and intrauterine growth restriction. Past obstetric complications included previous stillbirth, caesarean section and retained placenta.

Previous Reports have suggested that the death rate from AFE could be reduced by avoiding uterine over-stimulation and by prompt diagnosis of obstructed labour, and it is gratifying that these factors were not present in any of the cases in 1997–99. Recent Reports have suggested exploring ways of improving the treatment of women who survive long enough to be transferred to intensive care. In the present triennium, four of the seven women reached intensive care but, in two of those cases, death occurred soon after admission. In the other two cases, the women spent longer in intensive care and substandard features were identified in the anaesthetic care but these were not of critical importance to the outcome.

Although the number of deaths from AFE is low, it remains frustrating that we still have no clear idea how to prevent or treat this condition. Nevertheless, it is worth repeating the general recommendations made in the last Report. Rates of obstetric intervention in the form of amnniocentesis and induction and augmentation of labour should be kept as low as possible and research into the condition is still necessary.

## Amniotic fluid embolism register

A register of suspected cases who survive has been established. Such cases should be notified to Mr Derek Tuffnell, Consultant Obstetrician, Bradford Royal Infirmary, Duckworth Lane, Bradford, West Yorkshire, BD9 6RJ.

**Derek Tufnell has also seen and commented on this Chapter.**

CHAPTER 6

# Early pregnancy deaths

JAMES P NEILSON on behalf of the Editorial Board

## Early pregnancy deaths: key recommendations

- All clinicians, particularly those working in primary care and accident and emergency (A&E) departments, need to be aware of atypical clinical presentations of ectopic pregnancy and especially of the way in which it may mimic gastrointestinal disease.

- The possibility of atypical presentation should be taught to undergraduate medical and nursing students and highlighted in future textbooks.

- Urinary dipstick testing for beta human chorionic gonadotrophin (βhCG) should be performed in any woman of reproductive age with unexplained abdominal pain. The test is now rapid, easy, and sensitive.

- Laparoscopic surgery for ectopic pregnancy has probable advantages over open surgery. However, it should only be undertaken by staff with training and experience that meet RCOG requirements.

- Women with suspected ectopic pregnancies who have no signs of significant haemorrhage should not undergo surgery late at night if senior assistance is not immediately available.

- Difficult surgical cases should not be delegated to unsupervised junior medical staff.

- Cervical pregnancy may be associated with torrential haemorrhage. Care should be pre-planned carefully on a multi-disciplinary basis.

## Summary

Seventeen *Direct* deaths attributed to early pregnancy complications are listed in this Chapter. These include 13 deaths from ectopic pregnancy (12 tubal pregnancies and one cervical pregnancy), two deaths after miscarriage (including one hydatidiform mole) and two deaths after termination of pregnancy. There were also five early *Direct* deaths from sepsis associated with miscarriage counted and discussed in Chapter 7; Genital tract sepsis and 10 *Direct* deaths from pulmonary embolism before 24 weeks of completed gestation counted and discussed in Chapter 2.

These figures are tabulated with those from recent Reports in Table 6.1. Detailed interpretation of trends is inappropriate because definitions of gestational age have changed during this time. Also, a fine distinction has to be made as to whether deaths from miscarriage associated with infection should be included in this Chapter or in Chapter 7; Genital tract sepsis. The table does, however, have value in conveying a regrettable absence of progress.

**Table 6.1**    Causes of deaths in early pregnancy; United Kingdom 1985–99

| Triennium | Ectopic pregnancy (n) | Miscarriage (n) | Termination of pregnancy (n) | Total (n) |
|---|---|---|---|---|
| 1985–87 | 11 | 1 | 4 | 16 |
| 1988–90 | 15 | 6 | 3 | 24 |
| 1991–93 | 9 | 3 | 5 | 17 |
| 1994–96 | 12 | 2 | 1 | 15 |
| 1997–99 | 13 | 2+5[a] | 2 | 17+5[a] |

Note: Until the 1994–6 Report, early pregnancy deaths were defined as occurring before 20 weeks of pregnancy. In this, and the last Report, 24 weeks was used as the upper gestational limit. Thus, direct comparisons with data from previous triennia may be inappropriate.

[a] There were also five deaths from sepsis associated with miscarriage counted in Chapter 7

As in previous years, the major challenge is to reduce the number of deaths from ectopic pregnancy, especially those associated with substandard care. Overall, 11 (65%) of the 17 deaths counted in this Chapter were assessed as having substandard care. Eight of the 13 deaths from ectopic pregnancy were associated with substandard care.

## Ectopic pregnancy

Table 6.2 shows that the rate of deaths from ectopic pregnancies has not declined since the last Report. Further, the rate is higher than that calculated for 1991–93.

**Table 6. 2**    Deaths from ectopic pregnancies and rates per 1000 estimated pregnancies; England and Wales 1988–1990 and United Kingdom 1991–99

| Triennium | Estimated pregnancies (n, 1000s) | Estimated ectopic pregnancies (n) | Ectopic pregnancies per 1000 pregnancies | Deaths from ectopic pregnancies (n) | Death rate[a] |
|---|---|---|---|---|---|
| England and Wales | | | | | |
| 1988-90 | 2886.9 | 24775 | 8.9 | 15 | 0.5 |
| United Kingdom | | | | | |
| 1991-93 | 3139.5 | 30160 | 9.6 | 9 | 0.3 |
| 1994-96 | 2914.9 | 33550 | 11.5 | 12 | 0.4 |
| 1997-99 | 2873.3 | 31946 | 11.1 | 13 | 0.4 |

Note: comparative figures for 1985–87 not available; [a] per 1000 estimated ectopic pregnancies
Source: see Appendix 1, Table A1.3

In theory, establishing the diagnosis of ectopic pregnancy has never been easier. A combination of quantitative βhCG testing and transvaginal ultrasound allows sensitivities and specificities for the diagnosis of ectopic pregnancy that approach 100%.[1]

Commercially available dipstick tests for hCG are sensitive to values as low as 25 miu/ml, are simple to use and provide reliable results in three minutes. This test alone cannot diagnose ectopic pregnancy but does confirm the presence of an early pregnancy reliably. **These dipstick tests should be made readily available in general practices and A&E departments, as well as in specialist units in hospitals.** It is hoped that this simple measure will lower the threshold for testing and improve the diagnosis of ectopic pregnancy. However, the exact location of the pregnancy will continue to rely on ultrasound and, in some cases, will only be confirmed by laparoscopy.

The single major problem during this triennium (as in the last Report) was a failure to suspect the possibility of ectopic pregnancy in the first place and, therefore, to perform any sort of appropriate investigation. It is striking that a majority of the women who died from ruptured tubal pregnancies and who were known to have sought medical help before death had symptoms suggestive of gastrointestinal or urinary tract disease. Presumably, clinical presentation with more typical gynaecological symptoms (including amenorrhoea and vaginal bleeding as well as abdominal pain) is more likely to suggest the correct diagnosis and trigger the correct investigations and treatment. **There is a clear need to highlight the fact of atypical clinical presentation of women with tubal pregnancies to undergraduate medical and nursing students and postgraduate trainees in relevant specialties, including primary care, emergency medicine, general surgery and obstetrics and gynaecology.**

Five women who died presented with symptoms that suggested gastrointestinal disorder:

> A woman with a history of infertility developed diarrhoea and vomiting. Her period was late but her menstrual cycle was usually prolonged and she was apparently unaware that she was pregnant. Abdominal pain followed. She was found dead at home. Autopsy revealed a ruptured tubal pregnancy.

> Another woman complained to her GPs, on successive days, of abdominal pain. Her period was delayed and a pregnancy test proved positive. Abdominal pain with diarrhoea recurred before an arranged ultrasound scan could be done. The woman was noted to be pale and sweaty and hypotensive and an ambulance was called but she had a cardiac arrest with prolonged asystole in transit to the hospital. She was resuscitated in A&E and taken to the operating theatre. At laparotomy, three litres of blood were found in the peritoneal cavity from a ruptured tubal pregnancy. Unfortunately, major cerebral damage had resulted from prolonged asystole and the patient died in the intensive care unit (ICU).

> A woman presented to her GP with a short history of vomiting, diarrhoea and abdominal pain. There had been no history of abnormal vaginal bleeding or of a missed period. Despite this, a pregnancy test was positive on the day of consultation. It is not clear if the test was done by the GP or by the woman, or if that information was available at the time of the consultation. Whichever, the diagnosis of ectopic was apparently not considered and the patient collapsed

and died the following day. Autopsy revealed a ruptured tubal pregnancy with more than two litres of blood in the peritoneal cavity.

A very young and socially disadvantaged teenager was seen at home because of vomiting by her GP. The patient's mother was present during the consultation. There was no history of a missed period or of vaginal bleeding although the patient was noted to be pale. She was not referred to hospital and she collapsed later that day and died despite attempts at resuscitation in the A&E department. Autopsy revealed a ruptured tubal pregnancy.

It is difficult to elicit a sexual history from a young teenager with the mother present but the combination of vomiting and pallor, in this case, should have provoked further investigation.

A woman attended an A&E department on three occasions with abdominal pain. She was diagnosed as having constipation and discharged on each occasion. She died of a ruptured tubal pregnancy.

Ectopic pregnancy can also be mistaken for urinary tract disorder:

A woman with a history of infertility was known to be pregnant, but had not yet attended the antenatal clinic. She presented to her GP with abdominal pain, backache, shivering and dysuria. There had been no vaginal bleeding. Her abdominal tenderness was sufficient to make walking difficult. A diagnosis of urinary tract infection was made and antibiotic treatment was started. She collapsed and died of a ruptured ectopic pregnancy some hours later.

Three women with tubal pregnancies died while under the care of gynaecologists in hospital. Two of the women died as a direct consequence of laparoscopic procedures. In both of these cases, there seemed unnecessary delay (in hospital) in making the diagnosis despite high-risk features:

A woman who had undergone salpingectomy previously for an ectopic pregnancy and who was known to have a damaged remaining fallopian tube was admitted with a suspected further ectopic pregnancy. She had been amenorrhoeic for nine weeks, had a vaginal bleed and low abdominal pain. An ultrasound scan showed no evidence of an intrauterine pregnancy. Laparoscopy was undertaken several days after admission by a registrar and this proved a difficult procedure because the woman was overweight. Laparoscopy was abandoned for 'mini-laparotomy', which revealed an ectopic pregnancy in the residual tube, which was removed. For the rest of the following week, the patient experienced abdominal pain and vomiting. An abdominal X-ray revealed dilated loops of small bowel but the general surgical team did not think that there was evidence of intestinal damage. Eventually, laparotomy was undertaken when the patient was clearly very unwell. Three litres of intestinal fluid were free in the peritoneal cavity, having leaked from a hole in the ileum, presumably caused by the trochar before introduction of the laparoscope. The patient had a cardiac arrest during the operation. She was resuscitated but died later in the ICU.

This patient was overweight and that may have led to the delay in undertaking laparoscopy. If so, it was inappropriate to delegate to a trainee the surgical management of a case that was anticipated as potentially difficult. There was also inappropriate delay in making the decision to perform repeat laparotomy after the initial procedure, in a woman who was clearly becoming increasingly unwell.

> A woman was admitted to hospital with abdominal pain and vaginal bleeding. She had an intrauterine contraceptive device in place and a pregnancy test was found to be positive. There was no clear history of a missed period. It is not obvious from the records what was seen on ultrasound, if this indeed had been performed. Four days after admission, uterine curettage was performed and tissues were sent for histological examination. Because these showed no evidence of chorionic villi, and because the βhCG remained elevated, it was decided to perform a laparoscopy for a probable ectopic pregnancy. This procedure was performed by two specialist registrars, late one night, seven days after the patient's admission to hospital. Diagnostic laparoscopy confirmed the diagnosis of an ectopic pregnancy and attempts were made to perform laparoscopic salpingectomy. During this procedure, and presumably on introducing instruments into the peritoneal cavity, damage occurred to both the aorta and one common iliac artery. Despite laparotomy, massive transfusion, senior clinicians being summoned from home and repair of the damaged vessels, the patient died in the operating theatre.

The care in this case was substandard in a number of respects. It is difficult to understand why it took so long to perform a laparoscopy to confirm or exclude the diagnosis of ectopic pregnancy. Given that the patient had been in hospital for a week and that her clinical state was stable, there was no clinical justification for her operation being performed late at night. When major problems were encountered during the procedure, there was inevitable delay in summoning senior assistance from home.

The RCOG guideline *The Management of Tubal Pregnancies*[2] includes a systematic review of the evidence of effectiveness and safety of laparoscopic versus open surgery for ectopic pregnancy. From available trials, laparoscopic surgery is associated with less blood loss, lower analgesic requirements, shorter hospital stay and quicker postoperative recovery. Laparoscopic surgery is not recommended in the presence of profound shock, although that was not the case here (before surgery). The Guideline also contains explicit information about training requirements before undertaking such surgery. It is not known if the specialist registrars fulfilled these requirements or not.

In the following case, difficulties were encountered during open surgery:

> An epileptic woman with sickle cell trait and a 'low CD4 count' was admitted to hospital and diagnosed as having an ectopic pregnancy. She had multiple seizures before transfer to the operating theatre. General anaesthesia was induced by a senior house officer and surgery was undertaken by a junior specialist registrar, who encountered surgical difficulties because of dense pelvic adhesions. A more senior specialist registrar was summoned. The on-call consultant could not

be contacted but another consultant was consulted but did not attend. There was a ruptured tubal pregnancy. The procedure took more than two hours to complete and three units of blood were transfused in the operating theatre. Postoperatively, the patient developed pulmonary oedema which was treated promptly and correctly. However, she developed adult respiratory distress syndrome (ARDS) and disseminated intravascular coagulation and died some days later in the ICU.

Care was substandard in delegating the management of a manifestly difficult case to junior staff, who rapidly found themselves out of their depths. It seems likely that a very junior anaesthetist over transfused and infused the patient in theatre. The scale of lung problems postoperatively, however, does raise the possibility of gastric aspiration having occurred during the repeated seizures before surgery.

Three women were found dead at home. They were not, it seems, known to be pregnant and had not sought medical care. In each case, autopsy revealed a ruptured ectopic pregnancy with massive haemoperitoneum.

The final case of ectopic pregnancy represented a rare cervical pregnancy:

> A cervical pregnancy was detected by ultrasound in early gestation and feticide was performed by the injection of potassium chloride. This was followed by methotrexate treatment to try to prevent further trophoblast invasion. The patient remained in hospital for around a month and then went home but was readmitted subsequently with signs of infection. A decision was made to perform a surgical evacuation under general anaesthesia. The patient was apparently aware of the risk of haemorrhage but was keen to retain her uterus. Unfortunately, haemorrhage was torrential and, despite hysterectomy and transfusion, death occurred in the ICU.

Cervical pregnancy is a rare form of ectopic pregnancy, which obstetricians may never encounter during their professional careers. Little detailed information is available about this case, but general comments may be made. Because of the risk of life-threatening haemorrhage in this condition, the advice of interventional radiologists may be useful.[3] Opening the abdomen, before surgical evacuation, may also be wise to facilitate rapid hysterectomy, should that prove necessary.

## Miscarriage

Two women who died after miscarriage are counted in this Chapter and discussed here, as are one *Late* case counted in Chapter 15 and one case of sepsis after miscarriage counted in Chapter 7, from which similar lessons may be drawn. Four other women who died after septic miscarriage are counted and discussed in Chapter 7.

Under the heading 'miscarriage' are included women who had nonviable pregnancies, diagnosed by ultrasound, that would inevitably have resulted in miscarriage had surgical or medical intervention not occurred. Thus, one case of hydatidiform mole is included.

A woman with a long history of alcohol dependence had been admitted several times as an inpatient for psychiatric care, the most recent being shortly before her presentation to an A&E department with a major seizure. The seizure was attributed to alcohol withdrawal. The following day, a surgical evacuation of the uterus was performed for retained products, following a miscarriage at 13 weeks of gestation. A clotting screen was normal pre-operatively, and the procedure seems to have been straightforward. It is not clear from hospital records when the patient was discharged home but it was probably during the same day. She was found dead at home the next day. After autopsy, the death was ascribed to 'acute circulatory collapse' although there remains uncertainty about the exact pathway to death. Certainly, the pathology assessors were unconvinced that the amount of blood within the uterine cavity at autopsy could have caused death. It is not clear from available documents how much blood loss might have been 'revealed'. Other abnormal features at autopsy included early bronchopneumonia, extensive liver disease and some myocardial fibrosis.

Although the actual cause of death remains uncertain, it seems clear that a woman with such a complex medical history, including a recent major seizure, might have benefited from less abrupt discharge from hospital.

A homeless and very young teenager, who had run away from home following abuse, had an evacuation of uterus of retained products of conception after a miscarriage. The operation was complicated by perforation of the uterus. The patient appeared to recover from this, but was found, a few weeks later, in cardiorespiratory arrest, suffering from severe hypothermia, in a front garden on a freezing cold night. She died shortly after admission to hospital and, at autopsy, although some traces of morphine were found, no specific cause of death was determined. The balance of pathological opinion inclines towards an accidental overdose of morphine but this could not be accurately proven. This underage girl, who was also a regular injecting drug user, had at some time been known to social services but appeared to be out of touch with them at the time of her death. There is no indication that any thought was given to her future when she was discharged from medical care. No arrangements appear to have been made to offer her shelter or protection and, after discharge, she went to live in the open under a duvet. There was clearly a major failure in the provision of social service support for this vulnerable child and little consideration appears to have been given to her future care by hospital staff.

These two cases strongly highlight the need to consider each individual woman's particular needs rather than unthinking adherence to usual discharge routines.

The following disturbing case of sepsis following miscarriage and counted in Chapter 7; Genital tract sepsis also raises concerns about areas of the health service treating some people with a degree of complacency that borders on indifference:

A young woman from an ethnic minority group was found to have embryonic death early in her pregnancy. A decision was made to await spontaneous miscarriage. She underwent surgical evacuation of the uterus some two weeks later. She was discharged home but was readmitted shortly afterwards and it seems that she underwent a laparotomy because of suspicion of ectopic pregnancy. There was no ectopic pregnancy. She was subsequently admitted to the ICU where she remained gravely ill with ARDS and presumed sepsis, until she died.

This case was not reported to the Enquiry but was identified by screening procedures at the Office for National Statistics (ONS). The clinical details are thin in the extreme because the patient's case notes have gone missing in the hospital concerned. The consultant staff nominally responsible for this patient's care have no recollection of her.

Maternal deaths are thankfully rare in the UK and it is difficult to believe that, in an obstetrics and gynaecology unit in Britain with adequate pathways of communication and even minimal commitment to clinical audit, a death such as this can go apparently unnoticed. Possible reasons for this may include poor communications, institutional dysfunction or lack of concern for less articulate women from poor social circumstances. We cannot be sure whether some or all of these reasons applied in this case.

The deaths of four women after septic miscarriage are counted and discussed in detail in Chapter 7. These deaths include a case of embryonic death detected at 13 weeks, overwhelming sepsis after an amniocentesis for an abnormal Down syndrome serum screen result, a septic miscarriage at 20 weeks and septicaemia at 20 weeks associated with cervical cerclage and premature rupture of membranes.

In the next case, aspects of anaesthetic care and, in particular, the absence of a consultant anaesthetist during an anticipated high-risk procedure, demonstrated substandard care:

> A woman with a hydatidiform mole underwent suction evacuation under general anaesthesia. The operation was performed by a specialist registrar with a consultant gynaecologist in attendance. The anaesthetic was given by a specialist registrar. Further details are sketchy but the gestation seems to have been around 18 weeks. The possibility of hyperthyroidism associated with the mole had clearly been considered because the patient had started treatment with carbimazole two weeks previously. However, she was hypertensive and tachycardic in the anaesthetic room. These signs were attributed to anxiety. Beta-blockade was applied during the operation, which was uncomplicated. However, the patient developed pulmonary oedema at the end of the procedure in association with a 'thyroid storm'. She developed ARDS in the ICU and had signs of sepsis (source and organism undetermined) and died two weeks after evacuation of her uterus.

## Termination of pregnancy

There were two deaths that followed termination of pregnancy. In both cases, the processes leading to death were unclear. In neither case, could the death be attributed to substandard surgical technique. Care was not judged to be substandard:

> A woman with sickle cell trait underwent vacuum aspiration of an early pregnancy, without anaesthesia, and with no apparent difficulty. An intrauterine contraceptive device was inserted at the same time. The patient re-presented after three weeks with an acute illness diagnosed as thrombotic thrombocytopenic purpura. There was no objective evidence of infection or of retained products. She died despite intensive care.

> A young woman underwent termination of pregnancy by suction aspiration at 15 weeks of gestation in a private hospital. No problems were encountered during the surgical procedure or during anaesthesia but, shortly after the end of the operation, the patient's oxygen saturation dropped suddenly. She was resuscitated and transferred to a major hospital, after some delay. By the time of her arrival, there was evidence of disseminated intravascular coagulation. She died some days later, despite intensive care.

The history in this case is compatible with amniotic fluid embolism, although this would seem to be unusually early in pregnancy for such a complication. It is not clear from the autopsy report what strategies were used to identify fetal squamous cells in the maternal lungs. None was identified but these probably would not have been identifiable at such an early gestation in any case. The case is discussed in Chapter 5.

## Others deaths before 24 completed weeks of gestation

In all, 61women died before 24 weeks of completed gestation and, of those not counted in this Chapter, there were: ten *Direct* deaths from thromboembolism before 24 weeks of gestation, counted and discussed in Chapter 2; six *Indirect* cardiac deaths, counted and discussed in Chapter 10; and three *Indirect* deaths from suicide, counted and discussed in Chapter 11.

Eighteen *Indirect* deaths are counted and discussed in Chapter 12. Of these, four were diabetic, three had epilepsy, two had cerebral infarcts, two had probable HIV (one proven and one not tested for HIV but who had toxoplasmosis and a low CD4 count) and there was one case each of systemic lupus erythematosis, cystic fibrosis, asthma, liver disease, pneumonia, splenic artery aneurysm, and one woman had complications following an oophorectomy.

Eleven deaths were classified as *Coincidental* and are counted in Chapter 14 and there was one early pregnancy death from cancer included in Chapter 13.

**This Chapter has been read by Professor Lesley Regan, St Mary's Hospital, London.**

## References

1. Ankum WM. Diagnosing suspected ectopic pregnancy. *BMJ* 2000;321:1235–6.
2. Royal College of Obstetricians and Gynaecologists. *The Management of Tubal Pregnancies. Guideline No. 21.* London: RCOG; 1999. Available online at: http://www.rcog.org.uk/guidelines/tubal.html
3. Hanson E, Chitkara U, McAlpine J, El-Sayed Y, Drake MD, Razavi MK. Pelvic arterial embolization for control of obstetric haemorrhage: A five year experience. *Am J Obstet Gynecol* 1999;180:1454–60.

CHAPTER 7

# Genital tract sepsis

WILLIAM THOMPSON on behalf of the Editorial Board

## Genital tract sepsis: key recommendations

- The onset of life-threatening sepsis at any stage of pregnancy can be insidious and all doctors and midwives must be aware of the symptoms and signs and be prepared to institute immediate treatment to avoid serious consequences.

- A patient with prolonged rupture of the membranes who develops a fever and/or tachycardia should be carefully assessed by senior staff.

- In patients with spontaneous rupture of the membranes not in labour, vaginal assessments should be avoided or kept to a minimum and undertaken with appropriately aseptic precautions.

- There is clear evidence from controlled trials showing the benefits of prophylactic antibiotics for emergency caesarean section. This Report confirms that this policy is still not universally employed.

- When infection develops and the patient is systematically ill, urgent and repeated bacteriological specimens, including blood cultures, must be obtained. Advice from a microbiologist must be sought at an early stage to assist with the use of appropriate antibiotic therapy.

- There is some evidence in this Report of a failure to use the most appropriate antibiotics as recommended in hospital protocols.

- In severe cases of sepsis, doctors should be prepared, without delay, to give parenteral antibiotics before the diagnosis is confirmed.

## Summary

There were 14 deaths in this triennium directly due to genital tract sepsis and four others in which it may have played a significant part. These 18 deaths are four more than those reported in the previous triennial Report. Of the cases counted in other Chapters, one is classified as *Indirect* and counted in Chapter 12, as the infection most likely arose in the urinary tract. There was one death from peritonitis following a bowel perforation during an operation for an ectopic pregnancy counted in Chapter 6. There were also two *Late* deaths counted in Chapter 15.

Substandard care occurred in seven of the cases discussed in this Chapter.

The cases discussed in this Chapter have been divided into sepsis before delivery, puerperal sepsis after vaginal delivery and sepsis following surgery, as shown in Table 7.1. There were no cases of necrotising fasciitis in association with pregnancy, although such cases have been reported in all four previous triennial Reports.

**Table 7.1**  Maternal deaths from genital tract sepsis, rates per million maternities; United Kingdom 1985–99

| Triennium | Early pregnancy[a] (n) | Puerperal (n) | After surgical procedure (n) | Before or during labour (n) | Total (n) | Rate per million maternities |
|---|---|---|---|---|---|---|
| 1985–87 | 3 | 2 | 2 | 2 | 9 | 4.0 |
| 1988–90 | 8 | 4 | 5 | 0 | 17 | 7.2 |
| 1991–93 | 4 | 4 | 5 | 2 | 15 | 6.5 |
| 1994–96 | 2[b] | 11 | 3 | 1 | 17 | 7.3 |
| 1997–99 | 6 | 2 + 2 Late | 1 | 7 | 18 | 8.4 |

[a] Includes deaths following miscarriage, ectopic and other causes; [b] in 1994–96 these deaths were included in Chapter 6 Early pregnancy deaths

## Sepsis before delivery

There were five cases of sepsis occurring in early pregnancy, which are now counted in this Chapter. A further woman, whose death is counted and discussed in Chapter 6, Early pregnancy deaths, died of peritonitis following a bowel perforation at laparoscopy for an ectopic pregnancy. A further seven cases of antenatal sepsis occurred in pregnancies of greater than 24 weeks of gestation. In one of these cases, the most likely origin of the fatal infection was the urinary tract; this case is counted in Chapter 12 *Indirect* deaths.

There is a very significant increase in the incidence of fatal antenatal infections in both early and late pregnancy. There was only one case of sepsis before delivery in the previous triennial Report.

## Deaths before 24 weeks of gestation

In a case also discussed in Chapter 9 Anaesthesia, an older parous woman had a single puncture diagnostic amniocentesis. Within 24 hours of this procedure she was admitted to hospital with a pyrexia and lower abdominal pain. The following day she miscarried and an evacuation of retained products was undertaken. She suffered a cardiac arrest at the end of the operation and resuscitation was successful. Gram-negative rods were cultured from the products of conception and she was commenced on broad-spectrum antibiotics. She subsequently developed disseminated intravascular coagulation (DIC) and in spite of intensive therapy, including a subtotal hysterectomy, she died from multiple organ failure some days later.

It was suggested that the cause of death was amniotic fluid embolism but there was no pathological evidence to support this diagnosis. The most likely cause of death was a fulminating infection.

> A woman with learning difficulties was admitted to hospital with a septic miscarriage with a three-day history of diarrhoea and, on admission, she had a marked tachycardia. A manual removal of the placenta was performed under general anaesthesia and during the operation she was hypotensive. Shortly afterwards she collapsed with signs of septic shock. She was ventilated, stabilised, commenced on antibiotics and transferred to an intensive care unit (ICU) in another hospital some miles away. About two days later a laparotomy was performed because of free fluid in the abdomen and to exclude a uterine perforation. There was no evidence of organ pathology or abdominal sepsis. In spite of intensive management, she developed DIC and multiple organ failure and died a few days later.

The severity of this patient's condition was underestimated on admission and prior to the initial anaesthetic, which was undertaken by a junior anaesthetist. Furthermore, antibiotics should have been given some time prior to the manual removal of the placenta. The management of this case was clearly substandard.

> A parous patient was admitted with a short history of vomiting and lower abdominal pain at three months of gestation. An ultrasound scan confirmed that she had a missed embryonic death. A suction evacuation of the uterus was performed, which was followed by profuse bleeding. A laparotomy was undertaken, leading to a hysterectomy. She had a cardiac arrest at the end of the operation and was successfully resuscitated and transferred to ICU. In spite of massive transfusion and intensive management she had a further cardiac arrest from which she did not recover. The histology of the uterus and the clinical findings strongly suggested a fulminating streptococcal infection.

The GP failed to recognise the seriousness of her condition, ascribing her symptoms to a urinary infection. When the seriousness of her situation became obvious, the misdiagnosis was ascribed to the examination having been conducted in a room with the curtains closed. Once referred to hospital the management of this case with profound vaginal bleeding and DIC was left to junior staff and the clinical notes suggest that she was grossly under-transfused. Again, there was clear evidence of substandard care.

> A nulliparous woman who spoke little English had a missed embryonic death diagnosed by ultrasound. It was decided to await spontaneous miscarriage, although this was not according to the hospital protocol. She had an evacuation of retained products some two weeks later. This was unremarkable and she was discharged home the next day. Two days later she collapsed and was readmitted to hospital and a laparotomy was performed to exclude an ectopic pregnancy. However, the pelvic findings were normal. She was then transferred to ICU with a diagnosis of sepsis and acute respiratory distress syndrome (ARDS) and died several days later.

It is difficult to comment on the management of this case, as the medical records could not be located.

> A woman with a history of several unsuccessful pregnancies had a cervical cerclage performed at 12 weeks of gestation. At 20 weeks a second cervical suture was inserted because of bulging membranes and one week later a third suture was inserted. During the latter procedure the membranes were ruptured. Twenty hours later there was evidence of septicaemia with profound hypotension. The sutures were removed and the uterus evacuated. Her condition rapidly deteriorated and she developed DIC. In spite of intensive therapy she died within 48 hours. An autopsy confirmed uterine sepsis with mixed coliforms as the cause of the infection.

The decision to insert a third cervical suture after rupture of the membranes is considered by the *assessors* to have been inappropriate. Furthermore, the sutures should have been removed following the rupture of her membranes. This case highlights the potential dangers of this type of intervention.

## Deaths in pregnancy over 24 weeks of gestation

There were six cases of sepsis complicating later pregnancy counted in this Chapter and one arising from a urinary tract infection counted in Chapter 12 but discussed here:

> An older parous woman with a multiple pregnancy had normal progress until late in pregnancy, when she was referred to hospital with a brief history of vomiting and rigors. On admission, she had classical signs of septicaemia with extreme hypotension. There was no uterine tenderness but the fetuses were dead. Active resuscitation was undertaken and she was commenced on broad-spectrum antibiotics. An artificial rupture of the membranes (ARM) was performed and oxytocin was commenced. She then developed DIC and severe vaginal bleeding. A caesarean section was performed because of the deterioration in her condition. She had further vaginal bleeding and an unsuccessful attempt was made to treat this by arterial embolisation. She received large quantities of blood, plasma and platelets throughout. There was a significant delay of some two to three hours in obtaining platelets as they had to come from the blood transfusion service many miles away. Blood cultures reported group A haemolytic streptococcus. She developed multiple organ failure and died a few days post partum. Because this woman was stated as being allergic to penicillin she was not given the antibiotic on admission. When the culture confirmed that the organism responsible for the infection was a streptococcus a test dose of penicillin gave no reaction and she was then started on this antibiotic. An autopsy was not performed.

The source of the infection in this case was not determined. The surgical procedures undertaken were justified but were unlikely to influence the outcome, given the failure to arrest the coagulation failure. This case highlights the problem of treating severely ill patients with DIC without immediate access to a blood bank. However, it is unlikely that the delay in obtaining blood products would have influenced the outcome. The earlier use of penicillin is the other factor which might have helped but the staff could not be blamed for such a delay when it was stated in the notes that she was allergic to penicillin.

> A primigravida with no significant past medical history was admitted to hospital in mid pregnancy with an acute urinary tract infection. In spite of appropriate antibiotic therapy she developed an *Eschericia coli* septicaemia and was transferred to ICU. Intensive management was undertaken but her condition continued to deteriorate with multiple organ failure. A caesarean section was performed, as it was considered that the gravid uterus was contributing to haemodynamic compromise. However, shortly after this operation she had a cardiac arrest and did not respond to resuscitation. An autopsy confirmed that death was due to sepsis and there were multiple renal cortical abscesses.

This *Indirect* death is counted in Chapter 12, as the source of the infection was the urinary tract.

> A parous woman was admitted to hospital with spontaneous rupture of the membranes at 30 weeks of gestation. A sepsis screen was negative on admission. Twenty-four hours later she developed tachycardia, pyrexia and intrauterine death. A short time afterwards she had rigors and was transferred to the labour ward, where intravenous antibiotics were commenced. A vaginal examination confirmed that she was in labour and an epidural was sited. Approximately one hour later her condition rapidly deteriorated with pulmonary oedema and hypotension. She required intubation because of breathing difficulties and developed DIC shortly after delivery, when her blood pressure was unrecordable. In spite of active resuscitation she died within the hour. An autopsy confirmed that death was due to *E. coli* septicaemia following chorioamnionitis.

It was considered, from a review of the notes, that there was a delay in starting antibiotics. Furthermore, the antibiotics given were cefuroxime and metronidazole, which may have been suboptimal. It was also considered inappropriate to administer an epidural to a patient with pyrexia and evidence of chorioamnionitis. Earlier recourse to the expertise of an ICU might have influenced the outcome but this was not available on the same site as the maternity unit.

> An older multigravid woman, who was a poor attender at antenatal clinics, was admitted to a district general hospital (DGH) in mid pregnancy with a five-day history of passing fluid per vaginam and severe suprapubic pain. The diagnosis of ruptured membranes was not confirmed on examination and she was discharged home within 24 hours on oral antibiotics. She was readmitted the next day with obvious ruptured membranes and was transferred to a teaching hospital with neonatal ICU facilities. Within 48 hours she was pyrexial with tachycardia and complaining of abdominal pain. Intravenous

antibiotics were commenced and she delivered a stillborn infant. A general anaesthetic was administered shortly afterwards for removal of a retained placenta. It proved impossible to extubate her following the general anaesthetic and she was transferred to ICU with established ARDS. She remained critically ill and two days after delivery a hysterectomy was performed to eliminate a possible focus of infection within the uterus. Her condition did not improve during the next few weeks in ICU and she died from multiple organ failure. An autopsy showed infection with *Klebsiella* but this was probably acquired in the ICU and the underlying cause of death was most probably Gram-negative bacillary septicaemia secondary to intrauterine infection.

The management at the time of the first admission to the DGH was considered substandard. She presented with pain, pyrexia and tachycardia and was discharged home within 24 hours on oral antibiotics. A longer period of surveillance in hospital would have been appropriate. When transferred to the teaching hospital she was not seen or assessed by a consultant obstetrician for at least two days and then only when she had been transferred to ICU. There was some delay in recognising the severity of her condition and an early delivery might have influenced the outcome.

A parous woman had normal progress of her pregnancy until early in the third trimester when she was admitted to hospital with a short history of diarrhoea, vomiting and severe abdominal pain. There was extreme fetal bradycardia and it was assumed that she had had an abruption. An emergency caesarean section was performed, with the delivery of a live infant who subsequently died. The diagnosis of septic shock became apparent during the operation and she was commenced on antibiotic therapy and transferred to ICU. Group A haemolytic *Streptococcus pyogenes* was cultured from the placenta. She died several hours later from multiple organ failure.

The misdiagnosis of placental abruption when this woman presented with shock and fetal bradycardia was understandable; it did not contribute to the eventual outcome. This was considered to be a case of genital tract infection as streptococci were isolated from the placenta. There is no evidence of substandard care.

A primigravida from an ethnic minority with a short history of severe abdominal pain was admitted to hospital in the third trimester in a moribund state. The fetus had died. The clinical findings supported a diagnosis of septicaemia but despite energetic attempts at resuscitation she died within a few hours. Bacteriology at autopsy revealed positive culture for group A haemolytic streptococcus.

There appears to have been no substandard care in this case.

A parous woman with Ehlers-Danlos syndrome was admitted in the third trimester with a short history of severe abdominal pain, hypotensive and with a productive cough. She was a chronic alcoholic. It was assumed that she had a placental abruption and an emergency caesarean section was performed under spinal anaesthesia with delivery of a stillborn infant. During the operation, a haematologist reported that the blood film suggested severe sepsis. Her condition rapidly deteriorated and she developed DIC. As no ICU bed was available she was transferred some distance by ambulance but died on arrival at another hospital. The cause of death was probably septicaemia but no blood culture was taken and there was no obvious focus of infection. The autopsy was performed several days after death and was therefore of little value as regards the source of the infection.

## Sepsis after vaginal delivery

Two patients died from sepsis after vaginal delivery and are counted in this Chapter. There were also two *Late* deaths counted in Chapter 15 but described here. There is a very significant decrease in such deaths; there were ten cases in the previous Report.

> A parous woman died from generalised peritonitis five weeks after a normal delivery. She had spontaneous rupture of the membranes three days prior to augmentation of labour. She was discharged from hospital a day after delivery and was visited at home by the community midwives until two weeks post partum. Both mother and baby were reported to be well. She was then admitted to a medical ward three weeks after delivery with abdominal pain and vomiting and a diagnosis of atypical pneumonia (based on a shadow on chest X-ray). Her condition deteriorated and one week after admission a laparotomy was performed and two litres of fluid were aspirated from the peritoneal cavity. There was no obvious organ pathology apart from a thick exudate involving loops of small bowel and generalised peritoneal oedema. She subsequently developed pyrexia, extreme tachycardia and hyperventilation and two days postoperatively suffered a cardiac arrest and did not respond to resuscitation. An autopsy was not performed.

It was assumed that death was due to septicaemia but there were no details of cultures or antibiotic therapy. There would appear to have been a failure to recognise the severity of this patient's illness following her admission to the medical unit.

> A primigravida had an uncomplicated pregnancy and delivery by vacuum extraction. She was discharged home a few days post partum. Two weeks after delivery she was readmitted with pyrexia, slight vaginal bleeding and lower abdominal pain. On examination she was cyanotic and extremely hypotensive. Septic shock was diagnosed and she was resuscitated and given introvenous antibiotics. She was transferred to ICU and despite intensive therapy she developed DIC and multi-organ failure and died five weeks post partum. A high vaginal swab grew Group C beta-haemolytic streptococcus but blood cultures were sterile. An autopsy confirmed that death was due to puerperal infection and that there were retained products in the uterine cavity.

It was obvious that this patient was in a critical condition on admission to hospital and there was a 24-hour delay in her transfer to an ICU. Furthermore, there was a four-day delay between death and autopsy, which, with antibiotic therapy, meant a very poor chance of positive cultures from autopsy specimens. Group C streptococcal infections have been recorded as causing pneumonias, pericarditis, septic arthritis and a scarlet fever type rash.

There were two *Late* deaths from sepsis counted in Chapter15:

> A parous patient had a full-term normal delivery. Several weeks post partum she collapsed without warning and was transferred to A&E where she was declared dead. An autopsy showed severe pulmonary oedema and a moderate amount of haemorrhagic mucoid discharge and necrotic decidua within the uterus. A tampon was present in the vagina and cultures showed a mixed growth of Group B haemolytic streptococcus and *Clostridium perfringens* in various tissue samples, the blood and in the tampon. Death was due to septicaemia.

This *Late* maternal death occurred outside the recognised puerperium and is a classical case of 'toxic shock syndrome' rather than true puerperal sepsis.

> A parous woman, who spoke little English, was readmitted to hospital two months after a normal delivery with pyrexia and a four-day history of lower abdominal pain. A laparotomy was planned as there were signs of peritonism but she collapsed and died from a cardiac arrest prior to the surgery. The interval between admission and death was 12 hours. An autopsy revealed that she had a tubo-ovarian abscess, which had ruptured into the peritoneal cavity. Group A haemolytic streptococcus were isolated from a peritoneal culture.

## Sepsis after surgery

There was one case of sepsis after a caesarean section. There were three such cases in the previous Report. It may be speculative to suggest that, given the small numbers, this reduction is due to the recommended use of prophylactic antibiotics with caesarean section. In the following case, such a policy was not applied:

> A parous woman had a history of previous caesarean section, including one with abnormal adherence of the placenta. In this pregnancy, she had a known placenta praevia and an emergency caesarean section was performed under regional anaesthesia by a middle-grade doctor without consultant involvement. There was excessive blood loss at the operation and the uterus was closed with placental tissue still *in situ*. Transfusion with four units of blood resulted in a haemoglobin of only 7.1 g/dl. There was no record that antibiotics had been administered. She was discharged from hospital a week later and readmitted with vaginal bleeding and pyrexia a few days after this. She developed septicaemia and DIC and had further operations to control the bleeding without success. She died three weeks post partum from multi-organ failure. *Streptococcus faecalis* was isolated from high vaginal swabs and blood culture. Histology confirmed a placenta accreta.

The management of this case was clearly substandard. There was a poor appreciation of the potential risks given her past obstetric history and the caesarean section should have been performed by a consultant. Antibiotics should have been administered before and certainly immediately after the initial operation. There was also evidence that she had been under-transfused at or after the caesarean section.

## Comments

This Report demonstrates that the most common organism responsible for serious and life-threatening obstetric infections is the beta-haemolytic *Streptococcus pyogenes* (Lancefield Group A). The Lancefield Groups C and G streptococcus may also cause serious clinical syndromes but are less common. The Lancefield Group B streptococcus can be found in normal vaginal flora and is most commonly associated with neonatal septicaemia and meningitis, particularly in premature infants. Serious maternal infections may also occur with this organism.

All of these micro-organisms may be described as beta haemolytic streptococci in laboratory reports but it should be good practice to ensure that the Lancefield grouping is also reported.

In the seriously ill obstetric patient where sepsis may be implicated, it is advised that intravenous antibiotic treatment be commenced immediately. Bacteriological specimens, including blood culture, must be obtained prior to commencing such treatment but the results of the cultures will not be available. The most appropriate antibiotic treatment based on the organisms identified in this Report, would be the recently introduced penicillin derivative piperacillin/tazobactam in combination with the aminoglycoside, netilmicin.

**This Chapter has been read and commented on by Dr CH Webb FRCPath FFPRCPI, Consultant Microbiologist and Dr JG Barr PhD CBiol FIBiol FRCPath, Consultant Microbiologist.**

## CHAPTER 8

# Other *Direct* Deaths

ROBERT SHAW on behalf of the Editorial Board

## Summary

There were seven deaths due to other *Direct* causes. This is a similar number to that reported in 1994–96, although the causes of death vary. In four cases in this triennium acute fatty liver was confirmed at post mortem. Two deaths were due to genital tract trauma. One death was from septic shock following spontaneous rupture of the caecum (Ogilvie syndrome). The small number of cases by any individual cause makes statistical inference or comparison with previous Reports difficult. However, the overall maternal mortality was 2.8 per million maternities, which, as shown in Table 1.3 (in Chapter 1), is lower than in previous Reports.

## Acute fatty liver

In the first trimester nausea and vomiting are common and, unless persistent or severe enough to become hyperemesis gravidarum, can usually be managed conservatively. In the third trimester, however, these symptoms are uncommon and when they continue over several days, particularly accompanied by epigastric or abdominal pains, they can herald serious and life-threatening disorders. One such condition is acute fatty liver. In this triennium there were four deaths due to this uncommon cause:

> A primigravida was admitted in early pregnancy with hyperemesis. At 30 weeks of gestation she was readmitted with a history of vomiting but no abdominal pain. She was observed and discharged after a few days but she was readmitted two weeks later with vomiting and epigastric pain. She was mildly anaemic and had abnormal liver function tests. She was delivered by caesarean section but by then a severe clotting disorder had developed and she died shortly afterwards. Acute fatty liver and HELLP syndrome were confirmed at post mortem.

> A primigravid woman was seen by her GP over a period of a few weeks with vague symptoms. She was referred to hospital but discharged. She required readmission a few days later with vomiting and abdominal discomfort. Liver function tests were requested but not marked urgent. She then went into premature labour, requiring an assisted delivery, and later that evening the liver function test results came back as grossly abnormal. She was immediately reviewed by the medical team and transferred to a specialist liver unit. Her condition gradually deteriorated and she required several laparotomies to control bleeding but died several days later. The liver biopsy confirmed acute fatty liver.

A multiparous woman with severe social problems and a history of recreational drug use complained of vomiting for a week to neighbours and then had an antepartum haemorrhage (APH). An ambulance was called but she delivered a stillborn child during the transfer to hospital. In hospital she complained of further vomiting and abdominal pain and collapsed soon after admission. She was transferred to an intensive care unit (ICU) and soon became jaundiced and severely anaemic probably due to intra-abdominal haemorrhage. She died in the operating theatre. An autopsy showed acute fatty liver.

A young unmarried primiparous woman complained of vomiting from five months of pregnancy. She was visited several times by her GP and midwife over the next two months for sickness, headaches and vague abdominal symptoms. She was found dead in bed late in the second trimester of her pregnancy. An autopsy revealed acute fatty liver.

This last case was unusual in that she developed the problem in the later part of the second trimester.

A common thread in these four cases is an initial presentation with vomiting and vague abdominal pain or a feeling of being unwell. Three of the women were seen by medical and midwifery staff and two were admitted and then discharged from hospital. The additional symptom of associated epigastric and/or abdominal pain signalled the development of advanced liver dysfunction, coagulation disorder and haemorrhage. Early delivery, transfer to a specialist liver unit and consideration of liver transplantation may offer the possibility of survival. Nevertheless, no substandard care could be identified in any of these cases as the presentation in all of them was unclear and the diagnosis would not be immediately apparent. Patients with worsening pre-eclampsia or HELLP syndrome may well have similar features and indeed it could be argued that acute fatty liver is a variant of these disorders.

To help to recognise cases and ascribe an appropriate diagnosis clinical management advice is given in Box 8.1 below.

---

**Box 8.1     Acute fatty liver: clinical practice advice**

- Symptoms of vomiting and epigastric pain in women in the third trimester should be viewed as a potentially severe underlying disorder until proven otherwise.

- Liver function tests and full blood count (haemoglobin and platelets) are essential.

- Regular monitoring of blood pressure and urine tests for protein are necessary.

- When significant disorders of liver function develop, early delivery is advised and transfer of the patient to a specialist liver unit for subsequent management.

---

## Genital tract trauma

Instrumental delivery can cause tears in the vagina, cervix or perineum, resulting in considerable haemorrhage. The blood loss is often underestimated and, in a young woman, a fall in blood pressure and significant increase in pulse rate may not occur until imminent cardiovascular collapse.

A young single primigravida, booked for hospital delivery, went into labour early and delivered unattended at home. The child was stillborn and she was admitted to the maternity unit after delivery. There she had a primary postpartum haemorrhage (PPH). A large vaginal-wall haematoma was evacuated and the tear sutured. The total blood loss was not known and her postoperative observations were infrequent. Some hours later she had a cardiovascular collapse and senior staff were summoned. She was resuscitated and the bleeding from the vaginal tear was again sutured but by then a massive haemorrhage had occurred. Despite subsequent transfer to ICU she developed multi-organ failure and died some days later.

Estimation of blood loss at delivery is notoriously difficult and frequently it is underestimated. With genital tract trauma, severe and rapid haemorrhage can occur, which itself can hinder and obscure the site of bleeding during repair. It is advisable to measure the haemoglobin and packed cell volume in such cases and to have blood grouped and saved. Transfusion is necessary if the haemoglobin level is sufficiently low. After the repair, the pulse and blood pressure should be monitored and continued losses carefully noted.

Uterine rupture with revealed or concealed haemorrhage is nowadays likely to occur only in women who labour following a previous caesarean section:

A woman with a family history of venous thrombosis, whose previous child was delivered by caesarean section, developed a deep venous thrombosis in the late second trimester of her next pregnancy. She was anticoagulated and when the pregnancy went beyond dates, labour was induced. She required a vacuum extraction for fetal distress. Immediately after delivery she began to bleed vaginally. The consultant was called and a ruptured uterus was diagnosed. Laparotomy confirmed the diagnosis and uterine repair was undertaken. The next day it was clear that intra-abdominal bleeding was still occurring and a second laparotomy was performed with multiple bleeding points identified. Hysterectomy was performed and she was transferred to a specialist ICU. Despite extensive interventions including extra-corporeal membrane oxygenation (ECMO), the patient died.

This patient had a familial tendency to venous thrombosis and her anticoagulation for a deep venous thrombosis in this pregnancy complicated the management of her ruptured uterus and increased her risk of profound haemorrhage. Meticulous haemostasis at surgery is essential in patients on full anticoagulation and conversion to heparin allows easier reversal with protamine sulphate if required.

## Ogilvie syndrome

In 1948 Ogilvie reported spontaneous rupture of the caecum secondary to gross dilation without an obstructive cause (such as adhesions, torsion or diverticular disease)[1].

A woman had a caesarean section for a multiple pregnancy. Her postoperative recovery was not overtly abnormal, although some abdominal distension was noted. A few days after delivery she became acutely ill with a tense and tender abdomen. A laparotomy was performed and faecal peritonitis found from a perforated caecum. No cause for any obstruction was found or any other factors to explain the perforation. Despite all efforts, the patient died a day later of faecal peritonitis. This case is also described in Chapter 16; Pathology.

After postmortem examination, the cause of death was presumed to be Ogilvie syndrome: acute colonic pseudo-obstruction, characterised by acute massive dilation of the colon with no organic obstruction of the distal colon. It is an uncommon complication of many medical and surgical conditions, which, if left untreated long enough, can result in necrosis of the wall of the caecum. The resultant perforation and leak of caecal content produces a faecal peritonitis with a high mortality rate.

Current studies show that inhibition of parasympathetic nerves may be the mechanism involved. The clinical presentation is similar to that of paralytic ileus of the small bowel but abdominal distension may be more pronounced, with usually little or no abdominal tenderness, some abdominal pain and reduced or absent bowel sounds. A review of cases occurring after caesarean section[2] showed that intervention prior to rupture of the caecum significantly reduces mortality from this uncommon condition.

Careful observation of all patients who have undergone a caesarean section (or laparotomy) is essential to exclude paralytic ileus or intestinal obstruction from other causes. Auscultation of bowel sounds and recording the passage of flatus or stool are paramount in postoperative care so that if abnormalities occur appropriate investigation and management are instituted.

## References

1.  Ogilvie H. Large intestine colic due to sympathetic deprivation. A new clinical syndrome. *BMJ* 1948;ii:671–3.
2.  Tang PTM, Collopy BT, Somerville. Ogilvie syndrome with caecal perforation in the post-caesarean patient. *Aust N Z J Obstet Gynaecol* 1995;35:104–6.

CHAPTER 9

# Anaesthesia

Trevor A Thomas and Griselda M Cooper on behalf of the Editorial Board

## Anaesthesia: key recommendations

- Dedicated obstetric anaesthesia services should be available in all consultant obstetric units. These services should be capable of taking responsibility for regional analgesia, anaesthesia, recovery from anaesthesia and the management and monitoring of intravenous fluid replacement therapy.

- Adequate advance notice of elective high-risk cases must be given to the obstetric anaesthetic service. The notice must be sufficient to allow the consultation, investigation and assembly of resources needed for these cases to take place.

- When presented with problem cases requiring special skills or investigations, obstetric anaesthetists should not hesitate to call on the assistance of anaesthetic colleagues in other subspecialties, as well as colleagues in other disciplines.

- Invasive central venous and arterial pressure measurement can provide vital information about the cardiovascular system which can be life saving. Invasive monitoring via appropriate routes should be used particularly when the cardiovascular system is compromised by haemorrhage or disease.

- Care of women at high risk of maternal haemorrhage must involve consultant obstetric anaesthetists at the earliest possible time.

- Anaesthetists have a responsibility, as do all medical practitioners, to ensure that drugs are given in the correct dose, at the correct rate, by the correct route and by the most accurate means.

- It seems not to be widely appreciated that Syntocinon® (Alliance) can cause profound, fatal hypotension, especially in the presence of cardiovascular compromise. Administration should follow the guidance in the *British National Formulary*, *Martindale* and other standard formularies. When given as an intravenous bolus the drug should be given slowly in a dose of not more than 5 iu.

## Summary

The central assessors in anaesthesia reviewed the cases of all the women in this Report identified as having received an anaesthetic for this triennium, some 142 cases. In looking at the individual cases, the assessors were struck by the high standards of anaesthetic care generally provided, sometimes in difficult circumstances. In most cases the standard of record keeping was also high. However, there are areas of concern about the consistency of anaesthetic services between units. Reviewing the records showed that in some places the quality and quantity of anaesthesia service does not meet the declared standards of the relevant professional bodies.

In deciding the likely cause of death, the evidence had to be weighed up without the benefit of questioning all those involved in a patient's care. Much reliance was placed on the local assessors and their ability to make discreet enquiries. Sometimes, even after coroner's inquests, the cause of death was unclear. It was therefore a matter of judgement assigning a death as being a direct result of anaesthesia or whether substandard care contributed to the demise. Key points of the cases illustrated here result from the central assessors' judgement, bearing in mind that the purpose of the exercise is to learn from errors and improve patient care in the future.

The challenges presented to the obstetric anaesthetist are increasing in number, complexity and severity. Many sick mothers have received anaesthetics safely and anaesthetists are accepting an increasing responsibility for aspects of mother's care that fall naturally within their competence and control. Anaesthetists are trained to recognise and treat major haemorrhage that they encounter in many areas of their professional practice. Obstetric haemorrhage is sometimes more difficult to manage appropriately. Nevertheless, it is disappointing to record substandard aspects of anaesthetic care in seven deaths due to haemorrhage. These cases are discussed in Chapter 4; Haemorrhage, together with others. The contributions that anaesthesia services made to these fatalities are however discussed here.

Conduct of anaesthesia includes preoperative preparation, delivery of anaesthesia and postoperative recovery. In this triennium, there was one anaesthetic death ascribed as being directly due to the conduct of anaesthesia for caesarean section, in particular to the administration of oxytocin in a compromised patient. Two other deaths are ascribed to anaesthetics given after prolonged and complex care in the intensive care unit (ICU). In both these cases, the patient's condition was improving but further surgical treatment was needed. Death resulted from complications of anaesthesia for that surgery.

## Deaths due to anaesthesia

There were three deaths in this triennium that were directly due to actions or omissions of anaesthesia services or staff:

> A woman requested epidural analgesia during her labour. An epidural catheter was sited but a test dose of 4 ml bupivacaine 0.25% resulted in a high sensory and motor block within two to three minutes. Clear fluid aspirated from the catheter tested positive for sugar. A diagnosis of subarachnoid catheter placement was made.
>
> It was decided to use the subarachnoid catheter for labour analgesia. All subsequent injections of bupivacaine were given by an anaesthetist

and the quality of resulting analgesia was described as good. Seven hours later labour had failed to progress, in spite of oxytocin augmentation and it was decided to deliver the fetus by caesarean section. Anaesthesia was not adequate for caesarean section so a top-up injection of 2 ml plain bupivacaine 0.5% was given from a 20-ml syringe. The spinal block spread higher than expected. The woman experienced difficulty breathing and then lost consciousness. She developed a bradycardia of 30 bpm and the systolic blood pressure decreased to 60 mmHg. The patient was intubated promptly and given fluids, ephedrine, atropine and adrenaline/epinephrine. Cardiac output was restored but the blood pressure had increased only to 80 mmHg systolic when the baby was born apnoeic and pulseless. The paediatrician had not arrived and the anaesthetist was asked to intubate and resuscitate the baby. By the time the anaesthetist had completed the resuscitation the obstetrician had discovered an adherent placenta and the mother was losing blood. The obstetrician requested oxytocin (Syntocinon®) to improve uterine tone. The anaesthetist was reluctant because the systolic blood pressure was only 60 mmHg. After rapid infusion of intravenous colloid solution and further adrenaline/epinephrine, oxytocin 10 iu was given. Cardiac arrest occurred almost at once. Resuscitation followed accepted practice but was unsuccessful.

High spinal block, bradycardia and hypotension are recognised complications of spinal anaesthesia. The cardiovascular complications involve complex reflexes[1] that are still not widely understood. They are sometimes difficult to treat, especially when drugs with cardiovascular side effects further complicate the clinical picture.

Whether the use of hyperbaric bupivacaine would have limited the cephalic spread and avoided the high block is questionable. The literature would suggest not. However, using a 20-ml syringe to measure a 2-ml does not ensure great accuracy. Syringes of 2-, 3- or 5-ml capacity are available and employed because additional fractions of a millilitre of bupivacaine can affect the extent of a subarachnoid anaesthetic.

In this case, the patient was initially resuscitated effectively but the hypotension was not completely reversed when the anaesthetist was asked to resuscitate the baby. At the time the maternal blood pressure was 80 mmHg systolic. The baby was resuscitated quickly and effectively. However, the anaesthetist's full attention was distracted from the mother. In that time, the maternal systolic blood pressure had decreased to 60 mmHg. Uterine hypotonia occurred and the obstetrician asked for 10 iu oxytocin to be given. This is a common obstetric request during caesarean section.

The administration of oxytocin in the presence of a high spinal block, hypotension and recent bradycardia, accompanied by bleeding at caesarean section, produced a situation from which the patient could not be rescued. Oxytocin has peripheral and central cardiovascular receptor sites and complex cardiovascular actions.[5,6]

It is not widely appreciated that the dose recommended in the *British National Formulary*[2] (and other formularies[3,4]) is 5, not 10, units. The *British National*

*Formulary* states: 'Dose: caesarean section, *by slow intravenous injection* immediately after delivery, 5 units'. Oxytocin has a direct relaxant effect on vascular smooth muscle. Under normal circumstances there is a reflex tachycardia and increased cardiac output that accompanies the transient decrease in blood pressure, as shown in Figure 9.1. However, the hypovolaemic patient (or one with compromised cardiac function) may not respond in the normal way. In such circumstances, the drug may have lethal effects and among the contraindications to its use is severe cardiovascular disease.[2]

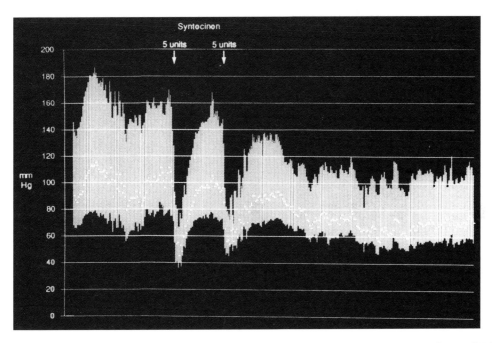

**Figure 9.1** Arterial pressure in a patient during caesarean section under spinal anaesthesia; note the decrease in blood pressure after five units of Syntocinon® on two occasions (courtesy of TH Clutton-Brock and GM Cooper)

Every medical practitioner administering any drug is responsible for ensuring that the drug, its dose and method or route of administration are correct and appropriate. A request from another practitioner does not absolve him or her from this responsibility.

The assessors appreciated the difficulties in this case. Anaesthetists should remember that their primary responsibility is to the mother[7] and that they must summon help at the first signs of unexpected reactions to treatment.

> The second patient received five anaesthetics, the first for a caesarean section during which she suffered a major obstetric haemorrhage. She then required several further operations to control the bleeding. During the fourth, abdominal packs were placed to control continuing venous bleeding and the patient returned to the ICU intubated and ventilated. She was successfully weaned from the ventilator and extubated 24 hours later. Two days later, removal of the abdominal packs was planned. The patient was taken to theatre from ICU with invasive cardiovascular monitoring in place. There is no record of any gastric secretion prophylaxis prior to this anaesthetic.

After preoxygenation anaesthesia was induced using propofol 120 mg and fentanyl 100 μg. Muscle relaxation was achieved with cisatracurium 14 mg. There was no mention of cricoid pressure. These two facts suggest that a rapid sequence induction technique was not used on this occasion. Pulmonary aspiration of fluid occurred. The aspirate was tested and gave an acid reaction. Surgery was completed successfully. The patient was extubated and returned to ICU. Her condition slowly deteriorated and she was re-intubated and required ventilation 24 hours later. Aspiration pneumonitis was subsequently diagnosed on X-ray appearances. She continued to deteriorate and died some 12 days later.

This patient was rescued from life-threatening problems, receiving anaesthesia without mishap on the first four occasions. There were many factors that could have contributed to the eventual organ failure but it is difficult to ignore the fact that her condition had been improving until the pulmonary aspiration. Given the patient's previous problems and the fact that she came to theatre from ICU for removal of abdominal packs, acid prophylaxis and a rapid sequence induction were indicated. There is no record that these precautions were taken. These omissions constitute substandard anaesthetic care.

A multiparous woman received a general anaesthetic for a caesarean delivery. She had suffered postpartum haemorrhages after earlier deliveries. Her blood was known to be difficult to crossmatch because of antibodies and she had failed to keep a blood transfusion service antenatal appointment to plan future haematological care. She was therefore a high-risk case. In spite of these known problems, blood was not crossmatched when labour began.

Because blood was not available when bleeding occurred at caesarean section, large volumes of colloid and crystalloid were needed to maintain cardiovascular stability. Carboprost was used to control bleeding, after which bronchospasm and crepitations were detected. Over-transfusion was diagnosed. Direct transfer from theatre to ICU was arranged. Treatment in ICU was successful in stabilising the patient for the first two to three days. However, after four to five days, she became anuric and she was transferred to another ICU for haemodialysis and further respiratory support including tracheostomy. Respiratory performance improved. The first tracheostomy tube was either blocked or became displaced. Attempts to change it were not successful and an endotracheal tube was introduced via the tracheostomy site.

The ICU did not have a small enough fibre-optic bronchoscope to perform an examination via the endotracheal tube that had been passed, so elective revision of the tracheostomy was attempted. During this procedure difficulties with the airway and ventilation were experienced. Jet ventilation was used in an attempt to overcome the problem. Surgical emphysema was detected. Eventually the airway was lost and death resulted.

At some stage, the endotracheal tube became extratracheal and jet ventilation probably caused the surgical emphysema. At post mortem, a number of tears were identified in the trachea and bronchi and surgical emphysema of the mediastinum and subcutaneous tissues confirmed.

Although death resulted from the difficult airway problem, substandard care was present in several aspects. Firstly, the failure to crossmatch blood for this high-risk mother when she was admitted in labour led to intraoperative difficulties which, in turn, contributed to the need for ICU admission. Secondly, there seems to have been little understanding that the adverse effects of carboprost include bronchospasm and pulmonary oedema. Thirdly, there was a failure to site a central venous pressure (CVP) line in theatre when it might have helped to differentiate between the possible causes of pulmonary oedema and to guide fluid therapy. Whether it would have changed the outcome is conjectural. Fourthly, in the second ICU there was no access to the fibre-optic endoscope of the size needed for endoscopy via a 6.0-mm endotracheal tube. This examination might have given a better understanding of the airway dimensions and condition before the tracheostomy revision was attempted. This knowledge may have allowed better preoperative preparation and may have prevented the death.

## Deaths to which anaesthesia contributed

In addition to the three deaths detailed above, there were a number of deaths that contain messages for anaesthesia services. In some, anaesthesia care was regarded as substandard. These deaths have been subdivided, although, inevitably there is overlap between the categories:

1.  Lack of multidisciplinary cooperation (seven deaths, one also counted in haemorrhage)

2.  Major obstetric haemorrhage (six deaths, one also counted in poor cooperation)

3.  Poor postoperative care (three deaths)

4.  Lack of appreciation of severity of illness (two cases are described here as illustrations but failure to recognise the severity of illness was present to some degree in most of the cases counted in categories 1, 2, 3 and 5; two others are counted in Chapters 5 and 6)

5.  Sepsis (two deaths).

### 1. Lack of multidisciplinary cooperation

Obstetricians failed to give adequate warning of impending problems to anaesthetic departments in at least six of the maternal deaths in this triennium. The lack of consultation with anaesthetic colleagues contributed significantly to a number of these deaths. The lessons from the following examples in this Chapter need to be widely disseminated. All team members need to be aware of the vital contributions that can be made by anaesthesia when adequate warning is given and the harm that can result when it is not. Obstetric anaesthetists must also remember that they have colleagues with different, but invaluable, skills provided that the anaesthetist calls on their help in good time.

> A morbidly obese woman became increasingly short of breath towards the end of her pregnancy. An initial diagnosis of pulmonary embolism was made but subsequently excluded. She developed a tachycardia of 120 bpm, oedema and proteinuria over a period of several days during which she was an inpatient. An elective caesarean section was planned but there was no anaesthetic consultation until the day before the planned operation. At that time, the anaesthetist obviously thought that cardiac problems might exist because echocardiography was considered but it was rejected, because obesity was thought to make the investigation unreliable. On the day of operation, invasive monitoring was thought necessary but it was abandoned after initial failures to site the lines. General anaesthesia was chosen because the obesity and shortness of breath made lying down difficult. However, an epidural catheter was placed successfully and tested. General anaesthesia was induced using a rapid sequence technique. The patient arrested almost immediately after injection of thiopental sodium and could not be resuscitated. At post mortem a cardiomyopathy was diagnosed.

This case is counted in Chapter 10; Cardiac disease, where further comments can be found. Care was substandard because there was no consultation with the anaesthesia service during the six days she was in hospital. Anaesthetic care was also substandard because further investigations should have been done preoperatively to properly evaluate her breathlessness. While it is true that obesity makes echocardiography more difficult and less informative, it might have been a helpful investigation and was worth attempting. Furthermore, perseverance with siting direct monitoring for this elective case could have involved attempts by other staff with more expertise. Direct arterial pressure monitoring might have improved the detection of problems and assessment of resuscitation efforts.

Having sited an epidural in such a difficult case, it is hard to understand why a regional technique was not at least attempted. Whether the use of the epidural would have changed the outcome is not possible to say, but at least the potentially safer technique would have been attempted.

The next four cases are described as examples of lack of consultation with, and involvement of, anaesthesia services. Criticism is of the failure to communicate, not of the anaesthetists involved:

> A woman with a multiple pregnancy developed proteinuria and subsequently hypertension. She was admitted as an emergency four weeks later, at 35 weeks of gestation with severe epigastric pain and pre-eclampsia requiring treatment with magnesium sulphate. She became unconscious because of a cerebral bleed but delivery and help from the anaesthetist were delayed for a further eight hours.

Other aspects of her care are commented on in Chapter 3; Hypertensive diseases of pregnancy, but it is obvious that a multidisciplinary approach should have been adopted as soon as she came into hospital.

> A multiparous woman had previous children who had died of pulmonary hypertension and she herself had the same diagnosis made during this pregnancy. A termination of pregnancy was offered but she declined. She was admitted to hospital late in the second trimester in severe right heart failure and transferred to the coronary care unit but when she started having spontaneous contractions she was sent to the labour ward. She had a spontaneous delivery but she arrested immediately after being given 10 units of Syntocinon®. Cardiopulmonary resuscitation was successful in restoring spontaneous rhythm and breathing resumed, but she died a day later in the coronary care unit.

This case is counted in Chapter 10; Cardiac disease. Substandard care was evident despite likely inevitable death. No consultations had taken place with the anaesthetic team. Monitoring of her cardiovascular status during labour should have included at least direct arterial blood pressure and central venous pressure. Pulmonary artery pressure measurements could also have informed the team caring for her. Anaesthetic services could have set up this monitoring. As in the first case in this Chapter and, as discussed in Chapter 10, the dose and method of administration of oxytocin were inappropriate.

> A woman had an uneventful multiple pregnancy until she was admitted to hospital near term with vomiting and rigors. On admission, she was obviously very sick with a pyrexia of 40.5°C, hypotension (systolic pressure of 70 mmHg), tachycardia (132 bpm), dehydration and ketosis. The babies died. Spurious high recordings were obtained on a noninvasive blood pressure machine, although her real blood pressure was barely recordable. It was not until more than three hours later that an anaesthetist was called because a midwife had difficulty taking blood. As the consultant anaesthetist arrived, the patient collapsed, was cyanosed and her blood pressure was unrecordable. Disseminated intravascular coagulation (DIC) was developing. A central venous line was inserted and further help obtained from intensivists. Despite caesarean section, supportive treatment and intensive care, the patient died of multiple organ failure three days later.

This case is counted in Chapter 7; Genital tract sepsis. It was only because the midwife could not obtain a blood sample that an anaesthetist was called. By then the patient was *in extremis*. This lack of appreciation of the need and value of multidisciplinary care is lamentable (indeed also the implication that the anaesthetic team are mere technicians). Thereafter, it was all too late. The practice of depending only on automatic blood pressure measurement rather than assessing the patient as a whole is to be deprecated.

> A woman who spoke little English had her labour induced and had a traumatic ventouse delivery with bleeding. Laparotomy was performed to tie off her internal iliac vessels but hysterectomy proved necessary. A massive blood transfusion was required. She had a prolonged period of care in ICU but eventually recovered. Some time later it was realised she had a vesicovaginal fistula that was repaired

as an elective procedure some months after delivery. Her preoperative condition seems to have been satisfactory but there was no record of electrolyte or liver function tests being performed. Anaesthesia proceeded uneventfully with stable heart rate and blood pressure. The operation took just under 90 minutes. The anaesthetist prescribed a postoperative fluid regimen of dextrose/saline 1000 ml eight-hourly. Subsequently the gynaecologist requested a postoperative urine output of at least 15 ml quarter-hourly. In order to achieve this, the senior house officer in gynaecology increased the prescribed intravenous fluids such that five litres of dextrose/saline were received overnight. The following morning the patient suffered a seizure and cerebellar coning. She was found to be hyponatraemic ($Na^+$ 122 mmol/l). She was intubated and ventilated but died a few days later without regaining consciousness.

This *Late* death is counted in Chapter 15. It is all the more poignant because she had survived a catastrophic postpartum haemorrhage. Following the subsequent fistula repair, the management of intravenous fluid therapy was clearly ill understood. Discussion with the anaesthetist might have prevented the unwise prescription change. What may not be widely appreciated is the increased susceptibility of premenopausal women to the effects of acute hyponatraemia.[8] Respiratory arrest and seizures occur at a higher plasma sodium in women (95% confidence limits, 95–130 mmol/l) than in men (95% confidence limits, 92–115 mmol/l) and at a significantly higher plasma sodium in menstruant women than in postmenopausal women.[9]

A woman had a medical history that included bicornuate uterus, uterine surgery to correct it, previous caesarean section and a recognised placenta praevia in the current pregnancy. She spent the last weeks of her pregnancy as an inpatient. She had a preoperative haemoglobin of 9.1 g/dl and was clearly a very high-risk patient. The obstetric service had more than a month to make the necessary consultations and arrangements to ensure consultant anaesthetist involvement for the planned elective caesarean section. However, contact with the anaesthesia service was delayed until the day before the planned operation because the surgeon did not anticipate problems. Two inexperienced trainees provided anaesthesia because there was no consultant available on the day of operation. A general anaesthetic was given using a standard technique. The case was apparently started with only one peripheral intravenous cannula sited. The case was uneventful until a major haemorrhage occurred. The woman suffered a blood loss, according to the anaesthetists, of 6.5 litres. In spite of the major blood loss and limited venous access, initial resuscitation was ultimately successful. However, the patient suffered 45 minutes of hypotension and the lack of CVP monitoring must have made it difficult to judge the adequacy of fluid replacement. The patient was transferred from theatre to the high-dependency unit, where she suffered further blood loss necessitating laparotomy. She died shortly after induction of anaesthesia for this surgery.

This case is counted in Chapter 4; Haemorrhage. It is included here because it illustrates so clearly how inadequate communication with anaesthesia services can lead to trainees treating cases and circumstances far beyond their experience and abilities. In this case, absence of a second intravenous cannula hampered fluid replacement and exposed the woman to a long period of hypotension. In addition, lack of a CVP line impaired recognition of blood loss. There was clearly an opportunity to site both before the woman left theatre. However, inexperience probably led to a false sense of security and the opportunity was not taken. Failing to do so hampered diagnosis and treatment of the continuing bleeding post-operatively.

The second anaesthetic was given in difficult circumstances. The woman had bled a large volume and the cardiovascular decompensation that followed induction was probably due to inadequate blood volume replacement. It might have been prevented if earlier haemorrhage and subsequent resuscitation had been better monitored. Poor anaesthesia care therefore contributed to this death.

Having made these comments, the main failure in the case was in communication and cooperation between specialties. Inadequate warning was given to the anaesthetic service. The caesarean section was an elective procedure with very high risk factors. Once the difficulty of providing a consultant anaesthetist was recognised it could have been delayed until senior anaesthetist input and full monitoring were available.

## 2. Major obstetric haemorrhage

Major haemorrhage is still one of the commonest causes of maternal death. It may complicate either caesarean delivery or other obstetric surgery, such as termination of pregnancy or removal of retained products of conception. Anaesthetists are trained to recognise the effects of major haemorrhage and to treat it appropriately. In a number of cases in this triennium they failed to exercise that skill. A small number of these women died in theatre, either during their initial operation or during surgical attempts to stop haemorrhage. Many of the women, however, were resuscitated in theatre and transferred to the ICU for further treatment. These transfers were often made directly from theatre, although in a small number of cases women were returned to postnatal or recovery rooms or wards because the severity of their clinical condition had not been recognised.

Assessments of cardiovascular stability were often based only on non-invasive blood pressure and pulse rate measurements. Estimation of blood loss at caesarean section or during evacuation of retained products of conception, is known to be extremely difficult and is often inaccurate. The severity of haemorrhage can be better judged by looking for the physiological responses to it rather than by trying to guess the amount of blood loss visually. Central venous pressure measurement, when made in conjunction with systemic blood pressure, pulse rate, urine output and visual assessment of the patient's pallor will give a better, more accurate assessment of the true cardiovascular state. Anaesthetists are skilled in the insertion and interpretation of CVP monitoring. When the internal jugular or subclavian routes are felt to be inappropriate, access may be gained from the antecubital veins. Failing to use this monitoring in the treatment of major obstetric haemorrhage is substandard care. In many cases, anaesthetists were called on to manage intravenous fluid replacement or resuscitate the mother.

Responsibility for substandard care in such circumstances must rest with the anaesthetic services.

In looking at some of the deaths attributed to haemorrhage, multifactorial causation is clear. Pathological process, poor obstetric management and care, poor interspecialty communication and inadequate anaesthetic response all appear in various combinations. The following two cases serve to illustrate most of these deficiencies.

> A woman suffered an early fetal loss and was anaesthetised for evacuation of retained products by a junior trainee anaesthetist. Following the surgery, she continued to lose blood per vaginaum. On return to theatre, she was again anaesthetised by a junior anaesthetist. Consultant input into her care did not begin for another hour. She eventually underwent hysterectomy. During the operation she suffered further major haemorrhage but blood replacement was limited to five units of blood. Maintenance of her blood pressure required methoxamine and noradrenaline/norepinephrine throughout the operation. Transfer to ICU was intended but while being moved moving to her bed she arrested. Although she was resuscitated from this arrest she died shortly after in ICU.

This case is counted in Chapter 7; Genital tract sepsis and also discussed in Chapter 6; Early pregnancy but anaesthetic services must carry some responsibility for this death. Management of a patient suffering continuing vaginal bleeding after evacuation of retained products of conception should not be left to a junior trainee. It took one hour for senior anaesthetic assistance to be summoned. This is substandard care.

Management of the patient subsequently seems to have followed widely accepted practice but inspection of the record would indicate that she received only five units of blood during a two-hour procedure during which she experienced major haemorrhage. Methoxamine and noradrenaline/norepinephrine were used freely during the same period. It would seem that the anaesthetists achieved acceptable blood pressure recordings by producing profound vasoconstriction. This may be an appropriate temporary measure in the face of major haemorrhage but is not, ultimately, the solution to the problem. There is a note indicating that the patient was peripherally shut down before the second anaesthetic began. The inference from the information available is that inadequate quantities of blood were given. There is no record of haematological investigations of haemoglobin or packed cell volume that might cast further light on these circumstances. However, the fact that the patient suffered a cardiac arrest during transfer from the operating table to her bed seems to indicate that the appropriate cardiovascular stability had not been achieved while in theatre.

> A woman who did not speak English had an urgent caesarean section and returned to theatre two hours later because of bleeding. She was tachycardic (140 bpm) and the coagulation screen was abnormal. After the second general anaesthetic she was extubated but her oxygen saturation varied between 85% and 93%. Two hours later, pulmonary oedema was diagnosed and she was reintubated. She had two more laparotomies for bleeding and died several days later.

Amniotic fluid embolism seemed the most likely diagnosis but it was not confirmed histologically. Although it would probably have made no difference to the eventual outcome, it represents substandard care not to have sought help and instituted CVP and arterial monitoring when this woman first returned to theatre with evidence of a coagulopathy.

### 3. Poor postoperative care

There were three deaths in this triennium in which poor postoperative care was a contributing factor, two of which are described here:

> A woman had a caesarean section in which anaesthesia was provided with a combined spinal–epidural technique. Within a few hours she developed a severe headache and hypertension. The anaesthetist treated this as a postdural puncture headache and gave a blood patch through the epidural catheter. She later developed slurred speech, constant vomiting and a hemiparesis followed by convulsions for which she received magnesium sulphate. She was transferred for computerised tomography that showed a subarachnoid haemorrhage. Despite intensive care she died some days later.

This case is one of several deaths from subarachnoid haemorrhage counted in Chapter 12. While the ultimate outcome is unlikely to have been different, the diagnosis of postdural puncture headache so soon after a spinal with an atraumatic needle is unlikely.

> The anaesthetist was not informed about a woman with severe hypertension (250/140 mmHg) and proteinuria until caesarean section was required at night. The patient was receiving hydralazine, labetalol and nifedipine. Her blood pressure decreased to normal values after induction of general anaesthesia. Magnesium sulphate was given during the procedure. The operation lasted one hour 45 minutes. Blood loss was estimated at 1500 ml to two litres, yet no blood was given. Fluid replacement comprised only 2000 ml crystalloid and 500 ml colloids were given during surgery. At the end of surgery her tachycardia persisted. Shortly after leaving the patient in recovery the anaesthetist was called back because the blood pressure was 48/23 mmHg. Transfusion with O negative blood was started. The nursing staff asked the anaesthetist to stay in recovery because they were concerned about the patient's condition. Nevertheless, the anaesthetist seems to have left recovery. Two hours after reaching recovery the woman suffered a cardiac arrest and attempts at resuscitation were futile.

This case is counted in Chapter 3; Hypertensive diseases of pregnancy. There were a number of aspects of substandard care, including the lack of senior involvement and poor fluid management. The anaesthetist's responsibility to the patient does not end with transfer to the recovery room. There remains a duty to ensure the patient's full recovery from their anaesthetic and operation. The duty can be discharged directly or by transfer to a site where that recovery can be monitored and completed. Abandoning the patient in recovery, having been alerted to her parlous state, represents gross substandard care.

### 4. Lack of appreciation of severity of illness

The following cases illustrate a common theme, showing how failure to realise the severity of illness meant that senior help was sought too late:

> A woman with learning difficulties had a septic fetal loss and required an anaesthetic for removal of a retained placenta. There was a two-day history of diarrhoea and the patient was tachycardic (125 bpm) and hypotensive (systolic blood pressure 60 mmHg). The clinical assistant discussed the case with a trainee in anaesthesia but both failed to realise the severity of illness or call for help. After three litres of fluid, the patient was still tachycardic and the systolic blood pressure was 100 mmHg. Antibiotics were given at manual removal but not earlier. The patient went to recover in a side room because of the pregnancy loss. Half an hour later, she lost consciousness, had difficulty breathing and her oxygen saturation was low. At that point, a consultant anaesthetist became involved and organised appropriate intensive care. After a laparotomy to exclude uterine perforation she developed multi-organ failure and died a few days later.

Had the severity of illness been recognised, experienced help would have been sought earlier. The seriousness of the mother's condition warranted better monitoring in a more appropriate environment, regardless of the sensitivities of fetal loss.

> Trainee staff cared for a patient undergoing caesarean section delivery because of pre-eclampsia. A consultant anaesthetist had been contacted during the caesarean section and gave advice via the telephone but failed to attend to assess the patient or supervise the care. The patient exhibited further hypertensive changes during arousal and, at this time, the anaesthetist noted that she was not tolerating the endotracheal tube. Following extubation, she was transferred to the postoperative high-dependency unit because there were no ICU beds available. Further telephone calls to the consultant anaesthetist on call only resulted in further telephone advice. Neurological changes were noted a few hours postoperatively. Intubation and transfer to the ICU occurred and there is no record to show whether control of blood pressure during intubation was undertaken at that time either. She died without regaining consciousness.

There seems to have been no recognition of the risks of hypertensive surges during intubation or extubation. Anaesthetic care was therefore substandard. These omissions may have been due to inexperience of the trainee anaesthetist. The decision to wake and extubate this patient was probably unwise. The lack of direct consultant input into her care was substandard care. The lack of an ICU bed is further substandard care.

Whether these deficiencies caused or exacerbated the cerebral bleed is a matter of speculation. However, it is possible that had appropriate standards of care been exhibited, the outcome may have been better.

## 5. Sepsis

The incidence of maternal infection during labour is in the region of 3%.[10] When septicaemia supervenes, anaesthetists should be involved in resuscitation. Additionally, sepsis can be associated with anaesthesia. The importance of constant vigilance and the use of strict asepsis during regional anaesthetic techniques cannot be overstated. These two cases illustrate possible associations between anaesthesia and sepsis:

> A primiparous woman had an uneventful spinal anaesthetic for caesarean section because of pre-eclampsia. She developed a pyrexia on the first postpartum day and was given antibiotics. She was otherwise well until some hours later, when she developed severe headache, vomiting and hypertension and became unrousable. She was transferred to intensive care and given magnesium sulphate. Computerised tomography showed cerebral oedema. Further supportive therapy was given but her condition deteriorated and she died a few days after delivery. At post mortem, acute purulent meningitis with sagittal sinus thrombosis was found.

This woman was appropriately treated for complications of pre-eclampsia and there was no finding of substandard care. The diagnosis of meningitis was a surprise: bacterial cultures in life and post mortem failed to grow any organism. She had received antibiotics because of a mild pyrexia on the first postpartum day.

Although there is good epidemiological evidence that the frequency of meningitis after lumbar puncture is no greater than in the ordinary population, the possibility that causative infective or chemical agents can be introduced at spinal anaesthesia has to be recognised. The onset of symptoms is similar to two previous reports after spinal anaesthesia in obstetrics where the patients survived.[11,12] Similarly, apparently aseptic techniques had been used. Whether meningitis was caused by the spinal or was an unfortunate coincidence is impossible to say. The case highlights the need for strict asepsis during regional anaesthesia and the need to consider, as the clinicians did, other rare causes of headache which might at first be thought to be due to dural puncture or pre-eclampsia.

> Another woman developed a pyrexia of 40°C and a tachycardia of 140 bpm following an intrauterine death. She requested and was given an epidural for analgesia for labour. She received excessive intravenous fluids to treat hypotension and developed pulmonary oedema. DIC developed, probably due to the intrauterine death. She became septicaemic and developed multi-organ failure and had to be transferred to an ICU at another hospital, where she subsequently died.

This case is counted in Chapter 7; Genital tract sepsis. The main criticisms are of the treatment of infection and the subsequent pathology. Nevertheless, it is worth thinking whether the possible complications or adverse effects of epidural block in a pyrexial patient were fully considered. Sympathetic blockade from epidural or spinal anaesthesia in these circumstances makes fluid and hypotension management more difficult because of impaired compensatory vasoconstriction and capillary permeability may also be compromised. Treatment in such circumstances is difficult and requires great forethought and care.

## Deaths or serious events occurring during anaesthesia

Some of the cases already described illustrate that death or serious events can occur during anaesthesia. The following cases are also included, not necessarily because there was substandard care but to reinforce the vigilance and standards required:

> A woman was known to suffer from pulmonary hypertension having had an atrial septal defect repaired many years previously. Echocardiography at 32 weeks of gestation estimated mean pulmonary artery pressures of 55 mmHg systolic but it is not known if her pulmonary hypertension worsened after this. She went into labour some weeks later. Epidural analgesia was used and direct arterial and central venous monitoring was instituted. Labour failed to progress and she required a caesarean section. She had a brief run of supraventricular tachycardia after delivery of the placenta, which spontaneously reverted to sinus rhythm, but seconds later she suffered an asystolic arrest from which she could not be resuscitated. She had only received one unit of oxytocin.

The poor outcome from pulmonary hypertension in pregnancy is well recognised. The care of this woman was good and illustrated interdisciplinary communication and early institution of invasive monitoring. Whether the appropriate risks were communicated to the woman is discussed in Chapter 10; Cardiac disease.

> A woman had a termination of pregnancy under general anaesthesia in an isolated clinic. At the end of the procedure, her oxygen saturation decreased from 98% to 83% and she became bradycardic and hypotensive. She was resuscitated with adrenaline/epinephrine and was intubated and ventilated. Before transfer to hospital, heavy vaginal blood loss was noticed. Fulminant DIC became apparent. She developed multiple organ failure and subsequently died.

The clinical signs were similar to those of amniotic fluid embolism. Resuscitation of this woman was prompt and emphasises the need for experienced personnel and appropriate drugs and equipment (as recommended by the Department of Health[13]) for the rare occasions when such complications occur in isolated sites.

> A woman had an amniocentesis for a one in ten risk of Down syndrome and had a spontaneous abortion the following day. She had a general anaesthetic, delivered from a facemask, and uterine evacuation to remove remaining products of conception. There was a sudden cardiac arrest at the end of uterine evacuation. Sinus tachycardia progressed to ventricular tachycardia to asystole. Cardiopulmonary resuscitation and adrenaline/epinephrine were successful in restoring cardiac output. She was transferred to ICU but died several days later.

It is not clear why this woman arrested. Before the evacuation she was pyrexial, but not tachycardic or hypotensive. During anaesthesia, her heart rate and blood pressure remained normal and the cardiac arrest was sudden. This might suggest amniotic fluid embolism (AFE). If the cause of the arrest were sepsis, one might postulate a myocarditis causing arrhythmia. Thereafter, the picture of DIC and multi-organ failure could fit either AFE or sepsis. It is unfortunate that there is apparently no histology of the lungs, uterus or heart, although it is by no means certain whether this would have been diagnostic with death occurring so long after the event as discussed in Chapter 18; Pathology. This case again illustrates the need for vigilance even for cases expected to be 'routine' or 'minor'.

**This Chapter has been seen and discussed with the National and Regional Assessors in Anaesthesia.**

## References

1. Kinsella SM, Tuckey JP. Perioperative bradycardia and asystole: relationship to vaso-vagal syncope and the Bezold-Jarisch reflex. *Br J Anaesth* 2001;86:859–68.
2. Drugs used in obstetrics, gynaecology, and urinary tract disorders. In: *British National Formulary*. London: British Medical Association and the Royal Pharmaceutical Society of Great Britain; 2001.
3. Parfitt K, editor. *Martindale: The Complete Drug Reference*. 32nd ed. London: Pharmaceutical Press; 1999. p. 1257–8.
4. Dollery C, editor. *Therapeutic Drugs*. 2nd ed. Edinburgh: Churchill Livingstone; 1998. p. 60.
5. Mukaddam-Daher S, Yin YL, Roy J, Gutkowska J, Cardinal R. Negative inotropic and chronotropic effects of oxytocin. *Hypertension* 2001;38: 292–6.
6. Cicutti NJ, Smyth CE, Rosaeg OP, Wilkinson M. Oxytocin receptor binding in rat and human heart. *Can J Cardiol* 1999;15:1267–73.
7. Association of Anaesthetists of Great Britain and Ireland and the Obstetric Anaesthetist's Association. *Guidelines for Obstetric Anaesthetic Services*. London; 1998.
8. Ayus JC, Wheeler JM, Arieff AI. Postoperative hyponatremic encephalopathy in menstruant women. *Ann Intern Med* 1992;117:891–7.
9. Ayus JC, Arieff AI. Brain damage and postoperative hyponatremia: the role of gender. *Neurology* 1996;46:323–8.
10. Lauretti GR. Infectious diseases. In: Gambling DR, Douglas M.J. *Obstetric Anaesthesia and Uncommon Diseases*. Philadelphia, PA: WB Saunders; 1998. p. 333.
11. Roberts SP, Petts HV. Meningitis after obstetric spinal anaesthesia. *Anaesthesia* 1990;45:376–7.
12. Lee JJ, Parry H. Bacterial meningitis following spinal anaesthesia for caesarean section. *Br J Anaesth* 1991;66:383–6.
13. Department of Health. Procedures for approval of independent sector places for the termination of pregnancy. London: DoH;1999. p. 25.

# *Indirect* deaths

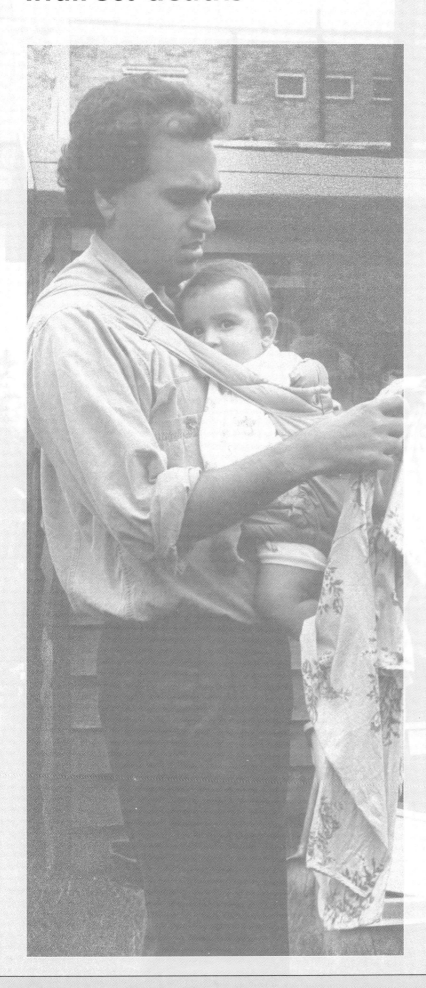

CHAPTER 10

# Cardiac disease

MICHAEL DE SWIET on behalf of the Editorial Board

## Cardiac disease: key points

- Heart disease is the joint most common cause of maternal death. It is still potentially dangerous in pregnancy even though disease patterns have changed.

- Women with pulmonary vascular disease have a very high risk of dying in pregnancy. Typical estimates of mortality risk are 30% per pregnancy in Eisenmenger's syndrome and 30–50% in primary and secondary pulmonary hypertension.

- Clinicians should be aware that women may minimise or deny symptoms relevant to heart disease.

- Oxytocin must be used with great care in women with severe heart disease.

- The possibility of endocarditis should always be considered in pregnant women with obscure febrile illness.

## Cardiac disease: key recommendations

- Women with severe cardiac disease require multidisciplinary care.

- Delivery must be planned in women with significant heart disease. At the very least this will involve discussion with the consultant anaesthetist(s) who will be responsible at the time.

- Tertiary centres accepting the care of women with medical complications in pregnancy must be staffed at consultant level by physicians with relevant specialised medical experience and knowledge of obstetrics.

- Prepregnancy counselling concerning the risks of pregnancy should not alienate the woman to such an extent that she does not come for antenatal care if she does become pregnant. These women need the best care that is available throughout pregnancy.

## Summary

There were a total of 35 deaths from heart disease in pregnancy in 1997–99. This compares with 39 deaths in 1994–96 (Table 10.1). However, with the decrease in mortality from other conditions, cardiac disease, although only an *Indirect* cause of death, has become relatively more important. Heart disease now equals thromboembolism (35 deaths) as a leading reported cause of maternal mortality and is considerably more frequent than the second *Direct* cause, hypertension (15 deaths).

**Table 10.1** Number and percentage of maternal deaths from congenital and acquired cardiac disease; United Kingdom 1985–99

| Triennium | Congenital | | Acquired | | | | Total cases |
| | | | Ischaemic | | Other | | |
| | (*n*) | (%) | (*n*) | (%) | (*n*) | (%) | (*n*) |
|---|---|---|---|---|---|---|---|
| 1985–87 | 10 | 44 | 9 | 39 | 4 | 17 | 23 |
| 1988–90 | 9 | 50 | 5 | 25 | 4 | 25 | 18 |
| 1991–93 | 9 | 24 | 8 | 22 | 20 | 54 | 37 |
| 1994–96 | 10 | 26 | 6 | 21 | 23 | 53 | 39 |
| 1997–99 | 10 | 29 | 5 | 15 | 20 | 56 | 35 |

Seven further deaths are mentioned in this Chapter, although they are counted elsewhere, one as a death due to haemorrhage, five as *Late* deaths and one in Chapter 12; *Other Indirect* deaths.

The overall pattern of heart disease has not changed significantly since 1991–93, with about 30% of deaths being due to congenital heart disease, 15% to ischaemic heart disease and 56% due to other acquired heart disease, particularly cardiomyopathy and myocarditis (Table 10.1). As usual, pulmonary vascular disease was an important cause of mortality and a significant number of deaths were due to endocarditis. Rheumatic heart disease is now uncommon as a cause of maternal mortality; in clinical practice it is most commonly seen in new immigrants to the UK.

Substandard care was present in a total of three cases.

## Congenital heart disease

There were ten deaths from congenital heart disease (Table 10.2). Care was substandard in two cases. One additional death, of a woman found dead in bed about 20 weeks after delivery, who had a floppy mitral valve is counted in Chapter 15; *Late* deaths.

In seven (70%) cases pulmonary vascular disease was the likely cause of death. There were three cases of primary pulmonary hypertension, another case of pulmonary hypertension (nature unknown), two deaths from Eisenmenger's syndrome and one from residual pulmonary hypertension following atrial septal defect closure. Pulmonary hypertension due to talc granuloma from intravenous drug abuse probably contributed to the death of another woman from abruption and haemorrhage. This case is counted in Chapter 4.

**Table 10.2** Maternal deaths due to cardiac disease; United Kingdom 1997–99

| Cause of death | Deaths (n) |
|---|---|
| *Congenital* | |
| Primary pulmonary hypertension | 3 |
| Pulmonary hypertension, cause unknown | 1 |
| ASD, Eisenmenger's syndrome | 2 |
| ASD closed; residual pulmonary hypertension | 1 |
| Bicuspid aortic valve; endocarditis | 1 |
| Coarctation repair; endocarditis | 1 |
| Previous ASD surgery, ? dysrhythmia | 1 |
| Total | 10 |
| | |
| *Acquired* | |
| Puerperal cardiomyopathy | 7 |
| Cardiomyopathy and myocarditis | 5 |
| Aneurysm of thoracic aorta and its branches | 5 |
| Myocardial infarction | 5 |
| Endocarditis; normal mitral valve | 1 |
| Heart failure, cause unknown | 2 |
| Total | 25 |
| Total of all cardiac deaths | 35 |

## Pulmonary hypertension

A middle-aged woman developed breathlessness in early pregnancy and was found to have primary pulmonary hypertension. She had already lost two of her previous children from primary pulmonary hypertension but had not herself been investigated prior to pregnancy. She was appropriately given a 50% risk of dying in pregnancy but elected to continue with the pregnancy. She was admitted late in the second trimester in labour and had a spontaneous vaginal delivery. The child survived but after being given an intravenous injection of ten units of oxytocin for the third stage, she suffered a cardiac arrest. She was initially resuscitated but died in intensive care on the next day.

This extraordinary case represents substandard care. Primary pulmonary hypertension is known to be familial in some cases and a gene responsible for some cases of primary pulmonary hypertension has already been cloned. The familial inheritance had already been demonstrated in this case by the death of two of the patient's other children. It was mandatory that she herself should have been assessed and kept under cardiological surveillance. It is likely that she had pulmonary hypertension months or even years before she became pregnant. If she had been assessed by echocardiography this would have shown evidence of pulmonary hypertension. Had she been counselled before pregnancy concerning the 50% risk of dying in pregnancy, she may well not have embarked on a further pregnancy.

There were further deficits in the management of her pregnancy. Patients with pulmonary vascular disease have a high risk of dying, particularly after delivery. A multidisciplinary team should plan their management. However, no anaesthetist was consulted about her until she arrived on the labour ward. No invasive monitoring was used. The dose of oxytocin used, ten units, was twice that recommended by the *British National Formulary* (BNF) (see also Chapter 9). The BNF also recommends that the drug be given slowly and that severe cardiovascular disease is a contraindication to its use. While the use of oxytocin may certainly be indicated in some patients with heart disease, it must be given slowly, preferably by infusion and in the recommended dose. If these aspects of serious substandard care had been avoided, the patient's life would not necessarily have been saved, but at least she would have had a better chance.

In another death from primary pulmonary hypertension the diagnosis was also made in pregnancy. The patient needed to be delivered early by caesarean section, because of increasing breathlessness, but she still died two weeks later despite exemplary treatment with pulmonary vasodilators including nitric oxide and epoprostenol (prostacyclin). One further patient was known to have primary pulmonary hypertension and died undelivered in the early third trimester following transfer from the regional cardiothoracic centre to the local maternity hospital. Insufficient details have been provided to comment further. Another mortality from pulmonary hypertension was also known to the assessors but they had insufficient details even to be able to comment on the cause of the pulmonary hypertension.

There were two deaths from Eisenmenger's syndrome. This is a form of congenital heart disease in which abnormally high blood flow through the lungs in earlier life is associated with a marked increase in pulmonary vascular resistance. Pulmonary artery pressure often exceeds systemic and then desaturated blood is shunted through the abnormal connection (typically atrial septal defect, ventricular septal defect or patent ductus arteriosus) to render the patient cyanosed:

> A woman who spoke no English had Eisenmenger's syndrome, which was diagnosed 18 months before her first pregnancy. Cardiac catheterisation had shown she had an atrial septal defect with pulmonary artery pressure of about 100 mmHg. She was warned of the risks of pregnancy. When she became pregnant, she was managed in a tertiary centre and was told through an interpreter that the mortality risk was 30–70%. She elected to continue with pregnancy. After delivery by elective caesarean section under general anaesthesia at 37 weeks, she initially did well but deteriorated after two days with increasing hypotension and desaturation. She died seven days after delivery despite maximal supportive therapy

> Another woman from an ethic minority group who had an arranged marriage and was known to have Eisenmenger's syndrome had her first pregnancy terminated at 25 weeks because the fetus itself had severe congenital heart disease. Her second pregnancy was complicated by spontaneous preterm delivery at 27 weeks and the baby suffered an early cot death during the index pregnancy. Also during the index pregnancy, she had a pulmonary embolus and initially opted for termination but then changed her mind. She was delivered very early by caesarean section because of concern about a further pulmonary embolus and pre-eclampsia. On the day of delivery she had a cerebral thrombosis, despite heparin prophylaxis. She died two days later.

There was no substandard care in this case, although it was questioned to what extent she was made aware of her very high risk by continuing with pregnancy. More likely, these two cases and the following case illustrate the desperation of some women, in particular from certain cultures, to produce a live child. Such women often make light of or deny cardiac symptoms. This had tragic consequences in a woman with transfusion-dependent thalassaemia, whose death from iron overload cardiomyopathy is described in Chapter 12.

> A further woman from an ethnic minority was known to have pulmonary hypertension despite surgery for an atrial septal defect, with an estimated pulmonary artery pressure 55 mmHg before pregnancy. She had extensive counselling between a district general hospital and a tertiary centre specialising in the management of heart disease in pregnancy. Because of her lack of symptoms, she was advised that the maternal mortality in her condition would be relatively low, i.e. 5%. During pregnancy, she was monitored very closely and was admitted at 32 weeks because of a history of cyanotic attacks. A few weeks later, she went into labour following spontaneous rupture of membranes and was delivered by caesarean section because of failure to progress. One unit of oxytocin was given for the third stage and, soon afterwards, she suffered a fatal asystolic cardiac arrest.

The tendency for women with pulmonary vascular disease to die soon after delivery has already been commented on. This woman had excellent care throughout her pregnancy. However, the prepregnancy counselling could be questioned. She did not have Eisenmenger's syndrome because she no longer had a shunt and, in any case, she did not have a pulmonary artery pressure that would have been great enough to cause shunt reversal. Nevertheless, the maternal mortality from Eisenmenger's syndrome is 30% per pregnancy and the nearest other condition for which figures are available, primary pulmonary hypertension, has a maternal mortality of 50%. Prepregnancy symptoms are not necessarily good predictors of outcome in pulmonary vascular disease and the expected mortality in this patient might therefore be thought to be nearer to 30–50% rather than 5%.

## Endocarditis

There were two deaths from endocarditis. There were no obvious foci of infection in either case. One woman had previously had aortic valve surgery. She had been assessed by her cardiologist before pregnancy and thought fit for pregnancy. However, once pregnant, she developed endocarditis with deteriorating cardiac function and died after caesarean section was performed early in the third trimester because of left ventricular failure. The other history was similar. This woman had had a coarctation repaired 15 years before pregnancy. She then had a large number of pregnancies. Just over halfway through the index pregnancy she developed endocarditis and was electively delivered by caesarean section because of deteriorating cardiac function a few weeks later. She died soon afterwards despite aortic and mitral valve replacement performed under the same anaesthetic as the caesarean section.

The final case of congenital heart disease had an atrial septal defect repaired as a young girl. Her pregnancy was uneventful until about seven months of gestation, when she woke gasping for breath and died. No abnormality was found in the heart at autopsy. Nevertheless, it is likely that this was a 'cardiac' death probably associated with dysrhythmia.

## Acquired heart disease

There were 25 deaths from acquired heart disease (Table 10.2). Substandard care was present in one case.

## Puerperal cardiomyopathy

There were seven deaths from puerperal cardiomyopathy. This is a dilated cardiomyopathy that typically occurs in the month before or after delivery. The condition is diagnosed when no other cause can be found for the cardiac dilatation. In one case, no details other than the death certificate are available and it is not discussed further. Of the other six cases, the first represents substandard care:

> A morbidly obese woman was admitted to hospital at the end of pregnancy, complaining of breathlessness. Pulmonary embolus and deep vein thrombosis were apparently excluded. The patient developed hypertension, proteinuria and tachycardia of 120 bpm. All these features were thought to be due to pre-eclampsia. Delivery by caesarean section was planned because of transverse lie. The anaesthetist had considered echocardiography but decided against the request because she was so obese. Invasive monitoring during the planned delivery had to be abandoned because of difficulty in siting the lines. During the induction of anaesthesia the patient suffered a cardiac arrest and died. Autopsy showed that she had a dilated enlarged heart thought to be due to puerperal cardiomyopathy. She also had a kidney tumour that may have been the cause of the hypertension and proteinuria, although pre-eclampsia is more likely.

The coroner's autopsy was unsatisfactory because no histology was performed. Care was substandard because no anaesthetist was involved until the day of delivery. Further preoperative evaluation in this case of elective surgery should have detected the cardiomyopathy, pulmonary embolism having been excluded. Echocardiography is such a valuable investigation in cases such as this, that it should not have been rejected because of concern about technical problems with obesity. Perseverance with siting the arterial and venous invasive lines should have involved more attempts or more experienced anaesthetists.

> One woman collapsed with a seizure after going out shopping early in the third trimester. An ambulance was called and she was found to have ventricular fibrillation. Resuscitation attempts in hospital, including caesarean section, were unsuccessful. Autopsy showed a dilated cardiomyopathy consistent with puerperal cardiomyopathy.

Another woman presented with breathlessness at term. The echocardiogram showed dilated cardiomyopathy. She was delivered by elective caesarean section under combined spinal epidural block. She received appropriate medical therapy and, since she was keen to go home and not in overt cardiac failure, she was discharged one week later. Five days later she was found by her husband unconscious and could not be resuscitated when she arrived in hospital. Autopsy confirmed the diagnosis.

Although the relatively early discharge could be criticised with hindsight, this certainly does not represent substandard care and the outcome might have been no different had she remained in hospital.

A woman who had suffered gestational diabetes collapsed when visiting her mother a few weeks after delivery. The ambulance crew could not revive her. Autopsy showed the typical dilated heart of peripartum cardiomyopathy with very little atheroma in the coronary vessels. Diabetes is unlikely to have been contributory.

The fifth case presented with collapse at the time of elective caesarean section. Echocardiography suggested a dilated cardiomyopathy. There is some uncertainty about the diagnosis, since at autopsy the heart was of normal size even though there was loss of myocytes with lymphocytic infiltration consistent with puerperal cardiomyopathy.

Another woman developed heart failure and died shortly after delivery. She had been transferred to a cardiac centre and was treated with intra-aortic balloon pumping while awaiting cardiac transplantation. She was labelled as having puerperal cardiomyopathy but there are no reports of echocardiography and no autopsy was performed.

## Other forms of cardiomyopathy and myocarditis

Five deaths are recorded in this category, including one where the cause of death is not certain. There were four additional cases counted elsewhere. Three of these were *Late* deaths, counted in Chapter 15. They were due to eosinophilic myocarditis, myocardial fibrosis and hypertrophic obstructive cardiomyopathy. The other case of myocarditis is counted in Chapter 12; *Other Indirect* deaths, since the primary condition was systemic lupus erythematosus.

A woman with a very unstable social background had had numerous previous pregnancies including several miscarriages. The most recent (successful) pregnancy had been complicated by heart failure, her sisters were known to have dilated cardiomyopathy and her mother had died following an attack of palpitations. She opted to continue the index pregnancy, having been warned of the risks. At three months of gestation she was admitted with ventricular tachycardia and was restored to sinus rhythm but, soon after, suffered a further cardiac arrest that was unresponsive to treatment.

Although there was little doubt about the cause of death, familial dilated cardiomyopathy, the autopsy was very unsatisfactory in that it was limited to an external examination of the body.

> Hypertrophic obstructive cardiomyopathy was thought to be the cause of death in a woman who collapsed unexpectedly four days after an uncomplicated pregnancy. She survived a further four days with assisted ventilation. Puerperal cardiomyopathy would have been another possibility but the diagnosis was changed to idiopathic cardiomegaly following an exemplary autopsy and subsequent consultation with a specialist cardiac pathologist.

> A woman with a history of palpitations preceding pregnancy attended a cardiologist because her symptoms persisted in pregnancy. Ambulatory monitoring showed runs of ventricular tachycardia. She was asymptomatic during these episodes. The echocardiogram showed some left ventricular dilatation with reduction in systolic function. She was not treated and died suddenly four weeks later. Autopsy showed a scarred left ventricle consistent with previous viral myocarditis.

Although the lack of treatment could be criticised, there is an understandable reluctance to use antidysrhythmic drugs in pregnancy and treatment would not necessarily have made any difference.

> A known heroin abuser collapsed near to term and the fetus was already dead when she arrived in hospital. Soon afterwards, she suffered a fatal cardiac arrest. At autopsy, the heart showed biventricular enlargement with foci of foreign refractile material invoking a foreign body histiocytic response with focal scarring, intracellular oedema and foci of acute ischaemia/necrosis.

These are the characteristic changes described in the hearts of those who regularly abuse heroin by intravenous injection. There was no evidence of endocarditis.

> The cause of death is uncertain in a woman who was found dead at home in her third trimester. However, she had been admitted to hospital with palpitations and collapse five years previously and was thought to have viral myocarditis. At a subsequent admission, three years previously, she was found to have mitral valve prolapse. Mitral valve prolapse is very rarely fatal but either of these diagnoses could have been the cause of sudden death. The autopsy was non-contributory.

## Myocardial infarction

There were five cases in this group. Substandard care was not identified. The women's ages ranged from 28 years to 42 years and were evenly distributed with a median age of 32 years. In three patients, infarction occurred between three and five weeks after delivery. The others died in the first trimester. All except one had risk factors. Three were smokers and, of these, one also had a history of previous deep vein thrombosis and one had a family history of early death from myocardial infarction. Another patient, who had insulin-dependent diabetes, had an infarct following diabetic ketoacidosis. Death was sudden, occurring in less than 24 hours in three patients. Autopsies were performed in all except one patient. There were no cases of abnormal coronary arteries or coronary artery dissection.

It is difficult to draw any conclusions from this series. It is likely that myocardial infarction will become more common as pregnant women become older and continue to smoke.

## Dissection of the thoracic aorta and its branches

This group of conditions has been included amongst the cardiac section of *Indirect* deaths since the triennial report for 1991–93, because dissection of the thoracic aorta is usually managed by cardiologists and cardiothoracic surgeons. There were five such deaths in 1997–99:

> A multigravid woman with known hypertension and renal impairment due to reflux nephropathy booked late. She was admitted because of hypertension in the mid trimester of pregnancy and then developed severe pain in the loin. This was thought to be due to hydronephrosis. In view of the severity of the pain she was electively delivered early in the third trimester. After delivery, she was managed in the intensive care unit (ICU) but she died the next day from a dissecting aneurysm of the aorta. Although the initial loin pain may have been due to dissection, an echocardiogram performed after she was delivered showed only a very small rim of pericardial fluid and was certainly not diagnostic of dissection.

It is difficult to see how the diagnosis could have been made before her final collapse. Even if the condition is diagnosed and treated promptly, such measures are not necessarily successful as the following case demonstrates:

> A pregnant woman with no risk factors and no hypertension developed severe back and abdominal pain while at work. On admission, she was profoundly hypotensive and became unconscious. Within two hours she had undergone transoesophageal echocardiography, which showed dissection of the thoracic aorta. She went to theatre for aortic root replacement immediately afterwards. She also had coronary artery bypass grafting but she could not be weaned off bypass.

Marfan's syndrome is a well-recognised cause of aortic dissection but surprisingly few cases have been recorded in the Confidential Enquiries into Maternal Deaths.

> A woman who was known to have Marfan's syndrome and whose brother had died at a young age from aortic dissection due to Marfan's syndrome booked early in her second pregnancy. Her first pregnancy had been uneventful and a magnetic resonance image (MRI) of the aorta a few months previously had been normal. She attended a tertiary centre where the medical antenatal clinic was not staffed by a physician with cardiological expertise. Near term, she was admitted as

an emergency with back pain and hypertension. Aortic dissection was diagnosed and, following delivery by caesarean section, she was managed conservatively on the ICU. Two days later she had a further episode of chest pain, further dissection and a fatal cardiac arrest.

This woman did not see a consultant cardiologist antenatally, although she was reviewed by an experienced registrar. Possibly he was falsely reassured by the normal MRI but the family history should have been a warning: families with Marfan's syndrome tend to 'breed true'. She did receive labetalol when she was admitted with back pain but had she been given effective beta blockade throughout pregnancy, with a drug such as propranolol, the shear stress on the aorta would have been less and it is possible that it would not have dissected. A physician who was more experienced in cardiology and in pregnancy might well have instigated effective prophylactic beta blockade. This case illustrates the need for informed, coordinated medical therapy to be available for pregnant women, particularly those with complicated pregnancies being cared for in tertiary centres.

Marfan's syndrome was also suspected at autopsy in a woman who died suddenly on the day after a normal delivery. She had no hypertension and her only past history was of previous surgery for pectus excavatum. She had dissected the aorta from the aortic valve to the iliac arteries. Unfortunately, no histology was performed but the pathologist commented that she was tall and thin with long thin fingers and toes, when making the diagnosis of Marfan's syndrome.

In retrospect, it is possible that the diagnosis might have been made during pregnancy but it is not known whether she had other extracardiac phenotypic features, such as lens dislocation, high arch palate or long patellar tendons.

At the end of a previously normal pregnancy a woman was admitted, collapsed, and was thought to have had an abruption. Some retroplacental blood was found at the subsequent caesarean section, although not sufficient to account for her severe shock. She was therefore transferred to the ICU of a neighbouring hospital. Echocardiography showed a pericardial effusion, which was drained and found to contain frank blood. Following drainage she improved temporarily and the haemopericardium was ascribed to a traumatic pericardiocentesis. She then collapsed again and, at thoracotomy, was found to have more clots in the pericardium, with inoperable bleeding from the aortic root. Autopsy showed a dissection 5 cm above the aortic valve.

This instructive case demonstrates that the most obvious explanation is not necessarily correct. All possibilities should be considered in seriously ill patients. The possibility of dissection is frequently not considered in pregnant women. Clinicians should remember that pregnancy causes arterial dilatation and that all blood vessels are more likely to rupture in pregnancy. The splenic and adrenal arteries seem to be particularly at risk in pregnancy.

## Endocarditis

Two cases of endocarditis have already been described in the section concerning congenital heart disease.

> A further death occurred in woman with a long psychiatric history who was delivered early by caesarean section because of pyrexia, intrauterine growth restriction and fetal tachycardia. She remained ill after delivery and took her own discharge twice before her final admission four weeks post partum with fatal septic shock. Autopsy showed endocarditis on an apparently normal mitral valve. The autopsy was unsatisfactory because no microbiological studies were performed and no attempt was made to find the source of the infection.

Endocarditis on a normal heart valve is very rare but well described. There have been 14 deaths from endocarditis in pregnancy in the last 15 years ; about 10% of all cardiac deaths are due to endocarditis, which should not be forgotten as a rare cause of pyrexia in pregnancy.

## Heart failure, cause unknown

> An obese woman prone to panic attacks was admitted with breathlessness at 18 weeks. Pulmonary embolus was suspected but not proven. Nevertheless, she was treated with heparin followed by warfarin. At about 20 weeks of gestation she was admitted with vaginal bleeding and the international normalised ratio (INR) was found to be 8.3. She was given vitamin K and heparin was substituted for warfarin. She miscarried. Six hours later she collapsed with chest pain and pulmonary oedema. The next day she had a fatal cardiac arrest. At autopsy, multiple platelet thrombi were found in the coronary arteries.

No cause was suggested for the platelet thrombi. However, in retrospect it seem likely that they were due to heparin induced thrombocytopenia, a condition where an allergic response to heparin causes platelet aggregation.

> Another morbidly obese woman weighing in excess of 150 kg with a body mass index of 62 was known to suffer from Wolff-Parkinson-White syndrome and was treated with flecainide throughout pregnancy. She also developed gestational diabetes. Two weeks after delivery she was readmitted with a methicillin-resistant *Staphylococcus aureus* hand infection. Three days later she died suddenly.

It is quite possible that the flecainide and/or a dysrhythmia due to Wolff-Parkinson-White syndrome were the cause of her death. However, the autopsy was totally inadequate, showing only left ventricular hypertrophy with no histological studies. This is discussed further in Chapter 18; Pathology.

The only death due to rheumatic heart disease is counted as a *Late* death in Chapter 15, since the patient, who was an immigrant to the UK, died from mitral stenosis, having developed rapid atrial fibrillation two months following termination of pregnancy.

## Conclusions

Heart disease is still potentially dangerous in pregnancy, even though disease patterns have changed.

Women with pulmonary vascular disease have a very high risk of dying in pregnancy. Typical estimates of mortality risk are 30% per pregnancy in Eisenmenger's syndrome and 30–50% in primary and secondary pulmonary hypertension. Tertiary centres should consider intensive monitoring including measurement of pulmonary artery pressure and treatment with epoprostenol (prostacyclin) and inhaled nitric oxide. However, there is no evidence that sophisticated management can reduce these risks.

These risks should be transmitted to the patient and her partners as clearly and humanely as possible preferably before pregnancy. However, it must be accepted that cultural pressures to have a child may be so strong that the woman will continue with her pregnancy whatever advice is given. Therefore, prepregnancy counselling should not alienate the woman to such an extent that she does not come for antenatal care if she does become pregnant. These women need the best care that is available throughout pregnancy.

Clinicians should be aware that women may minimise or deny symptoms relevant to heart disease.

The possibility of endocarditis should always be considered in pregnant women with obscure febrile illness.

Oxytocin must be used with great care in women with severe heart disease. The risk of postpartum haemorrhage must be balanced against the risk of oxytocin-induced hypotension and tachycardia. Neither situation is well tolerated in women with a fixed cardiac output or a right to left shunt. The haemodynamic effects of oxytocin are minimised when it is given by slow infusion. The recommended maximum daily dose of five units should not be exceeded.

Delivery must be planned in women with significant heart disease. At the very least, this will involve discussion with the consultant anaesthetist(s) who will be responsible at the time.

Tertiary centres accepting the care of women with medical complications in pregnancy must be staffed at consultant level by physicians with relevant specialised medical experience and knowledge of obstetrics.

**This Chapter has been seen by and discussed with David Williams MD MRCP, Consultant Physician in Obstetric Medicine at Chelsea and Westminster Hospital and Senior Lecturer in Obstetric Medicine in the Faculty of Medicine at Imperial College School of Medicine, London.**

CHAPTER 11

# Deaths from psychiatric causes

MARGARET OATES on behalf of the Editorial Board

## Psychiatric deaths: key summary points

- Psychiatric disorders are known to have caused or contributed to 12% of maternal deaths, 10% of which were due to suicide.

- Although the number of cases reported to this Enquiry suggests that death from mental illness is the second leading cause of maternal mortality, a recent study has shown that a large number of deaths were not reported and if these were included then deaths from psychiatric causes would be the leading cause of maternal mortality.

- Women who have had a past episode of severe mental illness following delivery have a one in two to one in three chance of recurrence.

- From the cases reported to this Enquiry, the risk of suicide is one per 100,000 maternities but if all the cases recently identified had been included the risk would be two per 100,000 maternities.

- Suicides in this group of women are characterised by their violent nature.

- There are marked social class differences between suicide and the other causes of maternal death.

- All the women who died from substance misuse were severely socially disadvantaged.

- Progesterone is not an effective treatment for depressive illness.

## Psychiatric deaths: key recommendations

- Protocols for the management of women who are at risk of a relapse or recurrence of a serious mental illness following delivery should be in place in every Trust providing maternity services.

- Enquiries about previous psychiatric history, its severity, care received and clinical presentation should be routinely made in a systematic and sensitive way at the antenatal booking clinic.

- The use of the term postnatal depression or PND should not be used as a generic term for all types of psychiatric disorder. Details of previous illness should be sought and recorded in line with the recommendations above.

- Women who have a past history of serious psychiatric disorder, postpartum or non-postpartum, should be assessed by a psychiatrist in the antenatal period and a management plan instituted with regard to the high risk of recurrence following delivery.

- Women who have suffered from serious mental illness either following childbirth or at other times should be counselled about the possible recurrence of that illness following further pregnancies.

- A perinatal mental health team that has the specialist knowledge, skills and experience to provide care for women at risk of, or suffering from, serious postpartum mental illness should be available to every woman.

- Women who require psychiatric admission following childbirth should ideally be admitted to a specialist mother and baby unit, together with their infant. In areas where this service is not available then a transfer should be considered.

- Substance misuse services, without the need for making an appointment, should be provided in antenatal clinics and to improve both the rate of engagement and the compliance with care.

- Future Enquiries must require the collection of information from psychiatric services in the case of a psychiatric case.

## Summary

First introduced in the last Report, this Chapter discusses all maternal deaths resulting from psychiatric causes notified to the Enquiry. These are important causes of maternal deaths and a major cause of maternal morbidity. Valuable lessons may be learned from the cases discussed in this Chapter, which may help to improve the care such mentally ill women receive.

**Table 11.1**  Chapters in which maternal deaths reported to this Enquiry caused by, or linked with, psychiatric illness are counted; United Kingdom 1997–99

| | Indirect | Late Indirect | Coincidental | Late Coincidental | Other Chapters | Total |
|---|---|---|---|---|---|---|
| Chapter no. | 11 | 15 | 14 | 15 | | |
| | | | | | | |
| Suicide | 13[a] | 15 | | | | 28[a] |
| Drug overdose | 1 | | 1 | 4 | | 6 |
| Alcohol | | | 2 | 1 | 1 | 4 |
| Drug reaction | 1 | | | | | 1 |
| Pulmonary embolism | | | | | 2 | 2 |
| Murder | | | 1 | | | 1 |
| Total | 15 | 15 | 4 | 5 | 3 | 42 |

[a] Death certificate information only available for one case

To enable comparison with earlier Reports, Table 11.1 shows a breakdown of the cases discussed in this Chapter, by the actual Chapter in which they are counted for statistical purposes related to the timing of death and whether it was considered to be related to the pregnancy. In terms of international definitions and comparisons for maternal deaths, those which are considered to be indirectly due to the pregnancy and which occur during pregnancy and up to 42 days after delivery are regarded as *Indirect* and counted in this Chapter. Those occurring later than this are regarded as *Late* and are counted in Chapter 15; *Late* deaths, although they have many common features and characteristics. Deaths from causes apparently unrelated to pregnancy are classified as *Coincidental* but valuable lessons can also be learned from these cases. Despite this allocation, the features of many of the cases are similar and it is only by bringing all the cases together for discussion in this Chapter that the full picture can be ascertained and the conclusions and recommendations strengthened.

Although these deaths are not recognised as maternal deaths by the International Classification of Diseases and thus not counted in the overall maternal mortality rate for other countries, in the United Kingdom, psychiatric deaths indirectly related to pregnancy are considered to be *Indirect* or *Late Indirect* maternal deaths. This means they receive the attention and recommendations they deserve in this Report. However, as a consequence, they inflate the UK maternal death rate when compared with other countries. The authors of this Report therefore recommend that other countries consider following this approach.

Overall, 42 women whose deaths are covered by this Report were identified as having psychiatric disorders causing or contributing to their deaths. In three of these notified deaths, including one from suicide, the details were unavailable and they are not discussed further. Fifteen women are counted as having an *Indirect* death. Thirteen of these women committed suicide during or with 42 days of pregnancy, although, in one case, despite numerous requests for information, only the death certificate details were available. This case has been included for statistical purposes in Table 11.1, but is excluded from any further evaluation. Another woman died from the side effects of her antipsychotic medication and a further woman died of an overdose of heroin. A further 15 women committed suicide after more than 42 days from delivery and are counted as *Late Indirect* deaths. There were also four *Late Coincidental* and one *Coincidental* deaths from drug misuse and four further cases associated with alcohol. In the cases of an overdose of recreational drugs or alcohol, it is difficult to know if death was intentional or accidental. Table 11.2 shows the timing, in relation to the pregnancy of these deaths.

**Table 11.2** Time of death in relation to pregnancy from psychiatric causes; United Kingdom 1997–99

|  | Pregnant (*n*) | Early[a] (*n*) | Late[b] (*n*) | Total (*n*) |
|---|---|---|---|---|
| Suicide | 6 | 7 | 15 | 28 |
| Overdose of illicit drugs | 2 | 0 | 4 | 6 |
| *Other:* |  |  |  |  |
| Pulmonary embolism | – | 1 | 1 | 2 |
| Murder | – | 1 | – | 1 |
| Alcohol related | 3 | – | 1 | 4 |
| Adverse drug reaction | – | 1 | – | 1 |
| Total | 11 | 10 | 21 | 42 |

[a] > 42 days after delivery; [b] < 42 days after delivery

### Cases counted in other Chapters

Of the six cases counted in other Chapters, an alcohol dependent woman died from an ectopic pregnancy whose symptoms may have been masked by her intoxication. This case is counted in Chapter 6. Another two women died of pulmonary embolism; one each is counted in Chapter 2 and Chapter 15, but both had received inpatient psychiatric care. Another case, counted in Chapter 14 *Coincidental* deaths and also discussed in Chapter 16; Domestic violence, was a woman who herself had psychiatric problems and was murdered by her schizophrenic husband.

Overall, cases reported to this Enquiry and in which known psychiatric disorders contributed to the death account for 12% of all maternal deaths. Taken together, the 28 reported deaths from suicide are the second leading cause of maternal death after thromboembolism and cardiac disease, as shown in Figure 1.2 in Chapter 1.

### Deaths from mental illness are actually the leading cause of maternal death

There has always been a large degree of under-ascertainment of deaths from mental illness or substance abuse to this Enquiry. Indeed, the CEMD only started to consider these deaths in detail in the last triennial Report. However, a recent Office for National Statistics (ONS) linkage study (described in Chapter 1) showed that over 40 extra deaths from suicide or deaths from violent causes and another eight where the coroner recorded an open verdict were not reported. In addition, eleven unreported women died from an accidental drug overdose. As it is not yet widespread practice for psychiatrists and community mental health or drug support teams to notify such deaths to this Enquiry, this degree of under-ascertainment is understandable. However, the results of the study show that deaths from suicide are not only the leading cause of *Indirect* death but also the leading cause of maternal deaths overall.

As it is not possible to evaluate the causes and circumstances of the unnotified deaths, this Chapter will base its conclusions on the cases that were made available to the Enquiry for this triennium. In future, the investigation of deaths from mental illness will be more comprehensive through improved reporting from other professionals, closer ties to the Confidential Enquiry into Deaths from Suicide and Homicide and the adoption of the ONS record linkage pilot procedure as a routine part of case ascertainment.

## Background

Mental illness associated with childbirth is common, both new episodes specifically related to childbirth and recurrences of pre-existing conditions. Ten per cent of new mothers are likely to suffer from a depressive illness,[1] of whom between one-third and one-half will be suffering from a severe depressive illness.[2] Two per cent of delivered women will see a psychiatrist during the first year after delivery,[3] four per 1000 will be admitted to a psychiatric hospital and two per 1000 will suffer from a puerperal psychosis.[4]

The incidence and prevalence of psychiatric illness in the first trimester of pregnancy is much the same as it is at other times, with approximately 15% of women suffering from a psychiatric disorder, mostly anxiety and depression. The incidence of serious psychiatric disorder in later pregnancy is lower than at other times.[4] All psychiatric disorders, including substance misuse, schizophrenia and obsessional compulsive disorders, will be present among the pregnant and recently-delivered population at least at the same rate as among the general population. However, it is known that the risk of suffering from severe affective disorders is elevated in women who have recently given birth compared with other women.

Despite the frequency of psychiatric disorder, suicide is a rare event during pregnancy and the postpartum period. It may be that pregnancy and the presence of an infant exerts a protective effect.[5] The 28 suicides identified by the Enquiry that occurred during this triennium and discussed in this Chapter have to be seen in the context of the over two million maternities: a suicide rate of approximately one per 100,000 maternities or two per 100,000 if the data from the record linkage study discussed previously are included.

Despite the drive over recent years to improve recognition and screening for postnatal depression in primary care,[6] there is little evidence that this has resulted in improved care. There has also been little improvement in the care for those suffering from serious mental illness in association with childbirth. The majority of women who suffer from these conditions still do not have access to mental health professionals with specialist knowledge and skills nor to a mother and baby unit, should they require admission for puerperal psychosis.[7]

Of great importance to the findings of this Enquiry is the risk of recurrence posed by childbirth to women who have a past history either of a previous severe postnatal depression, puerperal psychosis or a non-pregnancy-related condition such as bipolar illness, schizophrenia or obsessional compulsive disorder. Women with a past history of severe mental illness, be it puerperal or non-puerperal, face a risk of a recurrence of their condition of between one in two and one in three following delivery.[8] This risk of recurrence is at its greatest in the first 30 days post partum. Typically, these illnesses are of rapid onset and are of similar presentation and timing to previous puerperal episodes. The recommendation made in the last Report that 'a relatively simple procedure should be instituted in *every* antenatal clinic to identify women at risk of postnatal psychiatric illness and/or self harm' is strengthened in this Report to emphasise not only the identification but also the management of risk of a serious postnatal psychiatric illness.

## General features of the women

### Sociodemographic

The 39 deaths for which details are available occurred in women aged 15–50 years of age, with almost half occurring in women who were aged 30 years or older. The age at time of death is given in Table 11.3 and the cause of death by age is shown in Table 11.4.

Unlike deaths from other causes, the social circumstances of the women who committed suicide were more favourable than those who died from other causes. At least twenty-four of these women were married or in a stable relationship and at least six had higher professional qualifications. Several were healthcare professionals. In contrast, the women who died from the complications of substance misuse were younger, with half being under the age of 25 years. They were mostly single and all had marked social adversity.

**Table 11.3**   Age at death from psychiatric causes; United Kingdom 1997–99

| Age (years) | Pregnant (n) | Early[a] (n) | Late[b] (n) | Total (n) |
|---|---|---|---|---|
| < 19 | 1 | 0 | 2 | 3 |
| 20–29 | 7 | 6 | 6 | 19 |
| 30 + | 2 | 3 | 12 | 17 |
| Total | 10 | 9 | 20 | 39 |

[a] > 42 days after delivery; [b] < 42 days after delivery

**Table 11.4**   Age by cause of death from psychiatric causes; United Kingdom 1997–99

| Cause of death | Age (years) | | | Total (n) |
|---|---|---|---|---|
| | < 19 | 20–29 | > 30 | |
| Suicide | 0 | 14 | 13 | 27 |
| Illicit drugs overdose | 3 | 2 | 1 | 6 |
| Other | 0 | 2 | 4 | 6 |
| Total | 3 | 18 | 18 | 39 |

### Ethnicity

Three of the women who committed suicide were from ethnic minority groups. Two of these deaths were characterised by the woman or her family not accepting the help offered once the problem became obvious.

### Mode of death

The characteristic features of these deaths were commented on in the previous Report for 1994–6 and the main methods of suicide for this triennium are shown in Table 11.5. Of the 27 maternal deaths attributable to suicide and for which details were available, 24 were violent deaths. Ten women died by hanging, five by jumping from a height, four from cutting their throats or self-stabbing, two from gunshot wounds and three died, respectively, from self-immolation, drowning and an intentional road traffic accident. Only three women died by taking an overdose of psychotropic drugs. This stands in marked contrast to both attempted suicide and suicide at other times in women's lives, where the most common cause of death is the ingestion of psychotropic medication.

**Table 11.5**   Method of suicide; United Kingdom 1997–99

| Method of death | Pregnant (*n*) | Early[a] (*n*) | Late[b] (*n*) | Total (*n*) |
|---|---|---|---|---|
| Jumping from height | | 4 | 1 | 5 |
| Hanging | 4 | | 6 | 10 |
| Stabbing (cutting throat) | 1 | 1 | 2 | 4 |
| Burning | | | 1 | 1 |
| Gunshot | | 1 | 1 | 2 |
| Drowning | | | 1 | 1 |
| Road traffic accident (intentional) | | | 1 | 1 |
| Overdose of psychotropic drugs | 1 | | 2 | 3 |
| Total | 6 | 6 | 15 | 27[c] |

[a] > 42 days after delivery; [b] < 42 days after delivery; [c] information not available in 1 case

## Psychiatric diagnosis

As shown in Table 11.6, there was sufficient information in 35 of the 39 cases to make a definite or probable psychiatric diagnosis. There were nine cases of psychosis, ten cases of severe depressive illness and two cases of obsessive-compulsive disorder (OCD). One woman was suffering from a severe bereavement reaction, one a severe personality disorder and one suffered from an eating disorder. Four maternal deaths were related to alcohol misuse and seven were heroin users. In four cases of suicide, there was no evidence to suggest serious mental illness in the days before the suicide, although the mode of death in three cases strongly suggests that the woman was mentally ill (one self-immolation, one stabbing and one hanging).

**Table 11.6**   Psychiatric diagnosis and cause of death; United Kingdom 1997–99

| Probable diagnosis | Suicide (*n*) | Overdose illicit drug (*n*) | Other (*n*) | Total (*n*) |
|---|---|---|---|---|
| Puerperal psychosis/or depressive psychosis | 7 | | 2 | 9 |
| Severe depression | 10 | n/a | | 10 |
| Obsessive compulsive disorder | 2 | 0 | | 2 |
| Eating disorder | | 0 | 1 | 1 |
| Bereavement reaction | 1 | 0 | | 1 |
| Substance misuse | 1 | 6 | | 7 |
| Alcohol misuse | 2 | n/a | 2 | 4 |
| Personality disorder | 1 | | | 1 |
| Not ascertainable | 4 | | | 4 |
| Total | 28 | 6 | 5 | 39 |

n/a = not ascertainable

## Current psychiatric contact

As shown in Table 11.7, 33 of the 39 women were receiving help or had been referred for such help for their mental health problems in this pregnancy. Eighteen women were known to be in contact with psychiatric services during this pregnancy for mental illness or personality disorder. Nine of these women were inpatients at or shortly before the time of their death. A further four had been referred but not been seen at the time of their death. In addition to this number, six were being treated by their general practitioner for mental health problems, predominantly depression. Of the 11 women suffering from substance misuse, five had some contact with substance misuse services during the current pregnancy. However, for the latter group, there is information in most cases to suggest a failure to comply with treatment regimes. The lack of information provided by the substance misuse services to this Enquiry does not clarify the status of their care. Therefore, in all but six of the psychiatric maternal deaths, the mental health problems of this group of women had been identified.

**Table 11.7**  Highest level of psychiatric care provided during this pregnancy; United Kingdom 1997–99

| Level of care | Total (n) |
|---|---|
| Inpatient | 9 |
| Outpatient/community mental health team | 9 |
| Referral but not seen | 4 |
| GP treatment only | 6 |
| Substance misuse services | 5 |

## Previous psychiatric history

As shown in Table 11.8, 18 of the maternal deaths had a history of previous contact with psychiatric services, in eight cases as an inpatient. Three more women, at least, had been previously treated by their general practitioner for mental health problems. Nine of these 18 women had a previous history of severe postpartum mental illness for which they had been treated by a psychiatrist. All of those who died from the consequences of substance misuse had been in the past in contact with drug misuse services.

**Table 11.8**  Previous contact with psychiatric services for deaths from psychiatric causes; United Kingdom 1997–99

| When death occurred | Previous postpartum contact (n) | At other times (n) | Total (all contacts) (n) |
|---|---|---|---|
| Pregnancy | 0 | 3 | 3 |
| Early (before 42 days postpartum) | 5 | 2 | 7 |
| Late (42 days postpartum or more) | 4 | 4 | 8 |
| Total | 9 | 9 | 18 |

## The children

Twenty-four of the women had children prior to this pregnancy. No case of child death or infanticide was revealed to the Enquiry, although this information has not been actively sought to date. This has now changed for the next Report, as there are real concerns about the welfare of the surviving children, particularly in view of the violent nature of the deaths and severity of the illnesses. In 26 cases it can be surmised indirectly that the children were not harmed, usually because they were in the care of other people at the time. In the case of the woman who was murdered by her schizophrenic husband, who then killed himself, the absence of any mention of the infant is particularly worrying.

# Emergent themes in this Report

## Deaths associated with substance misuse

Eleven deaths in women who were drug or alcohol dependent are discussed in this Chapter. In contrast to the other women who died from suicide, these women are characterised by their high levels of social adversity, homelessness, poor uptake of services (particularly the substance misuse services), poor attendance for either psychiatric or antenatal appointments, and by their youth and single status. Many were also estranged from their families. Of particular concern was the relative absence of information given to the Enquiry concerning these cases. In some it was as if the woman never really existed, even though there was evidence in all cases of previous contact with substance misuse services. In no case was there any evidence to this Enquiry from either substance misuse or social services, neither was any information supplied about the wellbeing of the infant or older children at the time of their mother's death. Of these 11 cases, six occurred in pregnancy and five late in the postpartum year. There were no early deaths after delivery attributable to substance misuse.

*Drug misuse*
There were seven deaths in women who were drug misusers: one from suicide and six from a presumed accidental drug overdose. In one case, the woman committed suicide having taken heroin beforehand:

> This young, pregnant, heroin-dependent woman committed suicide by hanging. This took place on a significant public holiday, shortly after she was discharged from prison. On the day of her discharge, to an empty house and without any apparent support, she phoned her friends to say that she was intending to kill herself and did so, by violent means, the following day.

Although she had other children, and apparently had a partner, she died alone. Her friends did not respond to her threats nor did they check on her subsequently. Her body was found several days later. She had other children who were presumably living elsewhere. It may be that arrangements had been made for her transfer into the community at the time of her discharge, and that these may have been interrupted by the public holiday, but the lack of information provided suggests that even this may not have been the case. The absence of information from the GP, prison services, social services or substance misuse agencies does not allow us to know whether she received any care, nor what had happened to her children.

In another case, which also reminded the assessors of the film 'Trainspotting' a young girl was also known to social services:

> In this case, also described in several other Chapters in this Report, a very young girl, known to have a history of substance misuse, self-harm and sexual abuse, had run away from home and was sleeping rough. She died from hypothermia, probably under the influence of heroin. A few weeks earlier she had been in hospital for an evacuation of retained products following a missed abortion.

The extraordinary lack of information in this case makes it seem as if she never existed. Particularly noteworthy is the absence of any report from the social services, despite the fact that she was in their care.

One death from heroin overdose occurred during pregnancy:

> A multiparous married woman died from an apparently accidental overdose of heroin in the third trimester of pregnancy. She was known to have a long history of intravenous heroin use and arrangements had been made during pregnancy for her to access the substance misuse services and to transfer to a methadone maintenance programme. However she failed to attend.

There were four other *Late* deaths from substance misuse, all in the last three months of the postpartum year. In one, a young single unemployed girl living alone died from an accidental overdose of heroin. She was known to have abused drugs since a very young age and had a history of deliberate self-harm. Two further women died from a possible accidental overdose of heroin and the fourth, with a history of substance misuse, died from an accidental overdose of recreational drugs. The paucity of information from any of the healthcare workers or agencies involved in the care of these women makes it impossible to know whether anything more could have been done.

*Alcohol misuse*
Four deaths occurred in women who were alcohol misusers. In one *Late* case, for which few details were available, a woman known to have a problem with alcohol misuse died of alcohol intoxication and ingestion of unknown tablets. Details were available in the other three cases, which all occurred in pregnancy:

> A multiparous woman was noted by the midwives to have problems with alcohol and debts. She died from hanging in the third trimester having initially declined and then accepted offers of social and psychiatric help. She did not attend the appointments made for her and missed her last antenatal appointment.

Although the midwifery services had identified her problems and had made appropriate attempts to engage her in care, there is a lack of information from the

GP and from social services. It is difficult to know if anything more could have been done.

> An older grandmultiparous woman, whose case is counted in Chapter 6, died of a ruptured ectopic pregnancy. She was intoxicated at the time and had a long history of alcoholism, domestic violence and dysfunctional parenting. All her previous children were in the care of others. One of her children had fetal alcohol syndrome. At the request of her GP, contact had been made with the community psychiatric nurse prior to her death. There is a lack of information from the GP and from the psychiatric nurse.

The assessors are of the view that her the alcohol intoxication probably masked the symptoms of her ectopic pregnancy, preventing her from accessing medical care before it was too late.

> An unemployed woman died in the late first trimester due to inhalation of vomit at a time when she was intoxicated. She had a learning disability and a long history of drinking problems and epilepsy. A previous child had been fostered because of her inability to cope.

This woman was said to have a very supportive family and an excellent social worker but the lack of details available to the Enquiry makes it difficult to know whether more could have been done.

In these 11 cases of substance misuse, although five were in current contact with services, all had had previous contact for their substance misuse problem, which therefore could have been identified antenatally. The increased risk of suicide and accidental death is well established in both drug- and alcohol-dependent women. Their pregnancies and adjustments to motherhood are also known to be problematic. This, together with the established difficulty in attending outpatient appointments and regular compliance with treatment programmes, would suggest that maternity units, and antenatal clinics in particular, should provide open access to substance misuse advisors. The women could then be engaged at the time of their visit, perhaps improving the outcome for both mother and child.

**Previous history of psychiatric illness: risk of recurrence**

In nine deaths, where the past history had been recorded in the midwifery notes, it was referred to as 'PND' (postnatal depression) despite the evidence of previous severe psychiatric illness in relation to childbirth. In no case was there any evidence that the severity of the previous illness and indeed in-patient care had been ascertained. The use of the term 'PND' gave the impression that the illness had been less severe than it actually was.

In some cases, although the previous illness and the risk of recurrence had been noted (but not quantified), there appears to have been no recognition of the likelihood of the illness recurring at the same time and presenting in the same way as the previous illness. In the following case, the illness seems to have taken professionals by surprise:

> A multiparous woman died as the result of jumping from a height. She had previously had a rapidly deteriorating postpartum depressive

psychosis within days of the birth of a previous child, requiring admission to hospital and treatment with electroconvulsive therapy (ECT). The midwifery records reveal that the midwife had been very concerned about the possibility of a recurrence and had referred the woman to a psychiatrist during the antenatal period. She was given a prescription for an antidepressant to take at the first hint of a depressive illness starting after delivery and also given an open appointment with the psychiatric services. In the event, she became ill, with the same symptoms, on the same day after delivery as she had done previously, and killed herself on the same day after delivery that she had been admitted to hospital for her previous illness. The psychiatric appointment had been given for a few days following the patient's death.

This woman was at a one-in-two to one-in-three risk of a psychotic illness likely to recur around the same day as her previous illness and which would rapidly deteriorate as before. Antidepressant medication was unlikely to be effective in preventing such an illness. Offering a woman, rapidly losing contact with reality, an open appointment is not a realistic way of preventing deterioration. At the very least, frequent monitoring at home by a community psychiatric nurse and recognition by all parties of the likely time of onset of the condition might have prevented the tragic outcome. This is a case in which the midwives recorded the previous severe illness as 'PND' in the antenatal records.

In one case a past history of a postpartum psychosis was not recorded at all:

> In a *Late* death, an older multiparous woman died from being hit by a car after absconding from an inpatient psychiatric unit where she was being treated for a postpartum psychosis. She had previously suffered from a postpartum psychosis following the birth of another child some years earlier. There was no mention in her antenatal records of her previous psychiatric history and she had midwifery-led care and a home delivery. Shortly after this she became psychotic and required inpatient admission, during which time she expressed suicidal intentions.

In the absence of any psychiatric report to the CEMD, it is difficult to know whether she had been warned by her previous psychiatrist of the risk of recurrence. In the absence of any antenatal detection of this risk, it would not possible to take steps to avoid a postpartum recurrence. If her past history had been ascertained then her antenatal and postnatal care could have been planned in such a way that she was managed by the relevant health professionals during this high-risk period.

In one case very few details are available:

> In this case, a woman with a history of puerperal psychosis following a previous pregnancy was referred to her local psychiatrist but did not attend. She stabbed herself in the abdomen and took an overdose of tricyclic antidepressants early in her pregnancy. She never regained consciousness and died shortly after delivery.

In two *Late* cases, the psychiatric condition had been identified and the community mental health team was involved. However, the lack of specific focused treatment in the face of prolonged morbidity would suggest that the illnesses were not taken sufficiently seriously.

> An older woman with longstanding anxiety and obsessionality died by hanging. She developed an obsessive compulsive disorder (OCD) following the birth of her first child and was treated by her GP with antidepressants and partially improved. She conceived her second child whilst still symptomatic and was very ambivalent about the pregnancy. Her OCD deteriorated during the pregnancy and further following delivery. Although she was seen frequently by a community nurse, there was only very brief involvement by a consultant psychiatrist. The Enquiry had evidence that her symptoms were very severe and that her compulsive behaviour was severely interfering with her functioning at home and with her marriage. Despite the frequent contact with the community mental health team, there does not appear to have been any specific focused treatment nor an awareness on the part of the team as to how severely disabled she was. Fearing that her marriage was breaking down and that she might lose custody of her children, she hanged herself the day after she had told her husband and health professionals that she was thinking of ending her life.

This woman had severe chronic OCD with a postpartum onset and a predictable deterioration during her next pregnancy. This is an illness that required formal structured treatment in addition to the support that she received.

> Another older multiparous woman died by hanging late in the postpartum year. She had been treated for postnatal depression by her GP following the birth of her first child. This illness took a long time to resolve. During her next pregnancy she became depressed and was seen by the community mental health team, who noted that she had relationship problems as well. After delivery, she appeared to be well and was discharged by the community mental health team after a few weeks. Some months later, she was noted to have symptoms for anxiety but was not re-referred. Later in the postpartum year she was seriously injured in a road traffic accident and was noted to be depressed. Shortly afterwards, she killed herself after expressing suicidal thoughts to her husband.

Although her problems had been identified, she was probably discharged too soon by the community mental health team in view of the history of a prolonged recovery after her first postnatal illness. The recurrence of symptoms, particularly within the context of a severe life stress, should have alerted those involved in her care to the possibility of a relapse of her condition.

In two cases, the women were appropriately treated by their GPs for postnatal depression and seemed to be recovering satisfactorily. They then killed themselves by violent methods. Their suicides appear to have been triggered by events that may have been unknown to the professionals involved in their care.

> In the first case a single multiparous woman with mild postnatal depression was treated by her GP with antidepressants, apparently satisfactorily. Shortly before her death, some months after delivery, she

received enquiries about her social security payments. From the evidence to the Enquiry, it appears that she developed overvalued ideas that she might go to prison and lose her children.

This woman's GP and health visitor were not aware of her recent worries. However, this case is a reminder that women with a recent history of postnatal depression may remain vulnerable to adversity.

In the second case, a woman was appropriately treated by her GP for postnatal depression and appeared to be doing well shortly before she killed herself in a particularly horrific manner some months after delivery:

> This older multiparous woman died from self-immolation. She suffered from long-standing social and relationships problems and had previously taken an overdose in response to these some years previously. She was treated by her GP for mild postnatal depression with antidepressants and was seen regularly by him and her health visitor. Shortly after she was last seen, and said to be doing well, she set fire to herself. The final act appeared to have been precipitated by a crisis in a relationship.

There is nothing to suggest from the evidence that she received less than adequate care nor that such an act of desperation could have been anticipated. This case also serves to remind of the continued vulnerability to crises in women suffering from depression and chronic adversity.

A number of cases involved women in their first childbirth with a previous history of non-postpartum psychiatric illness. Again, the risk of a recurrence or relapse of the illnesses following childbirth appears not to have been recognised either by their psychiatrists or by their midwives. This led to the care being reactive rather than proactive. It again seems that the professionals involved in these women's care had been taken by surprise by the rapid escalation of symptom severity following the onset of the condition.

> A woman died by jumping from the maternity unit a few days after delivery. She had a long history of psychosis and had been an inpatient in a psychiatric unit within the previous year. She moved area during pregnancy but there is no evidence from the documentation that her psychiatric care had been transferred to her new area of residence during pregnancy. Her GP referred her to a new psychiatrist who did not obtain her previous records. He commented that she must be at risk of a postpartum recurrence of her condition but did not arrange to see her again and referred her to a community psychiatric nurse. The midwives were aware of her previous history but not of its severity, nor of the high risk of recurrence. There is no evidence that plans were made for her postpartum management. Shortly after delivery a relative warned the maternity staff that she was becoming psychotic and over the next few days they became increasingly concerned by her disturbed behaviour. Psychiatric assessment was sought but inadequate treatment given. In the hour before her death, the midwifery staff made multiple telephone calls for assistance to the psychiatric unit but before help arrived the woman jumped through a window and died.

In this case the psychiatrist failed to plan her care, appeared not to be aware that her risk of recurrence was between one in two and one in three, did not communicate with the midwives or obstetricians, nor put into place either prophylactic medication or an action plan in case of concern.

> An older woman, living in comfortable circumstances, was a *Late* death from an overdose of antidepressants. She had a long history of recurrent depressive illness prior to her first pregnancy. She suffered from a recurrence of her depressive illness after delivery but died before she was seen by the community mental health team.

Despite the length of her previous history, there was no record of this in her midwifery notes, nor had the possibility of a postpartum recurrence been considered. The GP was reassured by high levels of social support and an absence of a past history of deliberate self-harm. Nonetheless, the suicide note and careful planning of the overdose suggested that the intention was suicide.

> A young woman hanged herself in her first pregnancy, having had a psychiatric history of admission for a severe overdose in the preceding year. Towards the end of the second trimester, she was referred to a psychiatrist because of a short history of panic attacks and sleep and appetite disturbance. Her mental state was described in the notes as being distraught, rambling and with difficulty in concentrating. She was prescribed a selective serotonin uptake inhibitor antidepressant and a benzodiazepine, whose use are controversial in pregnancy. No plans were made for the psychiatrist to see her again. She was referred to a community psychiatric nurse, who saw her a few weeks later and noted that she had suicidal thoughts She committed suicide shortly afterwards.

Despite her evident psychiatric disturbance and recent past history of serious illness involving a life-threatening overdose and inpatient care, the response of the psychiatrist seems inappropriate. The long delay before being seen by a community psychiatric nurse, the absence of a management plan and correspondence with the obstetricians and midwives, represents less than optimal care.

## The importance of a family history

It is known that a family history of serious affective disorder is a risk factor for severe postpartum illness.[9] In two cases of early suicide after delivery, there was a family history of serious psychiatric disorder, despite the absence of any previous personal history:

> An older professional woman living in comfortable circumstances shot herself shortly after her discharge from the maternity hospital. She had been seen by a psychiatrist for depression while in hospital but was thought not to be mentally ill. It was noted at that time that her mother had suffered from severe postnatal depression. Despite good social support, she killed herself the day her husband returned to work away from home.

In the absence of detailed information from either the psychiatrist or the GP, it is difficult to know whether the initial assessment was adequate. However, early concerns about this woman's mental health following delivery, combined with a positive family history should, at the very least, have been communicated to the woman's community midwife and GP. Expert monitoring of her mental state following discharge might have detected the deterioration in her mental health.

In a second case, discussed later in this Chapter, there was a strong family history of psychiatric disorder and suicide. The woman and her husband decided not only to conceal this from health professionals but also from her extended family. If her GP had known of this, he might have taken more seriously her anxiety symptoms and insomnia following the birth of the baby.

In two cases, women died of causes other than suicide but, had the severity of the previous illness been noted, the high risk of early postpartum recurrence could have been predicted and perhaps prevented:

> In a very unusual case, a woman died from what the certificate of death describes as an adverse drug reaction to haloperidol, which she was prescribed while an inpatient for puerperal psychosis. She had a past psychiatric history of bipolar disorder and postpartum psychotic depressive illness, both necessitating inpatient stays. Again, this was recorded in her antenatal records as 'PND'. Shortly after delivery she became psychotic (at the same time as she had after the birth of a previous child) and was admitted to a psychiatric unit. She had an acute laryngeal spasm after taking haloperidol and required intubation in an ICU. She recovered from this but a few days later suffered a major gastrointestinal bleed and cardiac arrest from which she could not be resuscitated.

Care was substandard in a number of respects. Had the severity of her previous psychiatric illnesses been investigated at the booking clinic, the high risk of early postpartum recurrence could have been predicted and perhaps preventative measures taken. In the absence of any psychiatric evidence to the CEMD, it is not possible to know whether her supervising psychiatrist at the time of her previous illness had warned her of the risk of recurrence. Furthermore, an inadequate autopsy gave the cause of death as an acute reaction to haloperidol but other causes for the cardiac arrest or haemorrhage were not satisfactorily excluded.

> A woman died from a pulmonary embolism a few weeks after discharge from inpatient care for a postpartum depressive psychosis. She had had a psychotic postpartum depressive illness following the birth of a previous child. This too was recorded in her antenatal notes as 'PND'.

Again, if the severity of the illness had been noted then the high risk of early postpartum recurrence could have been predicted and perhaps prevented. As with the previous case, in the absence of any psychiatric evidence, it is difficult to know whether her supervising psychiatrist at the time had warned her of her risk of recurrence following future childbirth.

**Lack of specialist perinatal psychiatric services and mother and baby units**

In no case was the mentally ill mother seen by a specialist perinatal mental health service. None of the women who were admitted to hospital following the birth of their babies were admitted to a specialist mother and baby unit, nor does it seem that those admitted previously were. As described above, specialist experience and knowledge on the part of psychiatric staff may have meant, in certain cases, that they would have been familiar with not only the high risk of recurrence but also the rapidly escalating and changing picture of the women's illnesses. There is also the possibility of preventative action being taken and, in some cases, the illness might have been avoidable. However, even if this were not possible, for example in the case of very early onset psychoses, putting into practice a management plan and informing relatives and community midwives of the likely presentation could have meant earlier detection of the illness and perhaps even prevention of suicide.

Admission to a mother and baby unit, in some cases, might have made it more acceptable for the woman to stay in hospital until she recovered. A familiarity by the specialist staff of the rapidly changing and unstable clinical syndrome of bipolar affective psychoses following childbirth might have prevented premature discharge and repeated readmission, with a subsequent alienation of the patient.

> A woman with no previous history of psychiatric disorder died by jumping from a height. She had developed a manic puerperal psychosis a few days after delivery and was admitted to a psychiatric unit without her baby. She then became depressed with ideas of guilt and was discharged after a few weeks. She was readmitted for a few weeks of further treatment for a depressive psychosis shortly afterwards. She was then readmitted for a third time, for a short period of inpatient care, a few days later. A few weeks after this, and after seeing her psychiatrist, she declined any further contact and killed herself the same day. During her inpatient psychiatric care, there were documented reports of her threat to commit suicide by jumping.

In this particular case, admission to a mother and baby unit, together with her infant, might have made a difference to her outcome.

> Another woman, who also had a previous history of severe postnatal depression requiring inpatient care, died of a gunshot wound. She had a history of both attempted suicide and depression not associated with pregnancy and a family history of depressive illness. This history was described as 'PND' at the booking clinic. No antenatal referral to a psychiatrist was made. Antidepressant medication was initiated by the GP shortly after delivery and she was referred to a community psychiatric nurse. She was admitted for inpatient care twice, on both occasions without her baby, and killed herself shortly after returning home from her second in-patient stay.

In this case, the woman initially did not wish to be referred to a mental health team and perhaps that reflected upon her previous experience of being admitted without her baby. Admission to a mother and baby unit after the birth of her next child may have made a difference, leading to her staying for long enough to resolve her condition. As no information was provided by the psychiatric services to the Enquiry, it is difficult to know whether these issues had been addressed. Once again, those involved in her care should have known of the high risk of recurrence of her condition following the birth of another child.

> A woman with no previous psychiatric history was referred to a community mental health team with anxiety and depression a few weeks after delivery. Her condition deteriorated and then seemed to improve after she was prescribed antidepressant and antipsychotic drugs. She was admitted, at her own request, to a psychiatric hospital because of suicidal thoughts but was allowed to discharge herself against medical advice, in the early hours of the morning and then drowned herself in a river.

In the absence of any report from the GP or from the psychiatric hospital, it is unclear as to whether anything more could have been done. However, it is not good practice to allow a recently admitted postpartum woman to be discharged in the early hours of the morning. There is a possibility that this woman would have survived if she had been admitted to a mother and baby unit.

## Stigma and collusion

In a number of cases of maternal death, there is documented evidence that the woman herself declined psychiatric care, sometimes on a number of occasions and sometimes despite having had a severe, hospitalised previous episode. There is insufficient information to know whether the GP or the midwife explored this reluctance and sought the reasons for it. Again, perhaps the presence of a specialist service might go some way to reduce the fear of a woman accepting help in the face of serious mental illness. However, there is a suggestion in a number of cases that this reluctance to seek psychiatric help was accepted at face value and even colluded with:

> A woman who had previously suffered from a severe postnatal depressive illness requiring psychiatric care was reluctant to see a psychiatrist again. The midwife, GP and obstetrician were all aware of her history and the risk of recurrence was discussed during pregnancy. Her reluctance to see a psychiatrist was accepted and apparently not questioned. Plans were made to start progesterone suppositories after delivery. Within a few days of delivery she had clear symptoms of a developing a severe depressive illness and committed suicide a few days later.

Even in the presence of the woman's reluctance to see a psychiatrist, it would have been reasonable for the GP or the obstetrician to ask for some psychiatric advice during the pregnancy. Progesterone is not an effective treatment or prophylaxis for severe postnatal depression.[10] The use of the term 'PND' in the maternity records did not reflect the severity of her previous illness. Perhaps the availability of a specialist psychiatric service would have reduced the risk of refusal to seek appropriate help.

In another case, it was the woman and her husband who decided to conceal from all health professionals the strong family history of psychiatric disorder:

> This woman, also a death early after delivery, killed herself by jumping from a height. She herself had no previous psychiatric history but there was a strong family history of psychiatric disorder and suicide of which her GP was unaware. She started to develop symptoms a week after delivery and saw her GP with difficulty in sleeping and anxiety about the baby. She was prescribed progesterone suppositories and but committed suicide a very few days later.

From the information available in this case, it is difficult to know whether this was active secret keeping or whether 'did not disclose' equals 'was not asked'. The routine sensitive questioning of women at the booking clinic about past psychiatric and family psychiatric history may make it more difficult for people to actively keep secrets and may go some way to reduce the stigma of psychiatric disorder. It is restated that progesterone is not an effective treatment for a severe depressive illness.

## Even with the best care, prevention of suicide is not always possible

There are some examples among the maternal deaths of outstanding psychiatric care and documentation from the psychiatric team that reflects this:

> A woman whose husband accidentally died shortly before she discovered that she was pregnant committed suicide by hanging. From the booking clinic onwards she clearly revealed her intention to kill herself by hanging and that life without her husband was untenable. She was seen very rapidly by a psychologist, midwife, obstetrician, psychiatrist and social worker and she then retracted her suicidal statements. There was no evidence of a mental illness, only of a bereavement reaction. All those involved, including the midwives, tried their hardest to engage her with psychological help. There was excellent communication between all professionals. However, there was active family collusion and secret keeping, her family being adamant that she needed no help and angry at the intrusion into their privacy. She hanged herself a few weeks later, having made elaborate plans and putting her affairs in order. It is difficult to know what more could have been done.

Another woman killed herself by cutting her throat while pregnant. She had suffered from postpartum depression following a previous childbirth. In this pregnancy, a psychiatrist saw her late in the first trimester with a depressive illness. She was then seen daily by a community psychiatric nurse and weekly by a psychiatrist and was given the appropriate antidepressant treatment. When last seen before her death, she was said to be very much improved.

Again, it is difficult to know how much more could have been done and, indeed, whether most psychiatric services would have been able to provide such intensive care.

> Another woman, a *Late* death, died by cutting her throat. She was a young single woman with a history, since childhood, of severe personality disorder and serious self-mutilation and previous life threatening self-harm. She killed herself while an inpatient and detained under the Mental Health Act.

Although her psychiatric problems had become more frequent and intense after delivery, there was no evidence of a qualitative change in her condition and she had been in intensive inpatient care since her deterioration in the first few weeks post partum. Her psychiatric care appears to have been excellent, particularly in the face of such a difficult personality disorder. It is likely that her death was inevitable.

### Not all suicide is predictable

In some cases, there appears to have been no evidence of any mental illness prior to the death by suicide or no clear understanding of the final trigger for the act of suicide:

> A multiparous woman with no previous psychiatric history hanged herself some months after delivery. Shortly before her death, she had visited her GP complaining of stress over a neighbourhood dispute. She was said to be cheerful, smiling and not clinically depressed.

In a second *Late* death there was also no evidence of any mental health problems prior to her death:

> An older woman had conceived as the result of *in vitro* fertilisation. Shortly before her death, she visited her GP for the treatment of a minor physical condition and there was no evidence of any distress or depression as that visit. Shortly afterwards, she was found having died from an overdose of over-the-counter medication.

There is insufficient information to know whether postnatal depression had been missed in this case of a woman who was at theoretically increased risk by virtue of her age and assisted conception.

Two further *Late* deaths also seems to have occurred without any prior history depression:

> An older multiparous woman died by stabbing herself. She was a professional woman in comfortable circumstances with good family support. There is insufficient information to know whether signs of postnatal depression could have been missed.

> In another death, a woman with no past history of a psychiatric disorder was having some difficulties with her second family. She was seen by her GP frequently. On every occasion she was said to be in good spirits. Unknown to the GP, her family were aware that she had become depressed over the month before her death, by hanging.

No details are available for the case of a young woman who died by taking an overdose of paracetamol shortly after she discovered she was pregnant.

## Conclusions

Twelve per cent of all *Direct*, *Indirect* and *Late Indirect* maternal deaths were as the fatal consequence of psychiatric disorder and over 10% committed suicide.

The introduction to this Chapter shows that the deaths from suicide reported to this Enquiry are the second leading cause of maternal deaths, but that the number of unreported cases identified by a subsequent record linkage shows psychiatric causes to be the leading cause of death overall. Nevertheless, suicide is rare, particularly in pregnancy and the postpartum period. Numbers would suggest that the rate of suicide is one to two per 100,000 maternities.

In the absence of adequate information from psychiatric sources and in the absence of any control group, it is not possible to know whether the factors identified in these case studies can be generalised. It is equally impossible to know how frequently these risk factors are present in women who do not kill themselves.

Nonetheless, these psychiatric cases of maternal death may reveal important clues as to the common deficiencies in the management of serious perinatal mental illness. Addressing these problems would undoubtedly improve the care of the majority of women and may even prevent the death of some.

The major themes that emerge from these cases are:

- the importance of serious post partum illness

- the use of the tem 'postnatal depression' or 'PND'

- the importance of routine enquiry at booking clinic about previous psychiatric history

- the importance of communication

- the availability of specialist services

- access to substance misuse services.

## The importance of serious postpartum illness

The majority of the women who died after childbirth were seriously ill and already in contact with psychiatric services. Half of them had a previous psychiatric history and the majority died violently. The early deaths, in particular, were characterised by illnesses with very acute onsets within days of delivery. In many cases these women were older, living in comfortable circumstances and with good social support. These cases emphasise the need for focused expert surveillance and care. They underline that fact that support alone is insufficient to protect women from serious mental illness and that the profile of women who commit suicide following childbirth may be different from the profile of suicide at other times.

## Use of the tem 'postnatal depression' or 'PND'

This term should only be used to describe a nonpsychotic depressive illness of mild to moderate severity with its onset following delivery. It should not be used as a generic term to describe other mental illnesses. The use of the acronym 'PND' to describe cases, in this Enquiry, of very severe illness complicating previous childbirths, may have led to the likely severity of the recurrence being underestimated and opportunities for prevention missed.

## Importance of routine enquiry at booking clinic about previous psychiatric history

This should not merely be dismissed as 'PND' but an affirmative answer should be pursued by further enquiry as to the severity of the illness, its clinical presentation and the timing of its onset. Most women who have experienced a previous serious postpartum illness will be concerned about future recurrence. All those involved, midwives, obstetricians, GPs and psychiatrists need to acquire knowledge of the high risk of recurrence, to know that women with early onset conditions can quickly move from appearing to be merely anxious and depressed to being psychotic and suicidal within a few days. They also need to know that being mentally well in pregnancy does not necessarily reduce the risk of recurrence following delivery. Forewarned is forearmed and at the very least a period of skilled monitoring and management plans for early intervention could be instituted.

## Communication

It is apparent that psychiatric, midwifery and obstetric staff need to communicate with each other and with the general practitioner verbally and in writing about the care of women during pregnancy who are at risk of a postpartum mental illness.

## Availability of specialist services

None of the women who died had been managed by a specialist perinatal mental health team, nor had any been admitted at any time to a mother and baby unit. A specialist team would have been familiar with the distinctive features of the clinical syndromes and the risk of recurrence. They would have been able to offer care that did not necessitate separating the mother from her baby. Mother and baby units, in particular, may have gone some way to increase the acceptability of psychiatric care for this group of women.

## Access to substance misuse services

The last important theme to emerge is that substance misuse causes major problems in pregnancy both to the unborn child and to the mother. Its association with difficulty complying with routine services, appointments and treatment regimes is well known. Open access to readily available substance misuse services without the need for making appointments should be available, particularly in antenatal clinics, and might improve both the rate of engagement and the compliance with care.

## Psychiatric or social service information available to the CEMD

The quality and quantity of psychiatric information available to the CEMD was very poor. Despite the large number of women discussed in this Chapter being in contact with the psychiatric or substance misuse services at the time of their death, and the eight patients who were inpatients at that time, there was a lack of information from the psychiatric or social services in the documentation. In every case, there would have been a suicide audit and reports from the psychiatrist would have been requested by the coroner. The lack of this information makes it difficult to judge the adequacy of psychiatric care and may lead to the Enquiry being overly critical of psychiatric services. The new report forms for the Enquiry now actively seek this information and it is hoped that a more detailed and accurate assessment of these cases will be possible in future.

**The welfare of the children**

Another important theme to emerge concerns the children. Most of these women were already mothers and in only a very few cases was there any mention of the safety and wellbeing of the child. This is particularly alarming in the case of the violent deaths and substance misuse.

This Chapter has been seen and discussed with: Professor JE Cox MD FRCPsych, University of Keele, and Professor TJ Fahy MD FRCPsych, National University of Ireland at Galway.

# References

1.  O'Hara MW, Swain AM. Rates and risk of postpartum depression – a meta-analysis. *Int Rev Psychiatry* 19968:37–54.
2.  Cox JL, Murray D, Chapman G. A controlled study of the onset, duration and prevalence of postnatal depression. *Br J Psychiatry* 1993;163:27–31.
3.  Oates M. Psychiatric services for women following childbirth. *Int Rev Psychiatry* 1996;8:87–98.
4.  Kendell RE, Chalmers JC, Platz E. Epidemiology of puerperal psychosis. *Br J Psychiatry* 1987;150: 662–73.
5.  Appleby L. Suicide during pregnancy and in the first postnatal year. *BMJ* 1991;302:137–40.
6.  Cox JL, Holden JM, Sagovsky R. Detection of postnatal depression: Development of the 10-item Edinburgh postnatal depression scale (EPDS). *Br J Psychiatry* 1987;150:782–6.
7.  Royal College of Psychiatrists. *Perinatal Maternal Mental Health Services.* London: Royal College of Psychiatrists; 2000. Council Report CR88.
8.  Wieck A, Kumar R, Hirst AD, Marks MN, Campbell IC, Checkley SA. Increased sensitivity of dopamine receptors and recurrence of affective psychosis after childbirth. *BMJ* 1991;303:613–16.
9.  Dean C, Williams RJ, Brockington IF. Is puerperal psychosis the same as bipolar manic depressive disorder? A family study. *Psychol Med* 1989;19:637–47.
10. Lawrie TA, Herxheimer A, Dalton K. Oestrogens and progestogens for preventing and treating postnatal depression. *Cochrane Database Syst Rev* 2001; Issue 3.

# CHAPTER 12
## Other *Indirect* deaths

MICHAEL DE SWIET on behalf of the Editorial Board

## *Indirect* deaths: key recommendations

- Patients with known medical problems should be managed by consultant physicians with the necessary expertise. Ideally, these should be consultant obstetric physicians who can draw on their physician colleagues' assistance if necessary.

- When faced in an emergency with a medical problem that is outside their experience, consultants and other obstetric staff should be prepared to consult widely. Such consultations may often only require a telephone call.

- All obstetric decisions about pregnant women on the intensive care unit should have direct consultant input from the relevant consultant obstetrician.

- Anaesthetists should be consulted early when sick pregnant patients are admitted, particularly if there are problems concerning fluid balance and the siting of lines for monitoring and treatment.

- Women with epilepsy need specific specialist advice in pregnancy. The ideal treatment for pregnant women with epilepsy, which has already been instigated in some centres, is a dedicated clinic to encompass prepregnancy counselling and attended by an obstetrician, a neurologist/obstetric physician and a specialist midwife or neurological nurse.

- Women with epilepsy should also be made aware of the dangers of bathing during pregnancy. They should be advised to bathe only in shallow water with someone else in the house or, alternatively, to shower.

- All women should be encouraged to have HIV screening at booking.

- Pregnant women appear to be particularly susceptible to infectious diseases. Those who are not improving despite standard treatment should be admitted to hospital.

- The risk to the fetus from poorly treated asthma is much greater than any possible risk to the fetus of steroid drugs. Steroid therapy can and should be continued in pregnancy without harm to the fetus.

- Pregnancy is not a reason for withholding plain X-ray films of the abdomen, chest X-rays, some computed tomography scans or magnetic resonance imaging from sick women.

**Table 12.1**   Other *Indirect* causes of maternal mortality; United Kingdom 1997–99

| Cause | Cases (*n*) |
|---|---|
| **Infectious disease** | |
| Staphylococcus | 1 |
| *Streptococcus pneumoniae* | 2 |
| *Escherichia coli* | 1 |
| *Mycobacterium tuberculosum* | 1 |
| Varicella virus | 1 |
| Influenza virus | 2 |
| Human Immunodeficiency virus | 1 |
| Toxoplasmosis | 1 |
| Organism unknown | 3 |
| Total infectious diseases | 13 |
| | |
| **Endocrine, metabolic and immunity disorders** | |
| Diabetes mellitus | 4 |
| Systemic lupus erythematosus | 2 |
| Total endocrine, metabolic and immunity disorders | 6 |
| | |
| **Diseases of the blood** | |
| Haemoglobin sickle cell disease (Hb SC) | 1 |
| Thalassaemia | 1 |
| Haemophilia | 1 |
| Haemophagocytic syndrome | 1 |
| Total diseases of the blood | 4 |
| | |
| **Diseases of the central nervous system** | |
| Subarachnoid haemorrhage | 11 |
| Intracerebral haemorrhage | 5 |
| Cerebral thrombosis | 5 |
| Epilepsy | 9 |
| Miscellaneous | 4 |
| Total diseases of the central nervous system | 34 |
| | |
| **Diseases of the circulatory system** | |
| Splenic artery aneurysm | 1 |
| Intra-abdominal bleeding | 1 |
| Total diseases of the circulatory system | 2 |
| | |
| **Diseases of the respiratory system** | |
| Asthma | 5 |
| Cystic fibrosis | 2 |
| Pneumonia | 1 |
| Viral infection ? sleep apnoea | 1 |
| Total diseases of the respiratory system | 9 |
| | |
| **Diseases of the gastrointestinal system** | |
| Intestinal obstruction | 3 |
| Pancreatitis | 2 |
| Liver failure | 1 |
| Liver rupture | 1 |
| Total diseases of the gastrointestinal system | 7 |
| | |
| **Total *Other Indirect* deaths** | **75** |

## Summary

For the first time since the Confidential Enquiries into Maternal Deaths began, the number of *Indirect* deaths reported to this Enquiry is larger than the total number of *Direct* deaths. The rate for *Indirect* deaths is 6.4 per 100,000 maternities compared with 5.0 per 100,000 maternities for *Direct* deaths. As has been stressed in previous Reports, **the lessons that may be learned from these deaths are just as important as those for deaths due to *Direct* causes.**

In 1997–99, there was a total of 75 other *Indirect deaths* compared to 86 deaths in 1994–96. The reduction in numbers comes in part from 12 *Indirect* deaths due to cancer being counted in a new Chapter, Chapter 13; Cancer and other tumours. In addition, there were 13; *Late Indirect deaths* counted in Chapter 15; *Late* deaths. The causes of the *Indirect* deaths counted in this Chapter are shown in Table 12.1.

## Infectious diseases

There were 13 deaths due to infection other than arising from the genital tract. Deaths from genital tract infection are considered to be *Direct* deaths and are counted in Chapter 7. Five cases were associated with substandard care.

There were also three *Indirect* deaths from endocarditis considered in Chapter 10; Cardiac deaths. The deaths of a woman from meningitis due to group A streptococcus and of another from acute demyelinating disseminated encephalomyelitis are considered later in this Chapter, in the section relating to diseases of the central nervous system.

There was one further death from overwhelming *Streptococcus pneumoniae* pneumonia complicated by recurrent pneumothoraces but, due to intensive treatment, she lived for a few weeks after delivery and is therefore counted as a *Late Death* in Chapter 15.

The organisms concerned with the *Indirect* deaths this triennium were various: staphylococcus, *Streptococcus pneumoniae* (two cases), *Escherichia coli*, *Mycobacterium tuberculosum*, varicella virus, influenza virus (two cases), HIV and toxoplasmosis, which was almost certainly HIV related. In three cases the exact nature of the infection was not determined:

> A multigravid woman, early in her second trimester, had been ill for one week with chest pain, yellow sputum, wheeze and breathlessness. She had also had diarrhoea and vomiting. A locum GP called, heard crepitations and wheeze, diagnosed a chest infection and prescribed erythromycin and a linctus. The next day she was even more breathless and another locum GP was called. He diagnosed acute bronchitis and prescribed salbutamol. Within 48 hours she was found dead by her husband. Autopsy showed widespread broncho-pneumonia and *Staphylococcus aureus* was cultured from the pus.

This represents substandard care. A young pregnant woman who is deteriorating despite antibiotic treatment should be referred to hospital. In this case, admission may not have affected the outcome, since staphylococcal pneumonia often following influenza infection is notoriously virulent. But care was substandard nevertheless.

Two women did die subsequent to influenza infection, which is known to be more dangerous in pregnancy:

> One was a known asthmatic who was admitted to hospital early in the second trimester where a chest X-ray was compatible with atypical pneumonia, later shown by serology to be due to influenza. After a long illness managed in the intensive care unit (ICU), she went into very premature spontaneous labour and delivered a stillborn child. She subsequently died of acute respiratory distress syndrome (ARDS).

> The other patient was a smoker admitted late in the second trimester with pneumonitis. She deteriorated, developed ARDS and died some days after admission. Influenza type A was proven by serology.

In some other countries, influenza vaccine is recommended in pregnancy, particularly to patients who also have asthma. It is recommended that this practice should be considered in the United Kingdom.

Varicella pneumonia is also known to be more dangerous in pregnancy:

> A woman in the middle trimester of her pregnancy was admitted straight to the ICU with a diagnosis of varicella pneumonia. She died two days later, aciclovir only having been given just before her death.

This represents substandard care. The efficacy of aciclovir in treating varicella pneumonia is accepted and, indeed, many authorities would suggest that any pregnant woman who contracts varicella should receive aciclovir because of the increased risk of pneumonia, which seems to be particularly dangerous in pregnancy. This woman was ill enough to be admitted to ICU yet aciclovir was withheld because the drug had not been licensed for use in pregnancy, and then only on the basis of a telephone conversation between junior doctors and the consultant obstetrician. All obstetric decisions about pregnant women on ICU should have direct consultant input from the relevant consultant obstetrician. At the very least, the consultant obstetrician should have visited this woman who had been in the ICU for two days.

> In one very unusual case, a woman was found collapsed at home by her husband. Resuscitation was commenced by her husband and continued by the ambulance crew but she was in asystolic cardiac arrest by the time she got to hospital. At autopsy she was found to have acute phlegmonous gastritis, a fulminating pyogenic infection of the stomach wall, known to be caused by infection with *Streptococcus pneumoniae*.

Only one previous case has been described in association with pregnancy.[1] However, in view of the very rapid course of the illness, which could be pregnancy related, this case has been classified as an *Indirect* rather than a *Coincidental* death.

In a case also discussed in Chapter 4, a woman died of bronchopneumonia:

A severely socially deprived multigravid woman had a chaotic life style, a violent partner and mother-in-law and required much social services and child-protection support. She was anaemic throughout her pregnancy and had little money to buy food, her relatives spending it on alcohol. Despite this, she had a relatively uneventful pregnancy but had prolonged rupture of membranes and was eventually delivered by caesarean section for suspected brow presentation. The wound extended and she a major postpartum haemorrhage requiring extensive transfusion. She received antibiotic and thromboprophylaxis and was allowed home after one week. Two days later she was visited by her GP when she complained of productive cough. The chest was clear on examination and it was noted that she was continuing to smoke. She was readmitted several days later with an overwhelming chest infection and died on the ICU a few days later. Death was certified due to septicaemia.

In the absence of any other clinical details and of the autopsy report, it is difficult for the assessors to comment further, in particular with regard to substandard care. It is likely that the patient's lifestyle was an important factor. Septic pelvic thrombophlebitis may also have contributed to her death despite the prophylactic measures that had been taken.

Two women died of meningitis. One woman in the middle trimester of her pregnancy died from pneumococcal meningitis on the day of admission, having been treated for a dental abscess two days previously.

Purulent meningitis was also the cause of death in a woman who became very ill following delivery by caesarean section under spinal anaesthesia for pre-eclampsia. A few hours later, she became unresponsive with severe hypertension and she was treated with magnesium sulphate. She did not improve and a computed tomography (CT) scan showed cerebral oedema. A day later she was transferred to a neurosurgical centre, where imaging showed cerebral vein thrombosis, after which brain stem death was diagnosed. Autopsy confirmed the cerebral vein thrombosis but she also had an acute purulent meningitis. All bacterial cultures, both in life and post mortem, were sterile but antibiotics had been given at the time of caesarean section. Cerebral vein thrombosis was thought to be secondary to the meningitis. The relation of purulent meningitis to the spinal puncture is uncertain.

As occasionally occurs, one woman died of overwhelming *E. coli* urinary tract infection. She presented in the middle trimester and rapidly deteriorated with multiple organ failure despite excellent treatment in the ICU. In another case, *E. coli* urinary tract infection is likely to have been the cause of ARDS (as has been found on other occasions) but there was a large element of substandard care.

The patient was a very young girl who had been the victim of domestic violence in the past. She was also a poor attender at the antenatal clinic. She was seen by a consultant obstetrician in the accident and emergency department early in the third trimester, having been ill with a urinary tract infection for one week previously. A coliform was isolated from the urine at this time but the organism was not characterised any further. Throughout the remainder of her illness she was seen by no obstetrician more senior than a registrar. She was treated with intravenous fluids and antibiotics and attempts to insert a central venous pressure (CVP) line, which was indicated because of oliguria, failed. No anaesthetist was available to help or to assess her on the labour ward, so she was taken to the recovery room of the operating theatre. When the line was inserted her CVP was found to be 23 cm of water, which suggests mismanagement of intravenous fluid therapy. There was no ICU bed available at the hospital, so she was transferred to another hospital where she died from ARDS and sepsis some weeks later.

Substandard care was identified because of the lack of consultant involvement once the patient had been admitted. There was inadequate consultation with anaesthetists concerning the difficulties of fluid balance. The lack of involvement with anaesthetists was in part due to their unavailability on the delivery suite, a further element of substandard care.

> A woman from an ethnic minority group had an uneventful pregnancy complicated only by moderate anaemia resistant to iron therapy. About three weeks after delivery she developed a headache and her GP requested a domiciliary visit from a consultant physician. The consultant diagnosed tension headache. Three days later she collapsed and died from brain-stem infarction. At autopsy, a mass was found in the brain stem, only diagnosed as tuberculoma by histology.

This is a further case of substandard care in respect of the domiciliary visit performed by the consultant physician. In a woman who dies of raised intracranial pressure due to a brain-stem mass, it is likely that there would be physical signs to demonstrate more than tension headache three days beforehand.

There was one death from HIV and one from cerebral toxoplasmosis, almost certainly due to HIV. In a further death from malignancy, counted in Chapter 13, there was also a strong possibility of HIV infection but the woman declined testing. These are only the second, third and fourth HIV deaths reported to the Confidential Enquiries. However, it must be remembered that in some parts of the world, particularly sub-Saharan Africa, HIV infection is the most common cause of maternal mortality.

> A multigravid woman had no significant past medical history apart from a blood transfusion following abdominal surgery in another country some years previously. Although all the usual screening tests were performed, there is no comment about whether HIV testing was offered. She was admitted with a chest infection at 18 weeks. *Streptococcus pneumoniae* was isolated but she miscarried and deteriorated despite treatment. She was then found to be HIV positive. She required tracheostomy and the subsequent autopsy showed that this was complicated by oesophageal perforation and mediastinitis.

The oesophageal perforation represents substandard care. However, her lung infection was so overwhelming that it is unlikely that the perforation contributed much to her death. The general recommendation that all women should be offered screening for HIV in pregnancy was only introduced in 1999.[2] Had she been offered screening and been found to be HIV positive at booking, she should have been under surveillance and would have received sufficient treatment to prevent her death. However, in this case, the progress of her disease was very rapid so treatment might not have been effective.

> At booking, a patient coming from a high-risk country was found to be hepatitis B and C positive. She declined HIV screening. She received one week of inpatient treatment for pneumonia late in the first trimester and was readmitted two weeks later with vomiting. Her level of consciousness rapidly deteriorated and a CT scan showed intracerebral mass lesions. These were biopsied and were shown to be due to toxoplasmosis. She died soon afterwards.

Although not proven, it is overwhelmingly likely that the primary cause of death was HIV infection.

## Endocrine, metabolic and immunity disorders

Six deaths are recorded in this section, four relating to diabetes including three from hypoglycaemia, and two to systemic lupus erythematosus (SLE). In addition, one woman, whose death is counted in Chapter 2; Thromboembolism, is very likely to have had SLE.

A possible case of hyperaldosteronism, who died a few weeks after delivery, is counted as a *Late* death in Chapter 15. The diagnosis is in dispute, since the woman was found dead with no previous history suggestive of the condition. Hyperaldosteronism may deteriorate after delivery but the only evidence for the condition was an adenoma demonstrated at an inadequate autopsy. Many adrenal adenomas are nonfunctional 'incidentalomas'.

### Diabetes

There were four deaths from diabetes. The death of one further woman with diabetes, who had bronchopneumonia and possible hypoglycaemia, is described below in the section on respiratory disease. The death of a woman with diabetes from myocardial infarction is counted as a Cardiac death in Chapter 10.

> An insulin-dependent diabetic with retinopathy, nephropathy and neuropathy had been advised against pregnancy. She lived alone and was found dead towards the end of the first trimester of pregnancy. Her postmortem blood glucose was 2.1 mmol/l and it was assumed that hypoglycaemia was the cause of her death, no other cause being found.

The autopsy was inadequate in several respects including a lack of histology. Blood glucose results are notoriously unreliable after death. The glucose should have been analysed in the cerebrospinal fluid and the vitreous humor. The vitreous humor glucose was zero at the autopsy of a pregnant woman who was a known diabetic and who lost control of her car. She was dead on arrival in hospital because, during the ensuing accident, she lacerated her liver. Hypoglycaemia was also considered to be the cause of death in another insulin-dependent diabetic who died early in pregnancy. She appears to have had optimal input from her GP and the diabetes care team but she was known to have an eating disorder, had a morbid fear of obesity and was very resistant to any advice.

In another obese insulin-dependent woman with diabetes the cause of death is uncertain. There was concern that she might have had a pulmonary embolus following her previous pregnancy but the ventilation/perfusion scan was normal. This possibility arose again when she complained of breathlessness late in this pregnancy but the scan was again negative. Labour was induced because of diabetes and she had a normal delivery. Three days later she was found dead at home.

No autopsy details were available to the assessors. Obvious possibilities are pulmonary embolus or a coronary event relating to her diabetes.

### Systemic lupus erythematosus

Of the two cases of SLE, one was only diagnosed just before she died:

> This woman had given no cause for concern antenatally, apart from occasional epileptic seizures. She had had a generalised convulsion in her previous labour and was therefore taking sodium valproate. She was delivered by caesarean section because of poor progress and some concern about fetal wellbeing. The operation was uncomplicated. She was discharged a few days later but was readmitted two days later with pneumonia. She developed multi-organ failure. SLE was diagnosed but she died, despite treatment, following transfer to a national centre of excellence for the management of SLE.

> In the other case, a woman had a five-year history of SLE, first discovered because of miscarriages and the presence of anticardiolipin and double-strand DNA antibodies. She died five days following a spontaneous abortion because of congestive cardiac failure secondary to myocarditis. Myocarditis is a known feature of SLE.

A woman who died of multiple pulmonary emboli is counted in Chapter 2. At autopsy, she was found to have fibrin vegetations on the right side of the heart and pulmonary valves, further clot in the uterine and ovarian veins, central nervous system, splenic, adrenal and pituitary infarcts and renal disease. It is therefore quite likely that she also had SLE. A further possibility would be a primary thrombophilia such as antithrombin deficiency.

## Diseases of the blood

> An older multigravid African-Caribbean woman booked with known haemoglobin sickle cell (Hb SC) disease  Her previous pregnancies had been uncomplicated but the most recent had been several years previously. Most of her previous care had been with the haematology

department of the same local hospital. The patient herself said at booking that she was a mild case of sickle cell trait. It is not clear whether the obstetric staff did not know that she had Hb SC disease or did not appreciate the significance of Hb SC disease, granted that, as is usually the case with Hb SC disease, her haemoglobin level was 9–10 g/100 ml. She was induced post dates with prostin. Transfer to the delivery suite was delayed for reasons that are not clear and, by the time she did arrive there, she was noted to be breathless and tachycardic. Sickle cell crisis and pulmonary embolus were considered. She delivered vaginally soon after. It was thought that she had suffered a pulmonary embolus and she was heparinised in the local ICU. Sickle cell crisis was discounted by the local haematologist. She improved initially and was returned to the delivery suite on the next day. Following a lung scan, which showed multiple perfusion defects, she suddenly became desaturated and very ill. No ICU bed was available so she was transferred to theatre for ventilation and exchange transfusion. Her condition remained poor and she was transferred to a tertiary centre for spiral CT scan, on the assumption that she had suffered a massive pulmonary embolus requiring surgery. The CT scan was negative. She continued to deteriorate and died, despite haemofiltration. Autopsy showed no evidence of pulmonary embolus and death was certified due to multi-organ failure consequent to sickle crisis.

The fundamental problem in this case of substandard care was not realising the significance of Hb SC disease. This is a recurring problem, partly due to ignorance (i.e. lack of knowledge that Hb SC can cause fatal sickling) and partly due to false reassurance from the relatively high Hb levels characteristic of the condition. The patient may have contributed by her denial of any problems in the past and her increasing age probably contributed to the fatal nature of the crisis in this pregnancy. There seems to have been poor communication between haematology and obstetrics; the haematology department should have communicated the risk of sickling to the obstetricians. Perhaps it is significant that once she became ill the haematologists persisted in their incorrect view that sickling was not the main problem. The lack of resources (delivery suite beds, ICU beds, access to spiral CT scans) is also worrying.

A woman with known transfusion-dependent beta thalassaemia had been thoroughly assessed by her obstetrician before she became pregnant by ovulation induction, pituitary function having been impaired because of transfusion-associated iron overload. She had also had an essentially normal echocardiograph performed two years previously, with ejection fraction of 72%. The antenatal period was ostensibly uncomplicated. From the cardiac point of view she was managed with the help of a clinical assistant in cardiology. There was some confusion about the date of her previous echocardiogram, the cardiologist thinking that it had been performed just before pregnancy rather than two years earlier. Therefore another echocardiogram was not performed until about 24 weeks of gestation, when the ejection fraction had fallen to 62% with a normal-sized left ventricle. No further echocardiography studies were performed, perhaps because the patient only complained of occasional palpitations. However, in retrospect, her husband, who never came to hospital with her, said that by the end of pregnancy she had become severely breathless, needing to sit up in a chair rather than go to bed at night. Also, of course, the ejection fraction should increase rather than decrease in pregnancy. Her membranes ruptured prematurely and she was delivered by elective caesarean section under epidural block because of her small stature. Recovery had been planned in the ICU but no bed was available. She developed heart failure a few hours after delivery while on the labour ward, initially recovered after transfer to the coronary care unit but died from heart failure after two weeks of intensive therapy.

The major problem was that the patient did not tell her medical attendants how breathless she had become in the second half of pregnancy, although had she done so, the outcome would not necessarily have been any different. It has already been noted in Chapter 10 how patients with heart disease tend to deny their illness because of their desire to achieve motherhood. Care was considered to be substandard because of the lack of consultant cardiology involvement in a case that was so obviously at high risk from the onset. Further echocardiographs should have been performed once the decrease in ejection fraction had been noted. The unavailability of an intensive care bed after delivery also represents substandard care due to a lack of facilities.

A woman with known factor V and factor VIII deficiencies was monitored by haematologists and obstetricians throughout her pregnancy. In a previous pregnancy she had suffered a postpartum haemorrhage. There was an extensive family history of the condition. At delivery, she received fresh frozen plasma. Five days later she was admitted with a fatal brain-stem haemorrhage.

Without knowledge of the haematological monitoring performed it is impossible to comment on the quality of her care.

A woman became ill with high fever, haemorrhagic rash, hepatosplenomegaly and liver failure about one week after caesarean section for breech presentation. She developed pancytopenia and required assisted ventilation in ICU. She died three weeks after delivery, from subarachnoid haemorrhage and multiorgan failure. Autopsy confirmed the above features and also showed widespread haemorrhage. Bone marrow histology showed some haemophagocytosis. Although the haemophagocytosis was not as marked as usually occurs in haemophagocytic syndrome, this seems the most likely cause of death. Haemophagocytic syndrome is a rare condition with a very high mortality, thought to be associated with viral infection, typically cytomegalovirus or Epstein Barr virus. The bone marrow shows increased histiocytes with phagocytosis of red cells and platelets.

An additional case of thrombotic thrombocytopenic purpura in a woman with sickle cell trait is counted in Chapter 6 as an early pregnancy death, since the condition arose in conjunction with termination of pregnancy.

## Diseases of the central nervous system

### Intracranial haemorrhage

There were 16 cases of intracranial haemorrhage, eleven due to subarachnoid haemorrhage and five to intracerebral haemorrhage. In two of the cases of subarachnoid haemorrhage only death certification was available.

#### Subarachnoid haemorrhage

The ages of the patients with subarachnoid haemorrhage varied between 19 years and 39 years and were evenly distributed with a mean of 31.4 years. Six of the bleeds occurred antenatally, all in the second half of pregnancy at between 26 and 40 weeks of gestation. One case occurred in labour, one five days postnatally and one nine days after delivery by caesarean section. All of the bleeds were from aneurysm, except two where the source of bleeding is unknown since no autopsy was performed (one case) or the result of autopsy is unknown to the assessors (one case). Neurosurgery was performed (unsuccessfully) in two cases; the other women were either too sick or the aneurysms were deemed inoperable.

There were no cases of substandard care, though in one case where the bleed appears to have occurred soon after delivery by caesarean section, concern has been raised about the quality of postoperative monitoring.

> In a further case, concern was raised because a neurosurgical opinion could not be obtained at the local hospital. The woman was transferred to a specialist neurosurgical unit six hours later. It is doubtful if this delay affected the outcome.

> Another case occurred in a former abuser of cocaine. She was attending a rehabilitation programme at the time that she had her bleed. Cocaine abuse is a risk factor for subarachnoid haemorrhage but this is thought to relate to episodes of extreme hypertension occurring at the time that the cocaine is taken. Thus, the former history should not have been relevant unless she had gone back to her old habits.

The eleven deaths from subarachnoid haemorrhage represent a fall from the 14 deaths in the previous triennium. The autopsy rate was also better in this triennium, with 87% of the cases having a postmortem examination. In the previous triennium, only 29% of the cases came to autopsy. The pattern of mortality was not so clear in the previous triennium: eight of the 14 cases bled before delivery and six afterwards.

> The one woman who bled in labour did so at 7 cm dilatation when she had a seizure. She was treated in the first instance as if she had eclampsia and was then delivered by caesarean section. However, there were no other features of eclampsia and angiography showed that she had bled from an aneurysm. She died despite subsequent neurosurgery.

This single known death in labour during a six-year period in the United Kingdom does not give support to the concept that bleeding from aneurysm or arteriovenous malformation is likely during labour, granted the large number of women with these abnormalities who would have been undiagnosed and who came through labour unscathed.

### Intracerebral haemorrhage

Five deaths were ascribed to primary intracerebral haemorrhage.

One death occurred in an older woman who was found to have a massive cerebral haemorrhage when she collapsed at home two weeks after delivery by caesarean section. No cause for the haemorrhage was found at autopsy. Another woman became acutely unwell shortly after a normal delivery following a normal pregnancy. She was transferred to a tertiary centre where a CT scan showed a large intracerebral haemorrhage. She died two days later. She was hypertensive (blood pressure 170/95 mmHg) after the event but this may have been secondary to the rise in intracerebral pressure. She also had epigastric pain but these features do not seem sufficient to diagnose pre-eclampsia.

Pre-eclampsia/eclampsia was also questioned in the third woman who presented with epigastric pain and vomiting in the mid trimester of pregnancy:

> This woman rapidly became confused and may have had a seizure, although this is contested. The maximum diastolic blood pressure at this time was 90 mmHg. She was delivered by caesarean section and the subsequent CT scan showed intraventricular haemorrhage and hydrocephalus, which was fatal.

Again, there is insufficient evidence to ascribe this death to eclampsia. Acute hydrocephalus is unusual in the early stages of brain damage from pre-eclampsia.

> One antenatal case occurred in a young woman from an ethnic minority group who returned from her country to book in the last trimester. She complained of headaches at that time. Four days later she was admitted having had a convulsion. A CT scan demonstrated a massive intracerebral haemorrhage and she died despite an intraventricular drain.

The headache at booking may have been ignored but headache is quite common in pregnancy.

A further antenatal case occurred in a young woman who developed a very severe postcoital headache and then collapsed. Neurosurgery did not help her condition and massive intracerebral haemorrhage was demonstrated at autopsy.

One case of intracerebral haemorrhage due to haemophilia has already been described earlier in this Chapter in the section relating to diseases of the blood. A further case where the bleeding was from an arteriovenous malformation is counted as a *Direct* death in Chapter 3, since the primary cause was thought to be severe pre-eclampsia.

### Cerebral thromboembolism

There were five cases of cerebral thromboembolism in this triennium:

> In the first, a very young primiparous woman who did not smoke had a stroke and was found hemiplegic shortly after booking. She was transferred to a tertiary centre where she rapidly deteriorated and

died. She had a family history of vascular disease, with two close relatives having had a stroke in their fifties or a myocardial infarction in their thirties. An autopsy demonstrated a clot in the left middle cerebral artery but there is insufficient information to determine whether this clot was primary or secondary to embolism.

A multigravid woman consulted a neurologist because of headache. He diagnosed migraine and, because of circumoral anaesthesia during the attack, was concerned about brain-stem damage from vasospasm. He recommended a CT scan but she declined because she was pregnant. The pregnancy was uneventful and she was delivered by repeat caesarean section. She had some headaches after delivery. Three days after discharge she returned to hospital with a fatal middle cerebral artery infarct diagnosed by CT scan. No autopsy was performed.

There was some criticism of lack of communication between neurology and obstetrics but it is difficult to know how the pregnancy could have been managed differently. Although focal migraine is associated with greater prevalence of permanent vascular lesions, it is also difficult to know which particular woman with focal migraine is at risk. The demonstration of a focal vascular lesion might have promoted a thrombophilia screen which, if positive, might have resulted in thromboprophylaxis. However, such suggestions are very speculative.

Thrombophilia and antiphospholipid syndrome were also suspected in the case of another woman who had several previous miscarriages and a late second trimester stillbirth. She had also had a pulmonary embolus following a previous caesarean section. A close relative had also had several miscarriages. Several thrombophilia screens, including one in the index pregnancy, were negative. She booked early and was given low-dose aspirin. Antenatal progress was normal and she had a forceps delivery for fetal distress She was given subcutaneous unfractionated heparin thromboprophylaxis, 5000 units twice daily after delivery. A few days after discharge she was readmitted with blackouts and weakness of the arm and was shown to have a left carotid artery occlusion. She deteriorated and died a few days later.

It is very likely that this woman, and possibility her relatives, had some form of thrombophilia, even if it cannot yet be detected. Thrombophilia is known to be associated with early and late fetal loss, and venous, and in some cases arterial, thromboembolism. She had all of these. Even when thrombophilia has been diagnosed and characterised, it is difficult to know what level of thromboprophylaxis is appropriate for pregnancy. Twice daily injections of 5000 units of unfractionated heparin, even though currently recommended by the Royal College of Obstetricians and Gynaecologists for prophylaxis against deep vein thrombosis and pulmonary embolus,[3] is a small dose for puerperal women. Thus, some consideration should have been given to giving a higher dose, such as unfractionated heparin 7500 units twice daily or enoxaparin (low-molecular-weight heparin) 40 mg once daily. Whether this would have made any difference and whether an even higher 'therapeutic' dose should have been given, remain entirely speculative.

> A primigravid woman developed pre-eclampsia and HELLP syndrome in the mid trimester of her pregnancy. She had a hysterotomy, recovered from a stormy postoperative course and was discharged home. Three weeks later she developed an acute brain stem syndrome and was diagnosed to have basilar artery thrombosis by MRI.

This case is also mentioned in Chapter 3; Hypertension, but counted here because the primary cause of death was the basilar artery thrombosis rather than pre-eclampsia.

In view of the very severe early pre-eclampsia and the subsequent arterial thrombosis, it is likely that she also had some form of thrombophilia such as antiphospholipid syndrome.

> A woman who had been a moderate smoker before pregnancy developed severe pre-eclampsia with 4+ albuminuria and blood pressure180/90 mmHg in her first pregnancy. Labour was successfully induced near term and she was discharged home the next day, three postnatal blood pressure readings having been normal. She was apparently well when at home, although the community midwife did not measure her blood pressure. Ten days after delivery she was readmitted with a fatal right middle cerebral artery thrombosis.

This represents substandard care. Patients who have had such severe pre-eclampsia should not be discharged so soon after delivery. The blood pressure may well fall immediately after delivery, only to reach dangerous levels between postpartum days three and six. Once she had been incorrectly discharged, the failure to measure blood pressure in the community is also unacceptable. Whether or not treatment of postpartum hypertension (if present) would have made any difference is debatable.

## Epilepsy

There were nine deaths from epilepsy, a considerable reduction from the 19 deaths in the previous triennium. Again, there is no obvious reason for this decrease. In the last triennial Report, the concept of sudden unexpected death in epilepsy (SUDEP) was mentioned and this condition has received more publicity.[2,3] SUDEP is a syndrome where a person with epilepsy dies suddenly and no other cause of death is found. Often the person dies alone in their sleep. It is assumed that death occurs following a fit but since the deaths are not witnessed this is only an assumption. Risk factors that are pertinent to pregnancy include poor seizure control. This is particularly relevant since many women try to limit or even stop anticonvulsant therapy in pregnancy because of concern about adverse effects of drugs on the fetus. The possibility of SUDEP should be mentioned to all women who plan to stop anticonvulsant therapy. Fortunately, it is uncommon in those with well-controlled epilepsy. One death meets the criteria for SUDEP and one other may have been SUDEP but in this case an autopsy was not performed.

> In addition a patient with well-controlled nocturnal epilepsy was found dead at home very late in her pregnancy. She may also have had SUDEP but, since she had been treated for a cardiac arrhythmia in the past, there is the possibility that this was the cause of her death.

The autopsy report is unavailable but it is unlikely that these two conditions could be distinguished after death.

> A woman known to have epilepsy became pregnant while taking carbamazepine and clonazepam. She was referred by her obstetrician to a consultant neurologist but failed to attend and was sent no further appointments. The control of her seizures was good during pregnancy. The carbamazepine level was measured on one occasion and found to be at the upper end of the therapeutic range. She had a vaginal delivery and several days afterwards was found drowned after bathing her baby. It was assumed that she had had a fit. The postmortem carbamazepine level was subtherapeutic.

The care of this woman can be criticised, although it does not represent substandard care. Many women with epilepsy are disadvantaged and to send no further appointments after a single failure to attend denies them a fair chance of getting adequate therapy. Anticonvulsant levels usually fall during pregnancy and rise again after delivery. In this woman, the anticonvulsant level had fallen after delivery, suggesting that she had taken matters into her own hands and reduced dosing after delivery, possibly because she was disillusioned by the treatment she had (not) been given by the neurologist to whom she had been referred. Some specialist units are setting up specific 'epilepsy in pregnancy' clinics staffed by an obstetrician, midwife and/or specialist neurology nurse and consultant neurologist or obstetric physician. This is a very welcome development and must represent the best way of caring for such patients.

> Another woman was also found drowned in a bath very early in pregnancy. Her control was usually good. Subtherapeutic carbamazepine levels were again found post mortem.

Although anticonvulsant drug levels fall in pregnancy, largely because of increased liver metabolism, this probably does not occur as early as six weeks of gestation.

> A third woman was also found dead in the bath late in the first trimester. She had had poorly controlled epilepsy and control was much improved by the addition of lamotrigine to sodium valproate. She was seen early in pregnancy by a neurologist who recommended tapering valproate and increasing lamotrigine because of fears about the effect of valproate on the fetus. Her next follow-up appointment was in three months.

This represents substandard care. When patients are changing treatments and when their metabolism is changing because of pregnancy they need to be seen more frequently than every three months. No doubt the neurologist's clinic was overloaded but a four-week follow up would have been more appropriate.

Women with epilepsy should also be made aware of the dangers of bathing in pregnancy. They are, of course, aware of these dangers in general but there does seem to be a disproportionately large number of bathing-associated deaths in pregnancy, perhaps because of the additional risk of vasovagal syncope. It would better for pregnant women to shower.

A multiparous woman who had suffered from epilepsy since she was a child was treated with carbamazepine in pregnancy. Chlamydia infection was diagnosed early in pregnancy and cervical cerclage was undertaken at 14 weeks. However, there were no problems with epilepsy until late in the second trimester, when she was given dexamethasone because of the risk of preterm labour. She died later the same night from status epilepticus. Carbamazepine levels were therapeutic.

Standard medical texts suggest that corticosteroids may exacerbate epilepsy but these statements are not referenced. The manufacturers of dexamethasone did not have any records of similar cases. However, the time relationship between administration of dexamethasone and subsequent status epilepticus is suggestive and the case is reported here for the information of clinicians who may encounter other cases in the future.

A woman with known Charcot-Marie-Tooth disease (a muscular dystrophy) was admitted in her first pregnancy with antepartum haemorrhage early in the third trimester and was readmitted two weeks later with a prolonged convulsion. She was delivered by caesarean section and treated with diazepam for the presumed eclampsia because magnesium sulphate was not available. She did not get better and was transferred to intensive care where 'severe organic brain dysfunction' was diagnosed. She continued to require ventilation and died a few weeks after delivery from ARDS. Regrettably, no autopsy was performed.

The cause of her illness is obscure and her death has been counted under epilepsy for convenience; it certainly does not seem to have been eclampsia. The unavailability of magnesium sulphate gives cause for concern. Magnesium sulphate must be available on the delivery suites of all hospitals caring for pregnant women, although, as it happens, magnesium sulphate would have not been the correct treatment in this case. Magnesium sulphate is not a general anticonvulsant and should not be used for the treatment of seizures in pregnancy unless they are caused by eclampsia.

## Miscellaneous

### *Reactive cerebral gliosis*

A young woman had labour induced late in her pregnancy because of mild proteinuric pre-eclampsia. She behaved bizarrely after delivery and was eventually admitted four days postnatally to a psychiatric unit. She died suddenly a few days later.

A specialist neuropathologist reviewed the autopsy material. The brain showed no macroscopic abnormality but histological examination showed marked neuronal loss and reactive gliosis. Immunohistochemistry did not demonstrate prions. It was thought that the gliosis was likely to represent hypoxic/ischaemic damage occurring before delivery. This is not a recognised complication of mild pre-eclampsia. In the absence of any other explanation, undiagnosed nocturnal epilepsy causing intermittent cardiorespiratory failure was suggested as a cause.

### Acute demyelinating disseminated encephalomyelitis

> Late in her second trimester a multigravid woman was admitted, unconscious, to the accident and emergency department with a short history of diarrhoea, vomiting and epileptic seizures. An MRI scan showed the characteristic brain swelling of acute demyelinating disseminated encephalomyelitis and she died a few weeks after admission.

### Spina bifida; acute meningitis

> A woman with known spina bifida was admitted feeling unwell, thought to have spontaneous rupture of membranes and treated with oral antibiotics. The next day she started to have seizures and she had a cardiac arrest while she had her third fit in the imaging department. She aspirated and this caused pulmonary problems in her subsequent care in the ICU but she died from meningitis due to group A streptococcus. It was presumed that this skin organism, which does not usually cause meningitis, had entered through the meningo-myelocoele remnants relating to her spina bifida.

This represents substandard care. No anaesthetist was involved until after she arrested and aspirated during her third fit. An anaesthetist should have been contacted about this very-high-risk patient for advice about airway protection, before she went to the imaging department.

### Acute hydrocephalus, intraventricular cyst

> A woman was admitted with severe headache on two occasions at term. There were no neurological signs. During the second admission she collapsed, was resuscitated and successfully delivered by caesarean section. The subsequent scan showed hydrocephalus and brain-stem death was diagnosed two hours later. At autopsy, a benign intraventricular cyst was found in the region of the foramina of Monro. This is a very rare cause of death.

There was a *Late* death from meningioma but this was almost certainly present during pregnancy. It is known that meningiomas can enlarge in pregnancy.

Four cases of cerebral vein thrombosis are counted as *Direct* deaths in Chapter 2 relating to thromboembolism.

### Diseases of the circulatory system

There was one death from ruptured splenic artery aneurysm and one from suspected intra-abdominal arterial aneurysm:

> A woman with long-standing portal vein thrombosis developed hypersplenism, pancytopenia and oesophageal varices, from which she had repeated gastrointestinal haemorrhages. She became pregnant after extensive counselling about the risks of pregnancy. She was admitted late in the first trimester because of concern about the risk of bleeding again from her varices, with a platelet count of 20 x 10⁹/l. She

did not bleed from the varices but a few weeks later she suddenly collapsed and a laparotomy revealed an abdomen full of blood. The bleeding source was not identified and her bleeding could not be stopped despite excellent care. Autopsy showed that the bleeding had come from a splenic artery aneurysm that was fibrosed and calcified.

Splenic artery aneurysms are notorious for bleeding in pregnancy. Their cause is usually obscure. But in this case the long-standing nature of the aneurysm demonstrated by fibrosis and calcification make it likely that portal hypertension was the cause.

Two days after a completely normal pregnancy and delivery, a parous woman suddenly collapsed and died within minutes. At autopsy she was found to have about three litres of watery blood in the abdominal cavity. The source of the bleeding could not be identified but it was assumed that she had ruptured an aneurysm of a mesenteric, adrenal or splenic artery, as is known to occur more commonly in pregnancy.

## Disease of the respiratory system

### Asthma

There were five deaths from bronchial asthma:

A woman with long-standing brittle asthma who had twice been treated in ICUs became pregnant and stopped maintenance steroid therapy. Relatively early in pregnancy she was admitted to hospital with an exacerbation of asthma thought to be due to a chest infection. She required ventilation and initially improved. However she remained markedly febrile and then developed fatal rhabdomyolysis and hyperkalaemia. Autopsy was declined.

Although this does not represent substandard care, the healthcare system failed in its treatment of this patient. She should have been informed that steroid therapy can and should be continued in pregnancy without harm to the fetus. The risk to the fetus from poorly treated asthma is much greater than any possible risk to the fetus of steroid drugs. Because of the deterioration following withdrawal of steroids, the unexplained pyrexia and the rhabdomyolysis, it is possible that the patient had a form of vasculitis such as Churg-Strauss syndrome.

Death from asthma can be very sudden, as the following cases illustrate:

A woman who was known to have asthma, who was not taking regular medication, had an acute attack and attended a chest physician in the second trimester of her pregnancy. It is not clear what advice was given but two weeks later she suddenly became very breathless, collapsed, vomited and developed respiratory obstruction. She could not be resuscitated. Autopsy showed mucus plugging characteristic of acute severe asthma.

A woman with mild asthma, controlled by occasional inhalations of salbutamol, attended her GP in the middle trimester complaining only of generalised tiredness. She was reassured but her husband found her lifeless sitting in a chair when he returned later that evening. Autopsy showed marked bronchial occlusion by thick mucus consistent with an acute exacerbation of asthma.

Following a normal pregnancy and delivery a woman was discharged home; two days later she died suddenly at night. The autopsy showed a focal lymphocytic bronchiolitis. The bronchioles showed prominent smooth muscle and many subepithelial eosinophils. After international consultation with experts in lung pathology, it was agreed that death was due to asthma even though she had no previous history of the condition.

The cause of death is uncertain in the following case, which has been counted as an asthma death for convenience:

A woman with asthma, who had had a previous caesarean section and an ectopic pregnancy, was booked at home by the community midwife. Antenatal care was planned between the community and the hospital. However, she did not attend her hospital visit and it is not clear whether she had any more antenatal care. During the second trimester, while at home, she became acutely breathless and called for her salbutamol inhaler. She then collapsed and was taken to hospital by ambulance. She could not be resuscitated despite caesarean section on admission. There was some question of excessive bleeding. The autopsy, although technically perfectly satisfactory, was not helpful. The trachea and bronchi contained a large quantity of frothy mucus. Because of the history and numerous platelet thrombi, death was ascribed to disseminated intravascular coagulopathy related to pregnancy. There were no squames in the lungs to indicate amniotic fluid embolus. There were no autopsy features, such as mucus plugging, which might have suggested asthma as a cause of death.

Technically, this represents substandard care, since this high-risk woman never attended hospital before she died in the late mid trimester of her pregnancy. However, since there are no details of her state of health before her final illness, it is unclear whether any more hospital care would have made any difference.

## Cystic fibrosis

There were two deaths from cystic fibrosis:

One woman with cystic fibrosis had a significant decline in her respiratory function so that, even though she had had a previous successful pregnancy, her forced expiratory volume in one second ($FEV_1$) was only 36% of that predicted for a normal woman of her age and size. Termination had been advised and she attended for the procedure on two occasions but could not go through with it. During her pregnancy, which was managed between recognised centres for the care of cystic fibrosis and high-risk pregnancy, she became ventilator-dependent and died following caesarean section early in the third trimester.

Nutrition is also a problem in CF, and a young woman with CF became pregnant having had a previous gastrostomy and a Past Port because of problems with venous access. Her body mass index (BMI) had always been below 18. No details were available to the CEMD *assessors* regarding her respiratory function but her condition rapidly deteriorated in pregnancy. Termination was advised at her specialist centre but was declined and she died in early pregnancy

## Pneumonia

One death from bronchopneumonia is counted in this section, although five deaths from pneumonia are counted in the section above relating to infectious disease.

In this case, a parous woman with diabetes was admitted in early pregnancy for improvement of diabetic control. Two weeks later she died at home from bronchopneumonia. Since no details of her final illness are available, it is difficult to comment on the quality of her care. However, she did have a vague history of problems at home with her partner and she had to leave hospital early after her admission because of a domestic emergency. It is possible that domestic violence was a factor in this case.

## A possible case of sleep apnoea

A woman, already mentioned in the diabetes section of this Chapter, is included in this section because of the possibility of sleep apnoea:

She was a morbidly obese multigravid woman weighing 130 kg who was only 1.35 m tall, her body mass index being 71. Because of hypertension and gross proteinuria suggesting pre-eclampsia and because of diabetes she had been admitted for early delivery. This was deferred because the presenting part was not in the pelvis and she was not a good candidate for caesarean section. She remained in hospital and a few days later was found dead in bed in the early hours of the morning.

At autopsy, the pathologist noted that the fat on her abdominal wall was 10 cm thick. The autopsy showed no evidence of seizure such as might have occurred in eclampsia but did show inflammatory changes in the lungs consistent with viral pneumonia. Because of her obesity, it is suggested that this could be a case of sleep apnoea, with death precipitated by viral infection and respiratory embarrassment due to pregnancy. Hypoglycaemia due to diabetes remains another possibility.

## Diseases of the gastrointestinal system

There were three deaths from intestinal obstruction:

A woman with ulcerative colitis, who had previously had a colectomy, was delivered by caesarean section. She vomited for three days postoperatively and was hypotensive for a further few days, and intestinal obstruction was only diagnosed after she became oliguric. At laparotomy, intestinal adhesions were divided but she remained gravely ill; no intensive care bed was available. After much fluid therapy and significant hypoxia, she was eventually admitted to ICU, where she became septic and required a further laparotomy, eventually dying of multi-organ failure.

This represents substandard care. The delay in diagnosing intestinal obstruction particularly in such a high-risk case is unacceptable. The lack of intensive care facilities was also contributory and there was some criticism of the management once she had been admitted to ICU.

In another case of substandard care, a woman had an oophorectomy performed overseas in early pregnancy. Late in the first trimester she presented with severe epigastric pain and repeated vomiting. The senior house officer in the accident and emergency department made a provisional diagnosis of biliary colic. She was eventually admitted by the gynaecology senior house officer. On the day after admission she improved but on the next day her abdominal pain became worse and she vomited foul-smelling fluid. The diagnosis of intestinal obstruction was only made by the obstetric registrar one hour before her final cardiac arrest later the same day. Autopsy showed intestinal obstruction due to ischaemia of the terminal ileum secondary to adhesions from the previous oophorectomy.

This represents unacceptable substandard care. There was inability to recognise the severity of her illness, which was clearly not obstetric in origin. There was a total lack of involvement of senior staff in obstetrics or in general surgery, despite a formal request from the junior gynaecological staff. In addition, attempts at diagnosis were thwarted by reluctance to perform X-ray investigations in pregnancy.

An ethnic minority woman was admitted to hospital in the middle trimester with acute abdominal pain and vomiting. This was sufficiently severe to require a 'nil by mouth' regime, opiate analgesia and a surgical opinion. The symptoms improved and she spontaneously delivered a non-viable fetus. Her white cell count was elevated to $30,000 \times 10^9/l$ but she was very upset and insisted on returning home on the day of delivery, despite attempts by the midwifery staff to dissuade her. She collapsed and died at home the next morning. Autopsy showed peritonitis due to perforation subsequent to strangulation of the small bowel by a fibrous band. The fibrous band is likely to have arisen from a previous appendicectomy.

It is not clear to what extent the medical staff realised that this woman's admission symptoms were not due to preterm labour and therefore required explanation. But this case certainly illustrates the difficulty in diagnosing acute abdominal emergencies in pregnancy.

One woman died from ruptured liver. She developed epigastric pain in labour following a normal pregnancy with no evidence of pre-eclampsia. The pain became worse after delivery. Her oxygen saturation temporarily fell to 65%, although it was 98% 20 minutes later, despite continuation of symptoms. She was thought to have had a pulmonary embolus and was given heparin. Although considered, no ventilation perfusion (V/Q) scan was performed. Her condition deteriorated and her heart rate rose to 150 bpm. Laparotomy was performed a day after delivery at which time five litres of blood were found in the abdominal cavity. The blood was coming from the liver surface. She was transferred to a tertiary centre where another six litres of blood were found at a second laparotomy. She died shortly afterwards. At autopsy, no cause was found for the liver rupture despite an extensive search.

Although the fall in oxygen saturation was confusing and epigastric pain may be a presenting symptom of pulmonary embolus, this is unusual. Other causes, such as intra-abdominal bleeding, which would be made much worse by heparin, are more common. The medical registrar made the mistaken diagnosis of pulmonary embolus over the telephone without seeing the patient (although a consultant physician did see the patient and agreed with the diagnosis six hours later). This represents substandard care, as does the failure to obtain a V/Q scan. Clinicians should be reminded that young pregnant women can lose a considerable proportion of their blood volume and still appear relatively well before they finally collapse.

> A schoolgirl had appropriate antenatal care and was delivered by caesarean section. She took her own discharge three days afterwards. She was readmitted six days later with liver failure and died, despite transfer to a specialist liver unit.

A liver pathologist thought that the histology indicated a toxic aetiology rather than a pregnancy specific or any other cause. Paracetamol poisoning was a possibility.

> The cause of death is also uncertain in a woman with longstanding psychological problems including alcohol abuse. She was admitted with vomiting at 12 weeks of amenorrhoea and was found to have a missed embryonic death. She died two days later of multisystem failure. At autopsy, the liver did show fatty change but it was considered that this was more likely to be due to alcohol abuse than to pregnancy. The pancreas showed fibrosis, foci of chronic inflammation and pseudocyst formation. The most likely cause of events is therefore alcoholic pancreatitis leading to multi-organ failure.

Pancreatitis certainly was the cause of death in a woman with complete lipoprotein lipase deficiency.

> The patient had several admissions with abdominal pain in pregnancy and the diagnosis of pancreatitis secondary to hypertriglyceridaemia was made when a blood sample was noted to be lipaemic. Dietary advice was given but she required admission again in the last trimester very ill with further abdominal pain. She developed ARDS and was delivered by caesarean section immediately after she was intubated on

the ICU. The baby did well but the mother deteriorated despite transfer to a tertiary centre and finally died of staphylococcal septicaemia.

Complete lipoprotein lipase deficiency is a rare autosomal recessive disorder causing markedly elevated triglyceride levels from birth. Deterioration in pregnancy with pancreatitis are recognised features. Treatment of the hypertriglyceridaemia is with dietary restriction of fat and lipid lowering drugs.

## Conclusions

### Involvement of anaesthetists

Anaesthetists should be consulted early when sick pregnant patients are admitted, particularly if there are problems concerning fluid balance and the siting of lines for monitoring and treatment.

Minimum standards for the availability of anaesthetists on the delivery suite must be maintained.

### Patients with pre-existing disease

Patients with known medical problems should be managed by consultant physicians with the necessary expertise. Ideally, these should be consultant obstetric physicians who can draw on their physician colleagues' assistance if necessary.

All obstetric decisions about pregnant women on ICU should have direct consultant input from the relevant consultant obstetrician.

When faced in an emergency with a medical problem that is outside their experience, consultants and other obstetric staff should be prepared to consult widely. Such consultations may often only require a telephone call.

### Epilepsy

Women with epilepsy are often disadvantaged. They also need specific specialist advice in pregnancy. In the six years of this and the previous triennium there have been 28 deaths from epilepsy in pregnancy. Every effort should be made to contact patients with epilepsy, particularly if they fail to attend hospital or other appointments. More frequent follow up is necessary in pregnancy because of associated changes in metabolism.

The ideal treatment for pregnant epileptic women, which has already been instigated in some centres, is a dedicated clinic to encompass prepregnancy counselling and attended by obstetrician, neurologist/obstetric physician and a specialist midwife and/or neurology nurse specialist.

Women with epilepsy should also be made aware of the dangers of bathing in pregnancy. They should be advised to bathe only in shallow water with someone else in the house or alternatively to shower.

## Infectious disease

All women should be encouraged to have HIV screening at booking.

Pregnant women appear to be particularly susceptible to infectious diseases. Those that are not improving despite standard treatment should be admitted to hospital.

In some other countries, influenza vaccine is recommended in pregnancy, particularly to patients who also have asthma or other chronic respiratory diseases. Other established risk factors are chronic heart disease, chronic renal failure, diabetes mellitus and immunosupression. It is recommended that this should be considered by the Joint Committee for Vaccination and Immunisation (JCVI) in the United Kingdom. The vaccine is dead but it is prepared in hen's eggs and therefore should not be given to those with known anaphylactic hypersensitivity to egg products.

## Other

Fatal bleeding from cerebral aneurysm and/or arteriovenous malformation is very uncommon during labour. Women with these abnormalities do not necessarily need to be delivered by caesarean section.

Magnesium sulphate must be available on all delivery suites.

Steroid therapy can and should be continued in pregnancy without harm to the fetus. The risk to the fetus from poorly treated asthma is much greater than any possible risk to the fetus of steroid drugs.

Pregnancy is not a reason for withholding plain X-ray films of the abdomen, chest X-rays, some CT scans or MRI from sick women.

Clinicians should be reminded that young pregnant women can lose a considerable proportion of their blood volume and still appear relatively well before they finally collapse.

Hb SC disease is a dangerous sickling condition. The risk of sickle cell crisis is as great as in Hb SS disease.

**This Chapter has been seen and discussed by Catherine Nelson-Piercy MA FRCP, Consultant Obstetric Physician.**

# References

1.  Pedersen AS, Theilade P. Phlegmonous gastritis in pregnancy. *Ugeskrift for Laeger* 1993;155:1806–7.
2.  Nilsson L, Farnhmand BY, Perssson PG, Thiblin I, Thaman T. Risk factors for sudden unexpected death in epilepsy: a case–control study. *Lancet* 1999;353:888–93.
3.  Nashef L, Fish DR, Sander JW, Shorvon SD. Incidence of sudden unexpected death in an adult outpatient cohort with epilepsy at a tertiary referral centre. *J Neurol neurosurg psychiatry* 1995;58: 462–4.

## CHAPTER 13

# Cancer and other tumours

GWYNETH LEWIS, JAMES DRIFE, MICHAEL DE SWIET on behalf of the Editorial Board

## Deaths from cancer: key recommendations

- Clear and relevant information must be passed from the GP to the antenatal care team, at booking, concerning any past medical history including previous malignancies and abnormal cervical smears and any relevant family history.

- A clear medical and family history needs to be taken at booking to lower the threshold for the index of suspicion in women who complain of other symptoms during pregnancy.

- When any pregnant woman complains of episodes of vaginal bleeding in pregnancy, other than confirmed causes of haemorrhage, cervical cancer must be excluded by direct observation of the cervix and a cervical smear taken. This should be undertaken irrespective of her past medical history or reports of normal past cervical smears.

- Previous Reports have repeatedly stressed, and this Report does so again, that pregnancy is not a contraindication for radiological investigations for women with severe and unremitting pain, including chest pain, particularly if the pain is so severe it requires management by major analgesia or epidural analgesia.

- The importance of planned multidisciplinary care for women with cancer and other serious problems cannot be overstressed. Obstetricians, midwives, GPs, oncologists, surgeons, Macmillan nurses and palliative care services need to be involved, in conjunction with the woman and her partner, in planning a course of antenatal care that respects the wishes of the woman yet should optimise the outcome for the fetus.

- Delivery needs to be planned with care and, if possible performed at an optimum time with consultants in attendance. A paediatrician should be involved antenatally, not only to optimise the care of the baby but also to discuss with the parents what may happen afterwards about neonatal care. As the woman may require an elective caesarean section the anaesthetist should similarly be involved at an early stage in the pregnancy. A written and agreed care plan should be in her notes to pass this information on to colleagues who may have to attend for an emergency delivery.

- A summary of an excellent midwifery care plan developed for a particular woman in this Report gives a blueprint for others. Apart from providing routine care and support, the midwives also saw their role as including:

  o familiarisation visits to the special care baby unit

  o support to help the woman come to terms with her condition

  o liaison with other healthcare teams

  o provision of information for her and her family

  o provision of time for rest and privacy

  o ensuring that the complex set of hand-held notes were transferred to all the professionals involved in her care

  o teaching her partner parenting skills

  o being involved with the first course of post-delivery chemotherapy or treatment.

- Bereavement counselling and access to representatives of religious faiths should be offered on request or when appropriate.

## Introduction

In the past, this Report has included deaths from malignancy in several different chapters, *Indirect*, *Coincidental* (*Fortuitous*) or *Late*, depending on the timing of the death and whether the assessors considered the course, diagnosis or treatment of the disease was modified by the pregnancy itself. This division meant that the key messages derived from these deaths were scattered in a number of places throughout the Report and key recommendations may have been missed. This new Chapter therefore brings together all the 52 deaths from malignancies that were reported during this triennium. The aim of doing this is to strengthen the impact and recommendations that can be drawn from these cases. Whether a death was *Indirect*, *Coincidental* or *Late*, similar lessons can be learned about the management of these cases. It is the diagnosis and management, or lack of it, that is the most important factor in the case assessment.

Assigning a death from malignancy to any of the main internationally recognised maternal causes of death, *Indirect* or *Coincidental*, is also problematic. Although 12 cases in this Chapter are defined as *Indirect*, in that the course of the disease was modified by the pregnancy or pregnancy masked its effects, this definition does not currently accord with the International Disease Classification of Maternal Deaths (either ICD9 or 10). These extra cases help to artificially inflate the UK *Indirect* maternal death rate when compared with *Indirect* and overall maternal mortality rates from other countries.

The overall CEMD classification of these deaths is shown in Table 13.1.

**Table 13.1** Classification of causes of deaths from tumours or malignancy and type of death; United Kingdom 1997–99

| Cause | Indirect | Late Indirect | Coincidental | Late Coincidental | Total |
|---|---|---|---|---|---|
| Lymphoma or leukaemia | 2 | 5 | | 1 | 8 |
| Central nervous system: | | | | | |
|   Astrocytoma | 2 | | | | 2 |
|   Glioma | 1 | 1 | | | 2 |
|   Medulloblastoma | 1 | | | | 1 |
|   Tuberculosis | 1 | | | | 1 |
|   Hypothalamic | 1 | | | | 1 |
|   Meningioma | | 1 | | | 1 |
|   Neuroectodermal | | | | 1 | 1 |
| Melanoma | 2 | 1 | | | 3 |
| Cancer of cervix | 1 | 1 | | | 2 |
| Malignant omentum | 1 | | | | 1 |
| Cancer of breast | | 1 | | 2 | 3 |
| Cancer of ovary | | 2 | | | 2 |
| Ewings sarcoma | | 1 | | | 1 |
| Osteosarcoma | | 1 | 1 | 2 | 4 |
| Cancer of pancreas | | 1 | | 3 | 4 |
| Adrenal adenoma | | 1 | | | 1 |
| Cancer of lung | | | 3 | 2 | 5 |
| Cancer of gastrointestinal tract | | | 2 | 4 | 6 |
| Cancer of unknown origin | | | | 2 | 2 |
| Cancer of nasopharynx | | | | 1 | 1 |
| Cancer of bladder | | | | 1 | 1 |
| Total | 12 | 16 | 6 | 18 | 52 |

## Overview of cancer in pregnancy

The incidence of cancer in pregnancy is around one in 6000 live births. This is about 50% lower than the incidence in the nonpregnant population of a similar age.[1] There are several possible reasons for this. A woman who has already had cancer diagnosed may avoid pregnancy. A pregnant woman with occult cancer may have the diagnosis delayed because routine screening is not carried out or because symptoms are not investigated promptly (being attributed to the pregnancy) or because investigation is less thorough.

It is often thought that pregnancy accelerates the growth of cancer, particularly if the cancer is hormone-dependent. For many types of cancer, the numbers of cases occurring in pregnancy are too small for reliable epidemiological studies to be carried out. However, it appears that, for most types, pregnancy does not alter the incidence or prognosis compared with cancer diagnosed at a similar stage in the nonpregnant patient. Melanoma, unlike other cancers, is slightly more common in pregnancy than in the nonpregnant woman but, stage for stage, the prognosis seems to be unaffected by pregnancy. This is discussed in more detail below.

## *Indirect* deaths

There were 12 *Indirect* and 16 *Late Indirect* deaths from carcinoma, in which the pregnancy may have masked or affected the diagnosis or outcome. Some of these are discussed further to illustrate key points.

**A case where a lack of investigation in pregnancy may have affected the outcome**

> A woman who had previously had an abnormal cervical smear complained of vaginal bleeding or bloodstained discharge throughout her pregnancy. The abnormal smear result had not been conveyed to the antenatal team in the booking letter from the GP. On only one occasion, early in pregnancy, was an attempt made by a junior doctor to visualise the cervix and this failed. She then was cared for by a number of locum consultant obstetricians who did not appear to consider the diagnosis, despite several admissions for a presumed antepartum haemorrhage. The diagnosis was only considered just prior to delivery by lower-segment caesarean section, after which she was referred for terminal care. She died some months later.

This case has many disturbing aspects. Initially, the abnormal smear results should have been conveyed by the GP to the antenatal care team at booking. However, even without this information, the cervix should have been visualised and a smear taken, especially as the bleeding was severe enough to warrant a number of admissions for a suspected antepartum haemorrhage. A number of different locum consultants cared for her during pregnancy but none of them considered carcinoma as a possibility. It is possible that a prompt diagnosis when she first presented with bleeding may have changed the outcome. Once the possibility of invasive carcinoma was raised, the decision to perform a lower segment instead of a classical caesarean became questionable.

**Cases where the lack of investigation in pregnancy may have delayed the diagnosis.**

As in the last Report, in the opinion of the *assessors*, there were several cases of severe and unremitting pain reported during pregnancy that were not investigated fully. While the delay in diagnosis may not have made any difference to the outcome, earlier diagnosis may have made the women more comfortable.

> A young woman complained of severe leg and thigh pain from early in pregnancy. The severity of the pain was evidenced by the superficial scarring apparent on her legs from the repeated use of hot water bottles. After many weeks she was eventually referred by her GP for an orthopaedic assessment, which picked up the scarring on her legs but the consultant was 'disinclined to X-ray this young lass because of the risks that this may present to her unborn child'. A few days later she was admitted to the antenatal ward at the request of her GP because the pain was worse. Again, the orthopaedic surgeons prescribed pain-relieving drugs, this time including regular pethidine, and she was given a TENS machine. No investigations were ordered. A few days after admission, she felt numbness in both her legs and had to resort to a wheelchair. It was only when she became incontinent, unable to stand and her pressure areas were becoming mottled and discoloured that she was referred to the neurologists and magnetic resonance imaging (MRI) performed. This revealed an extensive

tumour. She died a few months after delivery, despite receiving all appropriate oncological care.

Another woman, who complained of increasing numbness and pain in her legs and back from early pregnancy, was eventually referred to a pain clinic where 'in view of her pregnancy and the fact she has responded to a lumbar epidural, further investigation or intervention was not arranged'. Some weeks later she was admitted with severe back pain and a swelling on her back. An MRI revealed a large tumour of the spine. She underwent an early elective caesarean section and commenced on radiotherapy but she died several months after delivery.

In both of these cases, the pain was severe enough to warrant regular pethidine or a lumbar epidural and both also had increasing numbness of the legs. The lack of investigation for the underlying cause represents substandard care.

A grandmultiparous woman with an extremely strong family history of ovarian carcinoma was admitted in early pregnancy with a large pleural effusion requiring a chest drain and antibiotics. No abnormality was found at bronchoscopy and a second opinion a few weeks later suggested that the effusion was due to post-pneumonic empyema and that she should be treated conservatively. Two months later she was admitted with a further effusion and anaemia requiring transfusion. A pleural biopsy was performed a week later and the results, which were not available for another week, suggested a possible metastatic adenocarcinoma with the ovary as the most possible site. After a spontaneous delivery of a live infant, but despite chemotherapy, her condition steadily deteriorated and she died a few months later.

Several aspects of this case cause concern. It appears that she received little formal antenatal care during her pregnancy as the obstetrician said she was 'medically ill'. There is no record of any midwifery involvement before delivery, although she was visited by the community midwife afterwards. It is difficult to establish the reasons for this but contributing factors may have been that she was illiterate and came from a travelling community that often faces discrimination. This case also demonstrates the need for a clear family history to be taken at booking. It is not clear whether she received antenatal care of any sort between her first and second hospital admissions. Although it would not have altered the outcome, particularly in view of her very strong family history, the diagnosis was delayed. Planned multidisciplinary care also appeared to be absent throughout.

In a case also discussed in Chapter 11, a grandmultiparous woman with little English and a history of depression booked late. Shortly afterwards she became forgetful, suffered several falls, was doubly incontinent and exhibited strange behaviour. The neurological opinion was that she was suffering from a psychiatric disorder and she was admitted under the care of the psychiatrists for treatment of an 'atypical depressive state'. A few days after discharge she was readmitted in labour and after delivery continued to exhibit very strange behaviour. An MRI scan revealed a large meningioma, which was operated on with no success.

Since meningioma is one of the tumours that are thought to grow faster in pregnancy it is particularly unfortunate that this tumour was missed.

There were also other opportunities for an earlier diagnosis:

> A woman who was referred for a neurological opinion for persistent headaches and an episode of facial numbness during pregnancy was considered to have migraine. Three weeks after delivery, a frontal glioblastoma was diagnosed, from which she died a few months later.

Although it would not have influenced the eventual outcome, the fact that the diagnosis was not made until after delivery, possibly due to a reluctance to carry out a full investigation because she was pregnant, meant that an opportunity to commence treatment immediately after delivery was missed.

> A young woman required several admissions during her pregnancy for anorexia, weight loss, abdominal pain and vomiting. Indeed, labour was induced early to assist in relieving the symptoms without any further investigation. However, the symptoms persisted and a few weeks later she was found to have carcinoma of the pancreas.

> Another woman complained of nausea, vomiting and persistent pruritus. She was considered to have obstetric cholestasis, having very abnormal liver function tests, but no other investigations were performed. After delivery her liver function was not checked again and she was discharged from care. Several weeks later she presented with acute ascites and a diagnosis of an adenocarcinoma, probably of pancreatic origin, was made.

> A woman who complained of persistent neck pain and tiredness throughout her pregnancy referred herself to a chiropractor for manipulation. Despite requiring regular analgesia by her GP her complaint was not investigated further. The diagnosis of disseminated nasopharyngeal carcinoma was made after delivery but even though it may have been possible to identify this earlier, the outcome was inevitable.

> A woman presented to her GP in the third trimester with pleuritic symptoms, which did not respond to antibiotics. She was referred as a matter of urgency as having a possible pulmonary thromboembolism but was discharged the same day after apparently normal blood gases but having had no chest X-ray or ventilation/perfusion (VQ) scan. Several days later she was admitted to hospital with severe pulmonary distress and a chest X-ray at this time revealed a hilar mass that was confirmed as a bronchial carcinoma. She rapidly deteriorated and died after an emergency caesarean section

Although the outcome would not have been changed by earlier diagnosis, the failure to fully investigate her earlier symptoms, which were compatible with a pulmonary thromboembolism, represents substandard care. Note that blood gases are not necessarily abnormal in pulmonary embolus, particularly if the embolus is small.

In an unusual case, a woman's pregnancy was undiagnosed until she delivered unexpectedly on an oncology ward. She had been ill for several years and had multiple intra-abdominal metastases. Her amenorrhoea was considered to be due to her chemotherapy because she had experienced amenorrhoea in several previous courses of treatment. In later pregnancy it was reported that she developed a huge complex mass from the midline of her abdomen. The computed tomography (CT) scan which, when reviewed by the CEMD assessors, clearly demonstrated a midtrimester pregnancy, failed to detect this. It was only when she was admitted to the oncology ward in severe pain occurring at regular intervals that midwife was called and she underwent what, in the circumstances, was a relatively straightforward delivery.

It is clear that her pregnancy was missed, despite the evidence on a CT scan. The good postnatal outcome for her baby is a testament to the prompt midwifery and postnatal care she eventually received.

## The importance of planned multidisciplinary care

In several cases, there was evidence of extremely good teamwork between the maternity team, the oncologists and surgeons, the paediatricians and support services, with clear multidisciplinary care plans drawn up and instituted. One case demonstrates this very clearly:

A woman was diagnosed with a brain tumour in the first trimester of pregnancy and immediately a multidisciplinary care plan was agreed between the oncologists, obstetricians, midwives and community services. Her partner also had several opportunities to discuss the possible outcome with the consultant obstetrician. As a result, a documented antenatal and delivery care plan was agreed between the woman, her partner, the obstetricians, anaesthetists, intensivists and paediatricians. She received supportive weekly visits from the community midwife throughout her pregnancy until she required hospice based care. A carefully planned elective caesarean section was eventually undertaken with the delivery of a live baby.

The report notes that several community midwives were extraordinary in the extra care and attention that they devoted to this woman.

A woman who was unaware she was pregnant until later in her pregnancy was admitted with shortness of breath shortly after booking. She was diagnosed as having metastatic carcinoma of unknown origin and spent much of the remainder of her pregnancy in hospital.

The excellent midwifery summary of her care during this time shows the careful thought that went into her care plan. Apart from providing routine midwifery care and support they also saw their role as including:

- familiarisation visits to the special care baby unit

- support to help the woman come to terms with her condition

- liaison with other healthcare teams

- provision of information for her and her family

- provision of time for rest and privacy

- ensuring that the complex set of hand-held notes were transferred to all the professionals involved in her care

- teaching her partner parenting skills

- being involved with the first course of post-delivery chemotherapy or treatment.

The above two cases act as a model for the standard of care that should be provided for all women. In another case, however, there was a cascade of substandard care and extremely poor liaison between the GP, oncologists, obstetricians and anaesthetists caring for a woman with what was clearly a terminal illness:

> In this case, a melanoma was diagnosed at about the same time as the woman's pregnancy and the oncologists wrote to the GP stating that they were very pessimistic about the outcome. The GP did not pass this information on to the obstetricians and as a result her pregnancy was managed by obstetric senior house officers in the antenatal clinic. They were both on the GP vocational training team and had little experience in either obstetrics or oncology. The fact that the woman had had extensive counselling from the oncologists about the possibility of a termination of pregnancy was also not passed on to the obstetric team. When the severity of her condition eventually became apparent, the community midwife started home visits, but she was only informed of the need to do this by the GP, not the obstetric staff. Continuing poor communications meant that the timing for the planned induction of labour was not optimal and the anaesthetists had not been involved in planning her care. She was profoundly ill before and during the induction and severe fetal bradycardia developed very quickly. There was then a further delay in carrying out a caesarean section while the anaesthetists, who had only just been informed of this case, needed to stabilise her before general anaesthesia. The baby died after delivery and the mother, who then experienced further delay in transfer to a high-dependency bed, died shortly afterwards.

This case demonstrates failings in communication from the beginning of her pregnancy until her death. Better communications would have led to more specialist obstetric antenatal care and support for her husband and family. Had the obstetricians and oncologists communicated with each other, plans for her delivery could have been made at a more optimal time and not when she was moribund. Had the anaesthetists been involved in planning the delivery and after care this may have resulted in an earlier elective caesarean section with a different outcome for the baby and a high-dependency bed available immediately after delivery for the woman.

## Other *Indirect* deaths

In other cases, care was not considered to be substandard but the virulence or size of the tumour was hastened by the physiological effects of the pregnancy. Some are described further.

### Lymphoma

Pregnancy does not adversely affect Hodgkins's disease or protect against it, but an acceleration of its progression in the puerperium has been suggested.[2] Non-Hodgkin's lymphomas are rare in pregnancy but seem to have a poor prognosis. A link has been suggested between pregnancy and Burkitt's lymphoma but, again, studies are difficult because of small numbers.

The overall ratio regarding lymphoma in previous triennia has been one death to two million births but in this triennium there were three cases.

> One woman, who was cared for in a midwifery-led unit, was found to have non-Hodgkin's lymphoma in the second trimester and was transferred for specialist care. It is worth noting that the midwives caring for this woman rapidly picked up a possible problem and referred her for immediate investigation. Another was diagnosed at a similar gestation and died shortly after delivery. A third woman, who had an uneventful pregnancy, had a precipitate delivery and retained placenta. She received prompt treatment for a subsequent postpartum haemorrhage but immediately became drowsy and disorientated. On transfer to ICU she was found to have an intracerebral tumour and non-Hodgkin's lymphoma was diagnosed from bone marrow aspiration. She died a few months later.

### Melanoma

A recent report from a Royal College of Obstetricians and Gynaecologists Study Group on hormones and cancer[1] discusses the results of a study based on the Swedish Cancer Registry from 1960 to 1990. This showed that, in pregnancy, the average ratio to observed to expected cancers was 0.49 for the ten most common sites. For melanoma, however, the ratio of observed to expected cancers was 1.1 (95% confidence interval 0.88–1.33). The effect of pregnancy on melanoma has been the subject of controversy. There have been suggestions that melanoma in pregnancy is likely to be diagnosed at a later stage than outwith pregnancy, and that lesions during pregnancy are more likely to appear at locations associated with a poorer prognosis. The latter suggestion has not been confirmed in recent controlled studies.[2]

Several controlled studies, however, have reported a decrease in survival rates for pregnant women compared with nonpregnant controls. Primary melanomas in pregnant women have been reported to be thicker than melanomas in matched women who were not pregnant. However, it is not clear whether this was due to late diagnosis or to a direct effect of pregnancy. When corrected for tumour thickness, survival after stage I primary cutaneous disease is the same in pregnant and nonpregnant women but women with stage II disease who have a recurrence during pregnancy may have a reduced survival rate.[3]

Three women died of melanoma. One has already been described in detail due to the substandard care she received. One death occurred some months after delivery and the third is described here:

> A woman who had a melanoma diagnosed in a previous pregnancy was found to have a recurrence in her next pregnancy, which was some years later. She was admitted to the oncology ward and had good multidisciplinary care from all specialities, with the aim of delivering her at a time that would improve the fetal outcome. Unfortunately, her condition deteriorated rapidly and she required an urgent caesarean section of a very premature infant who died shortly after birth. She died a few days later at home, having received excellent postpartum midwifery care in conjunction with the Macmillan nurses.

## Brain tumours

Pregnancy is known to have a dramatic effect on some types of brain tumour, including meningioma, which, as stated above, can rapidly enlarge during pregnancy. This is thought to be brought about by fluid retention and by the hormonal stimulation of responsive tumours.[1] Approximately 90% of menigiomas have high-affinity progesterone receptors and approximately one-third have oestrogen receptors.[3]

There were five deaths from cerebral tumours, three of which have already been described. In one further case, a medulloblastoma, the pregnancy was only discovered a week before death, but there had been no previous symptoms:

> A young woman, who had already had radiotherapy treatment for an astrocytoma, became pregnant and decided to continue with the pregnancy. She remained relatively well until the beginning of the third trimester when she developed spinal secondary deposits. A few weeks later she had an elective caesarean section and died shortly afterwards. The standard of her care seems excellent.

The autopsy report commented on the potential for pregnancy to influence the tumour.

# References

1. Drife JO. The contribution of cancer to maternal mortality. In: O'Brien PMS, McLean AB, editors. *Hormones and Cancer*. London: RCOG Press; 2000. p. 299–310.
2. Antonelli NM, Dotters DJ, Katz VL, Kuller JA. Cancer in pregnancy: a review of the literature (Parts 1 and 2). *Obstet Gynecol Surv* 1996;51:125–42.
3. Johnston SRD, Broadley K, Henson G, Fisher C, Henk M, Gore ME. Management of metastatic melanoma during pregnancy. *BMJ* 1998;316:848–51.

# *Coincidental* and *Late* deaths    Section

# 4

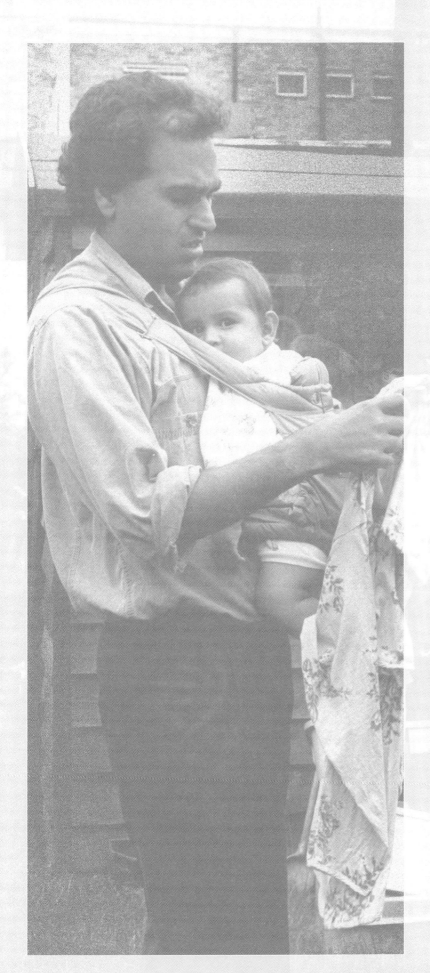

## CHAPTER 14

# *Coincidental (Fortuitous)* deaths

GWYNETH LEWIS on behalf of the Editorial Board

## Change of nomenclature

By international definition, deaths unconnected with pregnancy or the puerperium that occur before delivery or up to 42 days postpartum are regarded as 'fortuitous'. They are not considered to be maternal deaths and do not contribute to maternal mortality statistics. However, in the opinion of the authors, the term 'fortuitous' is seen as out-dated, inappropriate and insensitive, its general use in the English language implying a happier unexpected event. Therefore, for this and future Reports, the definition will be replaced with the term *Coincidental*. Even this word is an imperfect description for some such maternal deaths, which are related to pregnancy in the wider sense of public health and which may have important implications for appropriate health care delivery.

Although many *Coincidental* deaths are considered to be unrelated to pregnancy, it has long been standard practice to include them in this Report. These deaths may have important lessons for the management of certain non-pregnancy-related conditions, such as coincidental carcinomatosis (now discussed in Chapter 13) and they also identify some wider public health issues of which health professionals need to be aware. Deaths from domestic violence aggravated or directly caused by pregnancy (now discussed in Chapter 16) cannot be regarded as coincidental, nor deaths where women were ill advised or unaware of the correct use of car seat belts during pregnancy. However, for the purposes of comparative data, these deaths will continue, for the time being, to be counted as *Coincidental* and will be counted in this Chapter.

## Summary

In this triennium, 29 *Coincidental* deaths occurring during pregnancy or within 42 days of delivery or termination were notified to the Enquiry. These are shown in Table 14.1. In addition, there were 61 *Late Coincidental* deaths discussed in Chapter 15. The figures for the previous triennium were 36 *Coincidental* and 36 *Late Coincidental* deaths, respectively. This Chapter traditionally also contains descriptions of the small number of deaths for which, despite intensive investigations and assessments, no obvious cause of death could be found.

It is noteworthy that three of these deaths occurred in girls under the age of 16 years, all experiencing severe social exclusion and who presumably must have been in the care of social services at the time.

**Table 14.1** *Coincidental* deaths; United Kingdom 1997–99

| Cause of death | Total (*n*) |
| --- | --- |
| Neoplastic disease[a] | 6 |
| Undetermined | 4 |
| Other: | |
|     Cerebral haemorrhage early in pregnancy | 1 |
|     Alcohol | 1 |
|     Encephalitis | 1 |
| Unnatural: | |
|     Road traffic accident | 8 |
|     Murder[b] | 8 |
| Total | 29 |

[a] See Chapter 13; [b] see Chapter 16

## Domestic violence and murder

In the last Report, the issue of domestic violence against pregnant or recently delivered women was discussed for the first time. This Report has built on the previous findings and has actively sought out all cases in which domestic violence was proactively reported by the woman, whether she died as a result of this or not.

The prevalence of violence against pregnant or recently delivered women is demonstrated by the 45 cases in this Report in which domestic violence was a known feature and which was fatal for the eight counted in this Chapter. As none of these women were identified through routine questioning about violence in the antenatal period, and since routine questioning picks up other women too embarrassed or afraid to raise the issue themselves, this 12% will be an underestimate of the true prevalence of domestic violence in the 378 women in this Report. This is the first time that such data have been available. Since the reported rate is high and the issue of such importance, all cases of women disclosing domestic violence, as well as those who were murdered, are discussed in a new, separate Chapter: Chapter 16; Domestic violence. All healthcare workers are urged to read this new Chapter and to take account of the recommendations and further reading suggested.

## Road traffic accidents: seat belts in pregnancy

Seven women died as a result of road traffic accidents while still pregnant and one died after delivery. Another four cases are counted in Chapter 15; *Late* deaths.

Of the seven women who were pregnant, one was a spectator at a car rally, another was a pedestrian and a third was a pillion passenger on a motorbike. It is gratifying to note that all of the other four women were wearing seat belts and only one was not wearing it in the recommended position. In this case, the woman was wearing only a lap belt across her abdomen. Her fetus, which was in the breech position, was pushed up into her chest through a ruptured uterus and diaphragm. Another woman also suffered a ruptured uterus. In three of these cases, a perimortem or postmortem caesarean section was performed to no avail.

Of the five women who died after delivery, three were wearing seat belts. Of the two who were not, one was joyriding on the back of a milk float having consumed a considerable amount of alcohol and the other was severely depressed and is discussed in Chapter 11.

These cases continue to highlight the poor success rate for fetal survival in postmortem caesarean sections, which, unless performed immediately after the maternal death, are almost invariably associated with severe fetal anoxia and consequent stillbirth.

A recent survey[1] on pregnant women's knowledge and use of seat belts showed that, while 98% of pregnant front-seat passengers wore a seat belt, only 68% wore them in the back of the car. The survey also found that only 48% of women correctly identified the correct way to use a seat belt, with only 37% reporting that they had received information on the correct use of seat belts while pregnant. Although the survey was conducted just prior to the last CEMD Report, which highlighted the need for pregnant women to be informed of the correct way to wear a seat belt in pregnancy, its findings cause concern and the recommendations made in the last Report are therefore repeated here.

---

**Recommendations for use of seat belts in pregnancy**

All pregnant women should be given advice about the correct use of seat belts as soon as their pregnancy is confirmed:

'Above and below the bump, not over it'

Three-point seat belts should be worn throughout pregnancy, with the lap strap placed as low as possible beneath the 'bump', lying across the thighs with the diagonal shoulder strap above the bump lying between the breasts. The seat belt should be adjusted to fit as snugly as comfortably possible and, if necessary, the seat should be adjusted to enable the seat belt to be worn properly (Figure 14.1).

---

## Cases where the cause of death could not be established

There were three cases in which the cause of death could not be accurately ascertained:

> In a case also discussed in Chapter 6; Early pregnancy deaths, a homeless very young teenage primigravida who ran away from home following abuse had an evacuation for retained products of conception. The operation was undertaken by a senior house officer, who perforated the uterus. She appeared to recover from this and a few weeks later was found in cardiorespiratory arrest suffering from severe hypothermia in a front garden on a freezing cold night. She died shortly after admission to hospital and, at autopsy, although some traces of morphine were found, no specific cause of death was determined. The balance of pathological opinion inclined towards an accidental overdose of morphine but this could not be accurately proven.

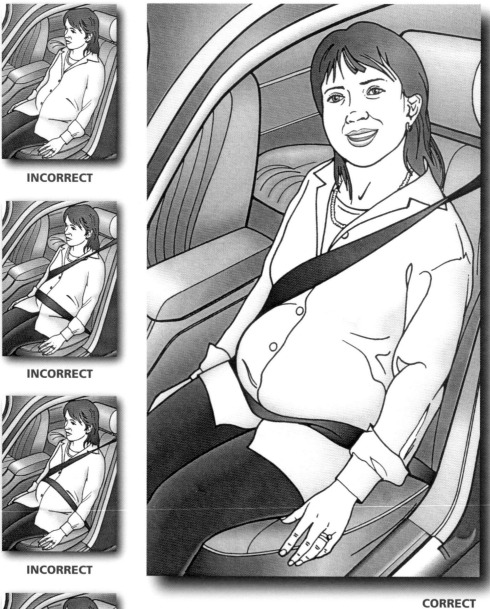

**INCORRECT**

**INCORRECT**

**INCORRECT**

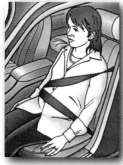

**INCORRECT**

**CORRECT**

## Seat Belts & Pregnancy

The shoulder belt should go over the shoulder, collar bone and down across the chest – between the breasts. Wear the lap belt as low as possible under the abdomen and the unborn child.

**ALWAYS WEAR A FULL SEAT BELT**

### Recommendations for use of seat belts in pregnancy

All pregnant women should be given advice about the correct use of seat belts as soon as their pregnancy is confirmed:

'Above and below the bump, not over it'

Three-point seat belts should be worn throughout pregnancy, with the lap strap placed as low as possible beneath the 'bump', lying across the thighs with the diagonal shoulder strap above the bump lying between the breasts. The seat belt should be adjusted to fit as snugly as comfortably possible and, if necessary, the seat should be adjusted to enable the seat belt to be worn properly.

**Figure 14.1** The correct and incorrect use of a seat belt in pregnancy

This underage girl, who also clearly was a regular injecting drug user, had at some time been known to social services but appeared to be out of touch with them at the time of her death. There is no suggestion that any care at all was taken over her future when she was discharged from hospital following the unsatisfactory operation. No arrangements appear to have been made to offer her shelter or protection and, after discharge, she went to live in the open under a duvet. There was clearly a major failure in the provision of social service support for this vulnerable child and little attention to her future appears to have been given by the hospital staff.

> Another young girl booked very late, having concealed her pregnancy for the first few months. She then failed to turn up for several antenatal appointments. She was rootless, living at a number of addresses and difficult to trace, although the midwives were usually able to track her down. After an uneventful delivery, she was discharged home but received little postnatal care as she moved again without informing anyone. She was readmitted in cardiac arrest, from which she could not be resuscitated, having collapsed during sexual intercourse. She apparently had a profuse vaginal haemorrhage during the attempted resuscitation and half a litre of blood was found in her abdomen at peritoneal lavage.

This is a puzzling case. The autopsy could not ascertain the precise cause of death. The obstetrician who attended the autopsy said that he thought there may have been air in the heart, although the autopsy report appears to rule this out. Unfortunately, the autopsy did not fully exclude all possible causes for the haemorrhage, including infection. Previous Reports have identified two confirmed cases of fatal air embolism during sexual intercourse, which is an exceptionally rare event due to air being forced into the blood vessels of an incompletely involuted placental bed. Although not proven in this case, it still raises the possibility that the early puerperium, when the uterus is not involuted and the cervix is open, may be a particularly risky time for sexual intercourse.

Another woman collapsed and died a week after a suction termination of pregnancy. Attempts at resuscitation were unsuccessful. The autopsy in this case was excellent despite the failure to find a definitive cause of death. In the opinion of the assessors this must, by exclusion, have been due to a cardiac arrhythmia.

## Other causes of death

These are detailed in Table 14.1. Two are described further:

> A very young homeless girl with a history of substance abuse and two previous pregnancies in her very early teenage years was admitted with rapidly deteriorating consciousness and a respiratory arrest in early pregnancy. She had not booked for antenatal care. She had a cerebellar haematoma evacuated and was transferred to the ICU. A few days later she 'self-extubated ' herself and inhaled gastric contents prior to reintubation. She died a few weeks later.

In the assessor's opinion, this girl's self-extubation constituted substandard care and the resultant aspiration contributed to her death.

Due to a very substandard autopsy, discussed in Chapter 18, which failed to ascertain the cause of death, the following case has, by convention, to be counted in this Chapter. The death could either have been attributable to hypertensive disease of pregnancy or have been a sudden unexplained epileptic death. Given the concerns raised about the quality of care she received, this case is also discussed in Chapter 3; Hypertensive disease in pregnancy:

> A woman who spoke little English and who had recently arrived in the UK received regular antenatal care, shared between midwives and her GP. At a visit in her third trimester she had oedema of her fingers and toes. Although her blood pressure was within normal limits, it had been steadily rising throughout her pregnancy. She also had a breech presentation. Despite these signs, her next appointment was given for three weeks' time 'according to the new protocol for antenatal visits'. After two weeks had elapsed, she fitted at home and was dead on arrival in the accident and emergency department.

Many features of this case cause concern. Given her puffy fingers and rising blood pressure, this woman should have been given an appointment for a week's time in any event, despite the new protocol. Although the notes say that she was given numbers to contact if she was concerned, her lack of English would have made this very difficult. When she collapsed, her relatives, who also had little English, had a difficult time explaining to the ambulance services what had happened. The autopsy and accompanying histology were very cursory and not performed until several days after her death, during which period a lot of valuable information had been lost.

## Reference

1. Johnson H, Pring D. Car seatbelts in pregnancy: the practice and knowledge of pregnant women remain causes for concern. *BJOG* 2000;107:644–7.

## CHAPTER 15

# *Late* deaths

GWYNETH LEWIS on behalf of the Editorial Board

## Introduction

*Late* maternal deaths are defined as deaths occurring in women more than 42 days but less than one year after miscarriage, abortion or delivery. The International Classification of Maternal Deaths (ICD10) only classifies *Late* deaths due to *Direct* or *Indirect* maternal causes, whereas this Report also includes *Late Coincidental* (*Late Fortuitous*) deaths from which educational, public health or other messages and recommendations may also be drawn. For this reason all *Late* deaths reported to the Enquiry for 1997–99 are counted, and some are discussed, in this Chapter but none is included in the overall maternal mortality rate as defined in Chapter 1.

Some *Late Direct* deaths may occur in women who have received prolonged care in an intensive care unit (ICU) following the initial event. It is possible that this Enquiry may have missed some of these deaths because the immediate cause of death, as given on the death certificate, is not usually directly related to the pregnancy-related event but relates to the final cause of death. These are therefore not currently picked up on death certificate data or currently notified by ICU staff, who may be unaware of this Report. The CEMD is currently working on a new record linkage system with the Office for National Statistics (ONS) in order that these cases may be picked up in the future.

*Late* deaths often contain important messages for maternal health. For example, the majority of maternal deaths from suicide occur in this period and there are a number of other *Direct* and *Indirect* causes, for example from pulmonary embolism, cardiac disease and malignancies. These cases, although the deaths are counted in this Chapter, are discussed in more depth in the relevant Chapters of this Report to consolidate the key messages and recommendations in a more appropriate manner. Thus, for example, *Late* deaths from pulmonary embolism are discussed in Chapter 2, heart disease in Chapter 10, suicide and drug misuse in Chapter 11 and deaths from cancer are discussed in Chapter 13.

## Summary

A total of 107 *Late* deaths were reported in this triennium, compared with 72 in the last Report. Thirty-four of these are discussed in Chapter 13. Completed reports were available for all but eight cases. *Late* deaths are further classified as *Direct*, *Indirect* or *Coincidental* (*Fortuitous*) although, as has already been stated, these are not included in the numerators for determining maternal mortality rates.

The interval between delivery and death for all *Late* deaths is shown in Table 15.1.

**Table 15.1** Interval between delivery or abortion and death, *Late* cases; United Kingdom 1997–99

| Days after delivery | Direct (n) | Indirect (n) | Coincidental (n) | Total (n) |
|---|---|---|---|---|
| 43–91 | 4 | 18 | 21 | 43 |
| 92–182 | 2 | 10 | 16 | 28 |
| 183–273 | 0 | 8 | 11 | 19 |
| 274–365 | 1 | 3 | 13 | 17 |
| Total | 7 | 39 | 61 | 107 |

## *Direct* causes

Seven *Late* deaths were considered to be directly related to maternal causes and are discussed in the relevant Chapters but counted here. Six cases of thromboembolism are discussed in Chapter 2, two other deaths from thromboembolism are classified as *Late Indirect* and there were two further deaths from thromboembolism that occurred so late after delivery that they are counted as *Late Coincidental*. The other *Direct* death, from hyponatraemia following an operation to correct vaginal trauma sustained during delivery, is discussed in Chapter 9; Anaesthesia, but is also briefly discussed here.

### Dilutional hyponatraemia

A *Late Direct* death occurred on an ICU, in a woman who had previously suffered complications at delivery. She had had an induction of labour, having had a previous caesarean section, but required a ventouse delivery after intravenous oxytocin in the second stage of labour. She suffered a large postpartum haemorrhage due to multiple tears in the vagina and required internal iliac artery ligation and hysterectomy. She then developed a vesicovaginal fistula, which was repaired some months later. During this latter operation, she developed cerebral oedema due to dilutional hyponatraemia following over-infusion and subsequently died.

This case represents a cascade of substandard care. Firstly, it was questionable whether she should have had labour induced, having had a previous caesarean section, and there was obviously major substandard care during delivery, leading to life-threatening postpartum haemorrhage. She then died after an operation to correct the vesicovaginal fistula, which had developed as a result of the delivery, as she had been over-transfused with five litres of dextrose/saline overnight.

## *Indirect* causes

There were 39 cases where the pregnancy may have indirectly contributed to the death. These are shown in Table 15.2 and some are discussed further in the relevant Chapters of this Report.

**Table 15.2** *Late* deaths: *Indirect* causes; United Kingdom 1997–99

| Cause of death | Total (*n*) |
|---|---|
| Neoplastic disease (see Chapter 13) | 16 |
| Suicide (see Chapter 11) | 15 |
| Diseases of circulatory system: | |
|    Thromboembolism (see Chapter 2) | 2 |
|    Mitral valve disease | 1 |
|    Myocardial fibrosis | 1 |
|    Myocarditis | 1 |
| Other: | |
|    Epilepsy ? encephalitis | 1 |
|    Pneumonia | 1 |
|    Haemophagocytosis | 1 |
| Total | 39 |

### Suicide

The largest category of *Late Indirect* deaths consists of those due to mental illness. In this triennium, 15 *Late Indirect* cases of suicide were reported. These deaths are discussed in full in Chapter 11; Deaths from psychiatric causes, where recommendations for the management of women suffering from postnatal depression or other mental illness are made. The birth/maternal death record linkage study identified a possible extra forty-five cases of suicide or death by misadventure occurring later in the first year after delivery, which were not reported to the Enquiry. This under-reporting is understandable in that these deaths, which occurred in the community, were not been recognised by this Enquiry until the last Report, and the relevant health professionals or coroners are not used to reporting to this Enquiry. With the new record linkage system in place, in future this degree of under-ascertainment should be reduced.

### Cardiac/circulatory disease

There were three *Late Indirect* cases of cardiac disease, which are also discussed in Chapter 10. One, associated with social exclusion, is described further here:

> A socially deprived woman with no English, who suffered from repeated episodes of domestic violence and who had mitral stenosis, was admitted with atrial fibrillation. She was found to be several months pregnant and an ultrasound scan revealed gross fetal abnormalities. She suffered a subsequent intrauterine death. After delivery she continued to suffer violence but refused help. Two months after delivery she was readmitted with atrial fibrilation and died.

This woman received excellent support services during her pregnancy but, when she allowed her partner to return after the birth of the child, further offers of help regarding her social circumstances were refused. It is not clear whether she was able to talk with the support services at this time through the use of an interpreter or whether her partner undertook the translation. The need to use an independent translator instead of the partner or family members has been a feature in a number of cases in this Report.

### Epilepsy ? encephalitis

A primigravid woman started having generalised convulsions in the first trimester of pregnancy, following a three-day illness characterised by vomiting, dizziness and visual disturbance. The fits were difficult to control and she suffered a cardiorespiratory arrest. Eclampsia was very unlikely by clinical criteria and termination of pregnancy did not result in any improvement. A brain scan was normal. She died several weeks later because of hypoxic brain damage with terminal bronchopneumonia. No autopsy was performed. The cause of her seizures remains obscure although there is a possibility that they may have been due to encephalitis.

There is no suggestion of substandard care in this difficult case.

## Late Coincidental deaths

Sixty-one *Late Coincidental* deaths are listed in Table 15.3. Sixteen are also included in Chapter 13; Cancer and other tumours. Some of the others, whose features cause concern, are described further.

### Hypertrophic cardiomyopathy

A woman who had been diagnosed as having hypertrophic cardiomyopathy following screening because of a family history had an unplanned pregnancy. She elected to continue with the pregnancy and was treated at a tertiary centre. After a relatively trouble-free pregnancy she required an assisted delivery and was transferred to ICU for observation. She was discharged home and died suddenly a few months later.

In this case, all appropriate medical care appears to have been given but what is not clear, given that her pregnancy was unplanned, was the extent of counselling she had received about the severity of her condition, particularly in relation to the risks of pregnancy, or the provision of contraceptive advice.

### Meningitis

A woman who had not attended for any antenatal care at all in her previous pregnancies and had also delivered twice unattended at home, including a previous stillbirth, booked late during this pregnancy and thereafter attended the antenatal clinic only very infrequently. She had been widowed early in the pregnancy and was caring for her family on her own. She died a few weeks after a normal delivery from streptococcal meningitis.

Although her death after delivery appears coincidental, in the opinion of the assessors the standard of her antenatal care was deficient. Despite the death of her partner during this pregnancy, her poor social circumstances and past obstetric history, no special midwifery or social services were offered during or after this pregnancy, and no midwifery contact or home visits were undertaken when she failed to attend her antenatal appointments. Although she had not sought care for her previous pregnancies, she made an effort to do so during this pregnancy. Given the death of her husband and a large number of recently bereaved children to care on her own, it is quite possible that she found the mechanics of getting to the clinic very difficult indeed and outreach midwifery and support services ought to have been provided.

**Table 15.3** *Late Coincidental* deaths; United Kingdom 1997–99

| Cause of death | total (*n*) |
|---|---|
| Neoplastic disease | 18 |
| Diseases of circulatory system: | |
|     Splenic artery aneurysm | 1 |
|     Subarachnoid | 7 |
|     Myocardial infarction | 2 |
|     Myocarditis | 1 |
|     Mitral valve disease | 1 |
|     Aortic aneurysm | 1 |
|     Cardiomyopathy | 1 |
|     Pulmonary embolism | 1 |
| Diseases of respiratory system: | |
|     Asthma | 2 |
| Infectious diseases: | |
|     Pneumonia | 1 |
|     Toxic shock | 1 |
|     Salpingitis | 1 |
|     Appendicitis | 1 |
|     Meningitis | 2 |
| Unascertained | 4 |
| Other: | |
|     Arachnoid cyst | 1 |
|     Diabetes | 1 |
|     Amyloid | 1 |
|     Epilepsy | 1 |
|     Ulcerative colitis | 1 |
| Sudden unnatural deaths: | |
|     Road taffic accidents | 3 |
|     Murder | 2 |
|     Drug overdose in known drug users | 4 |
| Total | 61 |

### Toxic shock

A young woman who was apparently fit and well after a normal pregnancy and delivery collapsed at a social occasion and was transferred to the accident and emergency department, where she was declared dead. Autopsy revealed she had been using a tampon and cultures showed a mixed growth of group B haemolytic Streptococcus and *Clostridium perfringens*. Although the initial pathologist ascribed the cause of death to puerperal sepsis, in the opinion of the *assessors*, this was a case of toxic shock associated with tampon use.

This case, also discussed in Chapter 7; Genital tract sepsis, highlights the possibility of toxic shock amongst tampon users, and women should be made aware of this rare possibility, which may occur more frequently when the uterus is not yet fully involuted.

### Salpingitis

A woman who spoke no English and who had gestational diabetes during an otherwise normal pregnancy had a spontaneous delivery and was discharged home shortly afterwards. She failed to keep the appointment for her postnatal check. Two weeks after this she was readmitted with a pyrexia and a tachycardia. She had a four-day history of lower abdominal pain. The differential diagnosis on admission was a possible ectopic pregnancy and she was observed overnight. The next morning she continued to complain of lower abdominal pain and a surgical opinion was sought. An exploratory laparotomy was planned but she collapsed and died of a ruptured tubo-ovarian abscess before this was performed.

In this case, the medical staff failed to consider severe sepsis as a cause of her pain, despite her having a tachycardia and pyrexia. The fact that she did not speak English might have affected the outcome, although it should not have done.

### Tetraplegia

A woman with tetraplegia who required long-term inpatient care became pregnant. She developed pressure sores that continued throughout her pregnancy. During her antenatal appointments she was found to be anaemic and was considered to be malnourished. She was on low-dose aspirin throughout her pregnancy. After delivery she had a pulmonary thrombosis, from which she recovered, despite having received inappropriate thromboprophylaxis as she was in a high-risk group. Her pressure sores did not heal and she continued to be anaemic. She did not always comply with treatment and refused blood transfusions but she eventually died of presumed amyloid.

**Sudden unnatural deaths**

Two women were murdered, both appearing to have suffered domestic violence in the past. Lessons from such cases are discussed in the section on domestic violence in Chapter 16. Deaths from overdose in drug-dependent women are discussed in Chapter 11.

# Other key issues

# Section

# 5

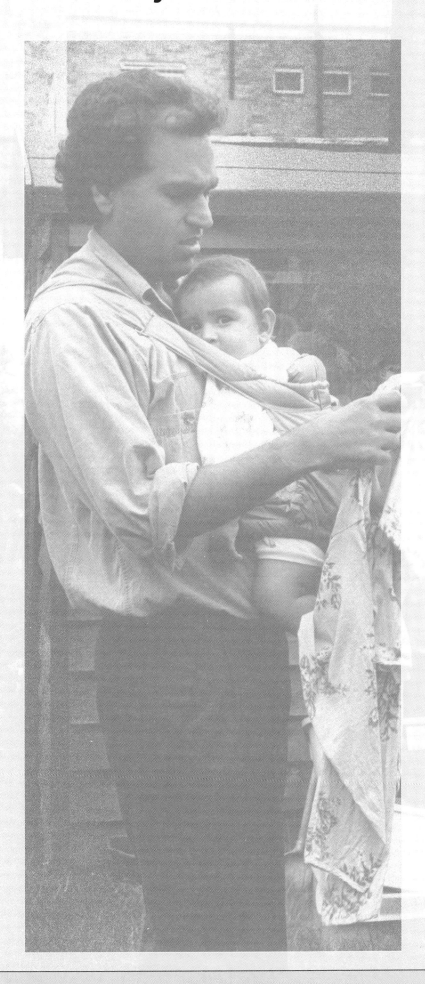

# CHAPTER 16

# Domestic violence

GWYNETH LEWIS on behalf of the Editorial Board

## Domestic violence: summary of key points

- 45 (12%) of the 378 women whose death was reported to this Enquiry had voluntarily reported violence to a health care professional during their pregnancy.

- None of the 378 women in this Report had been routinely asked about violence as part of their social history; thus, 12% is probably an underestimate.

- Eight women were murdered by partners or close relatives.

- 80% of the schoolgirls or young women under the age of 18 years whose deaths were considered by this Enquiry had suffered violence in the home.

- Many women reporting violence booked late or were poor attenders at the antenatal clinic. It was unusual for these women to be actively followed up.

- In many cases it appears that little or no help concerning the violence was offered to the woman.

- Family interpreters were used inappropriately.

- There was evidence of family 'secret keeping' in some cases.

## Domestic violence: key recommendations

- All health professionals should make themselves aware of the importance of domestic violence in their practice. They should adopt a nonjudgemental and supportive response to women who have experienced physical, psychological or sexual abuse and must be able to give basic information to women about where to get help. They should provide continuing support, whatever decision the woman makes made concerning her future.

- When a woman discloses violence this must be taken seriously. Women who are poor clinic-attenders need active outreach services.

- Local trusts and community teams should develop guidelines for the identification of, and provision of further support for, these women, including developing multi-agency working to enable appropriate referrals or provision of information on sources of further help.

- Information about local sources of help and emergency help lines, such as provided by Women's Aid, should be displayed in suitable places in antenatal clinic, for example in the women's toilets or printed as a routine at the bottom of hand held maternity notes or cooperation cards.

- Enquiries about violence should be routinely included when taking a social history. Obstetricians and gynaecologists should consider introducing questions about violence during the course of all consultations. In general practice and midwifery, this could be at the booking visit. There are a number of useful documents explaining how this can be achieved, through the use of sensitive questions.

- When routine questioning is introduced, this must be accompanied by the development of local strategies for referral. This should be accompanied by an educational programme for professionals, in consultation with local groups, and preferably delivered by those already working in this area.

- Where the woman is unable to speak English, an interpreter should be provided on at least one occasion. A partner, friend or family member should not be relied upon, especially if the index of suspicion is high.

- As does the RCOG,[1] this Report recommends that every woman is seen on her own at least once during the antenatal period, to enable the disclosure of such information.

## Background summary

Violence against women encompasses physical, sexual, emotional and psychological abuse. It is rarely an isolated event and can escalate in severity and frequency during pregnancy.[2] It is a serious and common offence. In the context of obstetric care it can cause recurrent miscarriage, stillbirths and maternal deaths. It is difficult to ascertain the prevalence of domestic violence as it remains largely unrecognised, but the last Report of the Confidential Enquiries into Maternal Deaths[3] estimated that:

- one in three women experience domestic violence at some point in their lives (perhaps one in ten in the last year),

- over one million incidents of domestic violence are recorded by the police each year (one in four of all assaults)

- about 30% of domestic violence starts during pregnancy

- two in five women who are murdered are killed by a current or ex partner.

In 1999–2000, 62% of women were murdered by a current or ex partner.[4]

## Domestic violence in pregnancy and the postnatal period

Studies have shown a variable incidence of abuse of pregnant women. A recent review article reports a range of 0.9%–20.2%,[5] but these studies mainly came from the USA or Scandinavia. Until now, there have been no published studies in the United Kingdom, although there are preliminary reports of rates between 1.8–5.8%.[6] Higher rates are elicited in response to direct questioning by health professionals[7] and repeated questioning, compared with questions only in response to clinical suspicion.[8]

Domestic violence is associated with death, severe morbidity, fetal death, miscarriage, depression, suicide, and alcohol and drug abuse. Apart from the personal costs to the woman of domestic violence, family life and relationships suffer. Children are often involved as a result of experiencing violence between their parents. Up to 36% of children of violent relationships witness their mothers being assaulted.[9] This has profound short- and long-term effects on the child.

Certain characteristics of domestic violence have been previously described[2,5,10] and these are summarised in Boxes 16.1, 16.2 and 16.3.

---

**Box 16.1   Indicators of domestic violence in the context of midwifery and obstetric practice**

- Late booking

- Poor/non attendance at antenatal clinics

- Repeat attendance at antenatal clinics, GP's surgery or accident and emergency department for minor injuries or trivial or non existent complaints

- Repeat presentation with depression, anxiety, self-harm and psychosomatic symptoms

- Minimalisation of signs of violence on the body

- Poor obstetric history (see Box 16.3)

- Unexplained admissions

- Non compliance with treatment regimens/early self-discharge from hospital

- Constant presence of partner at examinations, who may answer all the questions for her and be unwilling to leave the room

- The woman appears evasive or reluctant to speak or disagree in front of her partner.

---

**Box 16.2   Social indicators of women who suffer domestic violence**

The Yale trauma study[11] showed that victims of domestic violence are:

- 15 times more likely to abuse alcohol

- nine times more likely to abuse drugs

- three times more likely to be diagnosed as depressed or psychotic

- five times more likely to attempt suicide

than women generally.

Box 16.3    Physical manifestations of domestic violence in the context of obstetric and midwifery practice

Physical manifestations during pregnancy and postnatally include:

- gynaecological problems, such as frequent vaginal and urinary tract infections, dysparunia and pelvic pain

- frequent visits with vague complaints or symptoms without apparent physiological cause and recurring admissions for abdominal pain/reduced fetal movements or '? urinary tract infection'

- injuries that are untended and of several different ages, especially to the neck, head, breasts, abdomen and genitals

- repeated or chronic injuries

- postnatally, removal of episiotomy sutures.

There may also be a history of:

- repeated miscarriage or terminations of pregnancy

- stillbirth or preterm labour

- prematurity, intrauterine growth restriction/ low birthweight

- unwanted or unplanned pregnancy.

## Identification of domestic violence

The Royal Colleges of Obstetricians and Gynaecologists,[1] Midwives[12] and General Practitioners[13] have all published guidelines for the detection and management of women who may have been abused, as have other organisations including the Royal College of Nursing[14] and the Community Practitioners and Health Visitors Association.[15]

The use of simple screening questions, for example at antenatal clinics and where there may be an index of suspicion, is recommended. The last Report, as does this one, recommended that routine questions be asked about violence as part of the social history taken at booking, in line with the recommendations from the RCOG. Evidence from practice where this has been followed suggests that most women do not mind being asked when it is explained to them that the same enquiry is being made of all women because domestic violence is so widespread and often hidden. Since the publication of the last Report, the Department of Health has published a resource manual for healthcare professionals, which gives guidance on how best this might be achieved.[16] The Department of Health has also published an interagency guide on working together to promote the welfare of children.[17]

In response to the recommendations in the last Report, two recent surveys have been undertaken to benchmark the extent to which health services have policies, protocols and guidelines for good practice and to document current responses by healthcare professionals. One, a survey by Women's Aid,[18] found that only 27% of health authorities had written policies or protocols with regard to domestic violence and a further 15% had no written policy but an agreed practice. Twenty-nine per cent of NHS trusts had written policies and a further 15% had an agreed but unwritten practice. Less than half the trusts who responded had a designated member of staff with responsibility for domestic violence and, where such a role existed, it tended to be only for a specific department and not for the trust as a whole. In contrast, 86% of trusts thought that they should have a written policy. Only 9% of primary care groups and primary care trusts had a written policy.

The other study surveyed current policies and practice in maternity units in relation to domestic violence.[19] Eighty seven percent of the NHS Trusts providing maternity care in England and Wales responded. Of these, only 12% had a written policy and routinely asked questions about domestic violence. A further 30% had some sort of agreed practice. Less than half of maternity units routinely offered women an appointment without their partner. Just over half had printed information available in the clinic, and only one-quarter had information in the toilets which might be considered the best place to reach a woman safely and effectively with information on how to get help. Only three units had undertaken any audit of their DV practices.

## The findings of this Report

Forty-five of the 378 women whose deaths were investigated this triennium self-reported a history of domestic violence to a healthcare professional caring for them. This represents 12% of all cases. This percentage is undoubtedly an underestimate of the true prevalence of violence to this group of women, as in none of the 378 cases was a history of violence actively sought through routine questioning as part of the social or family history at booking.

Domestic violence was fatal for eight of these women. It is also possible two other women died as a direct result of violence. Half the girls or young women aged under 18 years of age who died were in violent, dependent relationships and four had been sexually abused in the past. All except one girl aged 16 years or under had also been abused, mainly by a family member. Four women were living in refuges. In some cases the women received excellent care but in others it seemed sadly lacking.

Currently, routine reporting of such cases to the CEMD does not always take place, although the association between pregnancy and increasing domestic violence is well known. The cases described in this Chapter should be regarded as being representative of other cases of murder and domestic violence that have not been reported to the CEMD. With new data linkage systems it is hoped that more such cases may be identified in future. From the cases that were reported, the warning signs were all too obvious in most cases. Several features of the cases illustrate the already described features of domestic violence as shown in Boxes 16.1, 16.2 and 16.3, and some of these features will be illustrated by the cases in this Report.

# Murder

Murder by a partner or ex-partner is the extreme end of the spectrum of domestic violence, and is an extremely important, but often overlooked, cause of maternal and child morbidity and mortality. In a recently published study from the USA,[11] investigators found murder to be the leading cause of death (20%) among pregnant or recently delivered women living in Maryland but only the fifth most common cause of death among nonpregnant women of the same age. An accompanying editorial called for the introduction of the American College of Obstetricians and Gynecologists recommendation that 'women should be routinely asked about violence as part of their case history'. This was also a recommendation in the last CEMD Report. The editorial accompanying the US article said that 'threats from a (pregnant) woman's social environment, like homicide, may be found to be more deadly than those from her biological environment'. While not directly comparable to the United Kingdom, particularly in respect of the availability of firearms, the American results underline the recommendations made in this Report.

Because some of the cases in this Report are still *sub judice*, it is not possible to give details of the exact circumstances but they underline the need for vigilance, especially when there may be a high index of suspicion.

Ten women who were murdered were reported to this Enquiry, two being counted in Chapter 15, as they occurred some months after delivery. Two of these women were killed in acts of terrorism and are not discussed further. In all but one of the other cases, family members, partners or ex-partners appeared to have been implicated or found guilty.

In four cases, full details of the woman's care were not available to the Enquiry. Of these, one woman was murdered a few months after delivery by her partner, who had subjected her to numerous episodes of domestic violence in the past, and who was under a restraining order by the police. In another case, a young woman was murdered and dismembered by her husband during the early stages of pregnancy. In a further case, the transient partner of a pregnant woman was eventually aquitted of her murder. One case is still *sub judice*.

### Ethnic minority women

In three of the eight murders the woman was of either Indian or Pakistani ethnic origin. Only a few details are available for the first case, in which a pregnant primigravid Indian woman, reported by the midwives as having an apparently good relationship with her husband, was murdered by a hired assassin. The reasons for her murder remain circumstantial and the family gave no details to the police. In the two other cases there was also collusion on the part of the family or by the woman with her husband for fear of further attack:

> In a well-publicised case, a young Pakistani woman was murdered by her brother and mother to save their family from the disgrace of an illegitimate child. She had been sent back to Pakistan at the age of 15 years on the pretext that her grandparents were sick and led into an arranged marriage to a man whom she did not know but who wanted

to enter the United Kingdom. His visa was denied and she returned home. A few years later she became pregnant by a man she wanted to marry. She refused to consider an abortion despite heavy pressure from her family. The midwives involved in her subsequent antenatal care were very aware of the potential risks she faced and had taken every step to offer help and support. She was given their out-of-hours emergency telephone numbers and a place of refuge, if she felt in immediate danger, was also arranged. However, at her last visit the woman said that she had had a long talk with her mother and now believed she was now out of danger.

At her trial, the mother expressed the view that the murder was written in her fate. This case shows the tensions that can occur within a devoutly religious family when the behaviour of a 'Westernised' daughter appears to challenge the religious traditions of her parents and siblings. Other women in similar situations have suffered greatly and been subject to attempted murder and abductions. While it appears that nothing more could have been done in this case, her midwives acting in an exemplary manner, it highlights the need for cultural awareness and sensitivity among midwifery and obstetric staff. They may need to share their concerns with advocates from the particular minority groups involved, or, in extreme cases, assist the woman to seek the protection of the local police, who may have specific schemes to help women in similar circumstances.

> Another primigravid Pakistani woman separated from her husband during pregnancy following several episodes of severe domestic violence, which she disclosed during an antenatal visit. She was offered extra antenatal visits and social support during her pregnancy, which she accepted. After she was delivered her husband returned home and a further referral to social services was made. Further contact with social services was refused and the woman was murdered a few days later.

In this case, although all the relevant services seem to have been involved in the antenatal period, there appears to have been a breakdown in communication in the postnatal period. This case also highlights weaknesses in the information provided to the Enquiry by staff involved in this case, who stated ' all appropriate support given to help with social problems'. This appears questionable as the woman was murdered. In all the reports it receives the Enquiry looks to local staff to offer some insight into how other cases might help change local professional practice in future.

## Family collusion and mental illness

> A woman and her partner both had histories of psychiatric disorders. He was known to be schizophrenic and was cared for by his own family in times of crisis. Both were poor attenders at their respective psychiatric clinics, although when the woman became pregnant she was a regular attender at the antenatal clinic. She was referred to the psychiatric services during pregnancy for bulimia and incidents of minor self-harm. She had a normal delivery, after which her partner exhibited some agitation on the postnatal ward and needed to be

removed by his family, who stated that he had not been taking his medication. There were regular community midwifery visits for the next three weeks, but one-to-one communication with the mother was said to be difficult due to the constant presence of other family members in the room. Ten days after the woman was discharged by the community midwives she was stabbed to death by her partner who then killed himself.

The psychiatric details of this case are sparse and it is not clear whether this outcome could have been predicted but the very close family presence may have masked or underplayed the seriousness of the situation.

## Cases in which domestic violence may have directly contributed to death

### Use of relatives as interpreters

Domestic violence also may have played a part in two other women's deaths. One was a *Late* cardiac death, counted in Chapter 15, which highlights a number of areas of concern:

> A woman who spoke no English and required her children to interpret for her was subject to regular assaults by her husband for a number of years and had been admitted to hospital on several occasions as a result. During one of these admissions she was diagnosed with mitral stenosis. When she became pregnant again she booked late and the fetus died shortly afterwards due to lethal abnormalities. She herself died of atrial fibrillation, some months after delivery, which, in the opinion of the assessors could have been precipitated by an episode of domestic violence.

After her delivery the postnatal notes indicate that she had complained of further violence on a number of occasions. As her teenage children were used as interpreters it may have been difficult for the healthcare workers to accurately judge the severity of the situation and the need to offer specific help in dealing with her concerns for her safety. There is no evidence that anyone actively tried to help this woman, who was clearly at risk, with her notes stating she had required operative procedures to fix broken bones in the past. This woman definitively required access to an expert and independent translator.

### Warning signs ignored

In the other case, which is counted and discussed in Chapter 4; Haemorrhage, warning signs were also ignored:

> This woman lived in very deprived circumstances, used intravenous drugs, had a violent partner and died of abruption. She also had pulmonary hypertension, which required inpatient care during her pregnancy, but when asked to stay she always left hospital against advice, supposedly because she was needed at home. When asked

about bruises that had been noticed on her body, her partner gave the explanation that she bruised easily. On her final admission, in extremis from haemorrhage, large areas of fresh bruising were noticed on her arms, abdomen and chest.

In the opinion of the assessors, it is quite possible that the abruption may have been precipitated by violence. Although warning signs were present during her pregnancy, it appears no one offered her support and help for the abusive relationship. It would appear that the partner's reply, that 'she bruises easily', was accepted by those caring for her. Her bruising, poor home circumstances and early self-discharges from hospital all pointed to her being in a dependent and abusive relationship. When an index of suspicion was raised it appears the only action taken was to ask her partner why she had the bruises and not provide a confidential setting in which to ask the woman herself.

## Key features of other cases of domestic violence

### Self-discharge from hospital

In a number of cases, women in known violent relationships and who were admitted during pregnancy for medical care for other conditions took their own discharge for similar reasons to the previous case. The reasons for their self-discharge were that they were needed urgently at home. One woman, who kept discharging herself, cited a number of domestic emergencies as the reason for this. In this case there was high index of suspicion of violence throughout her pregnancy but it is not clear if the woman was offered further help.

### Poor clinic attendance

As described in Chapter 1, a significant number of women who were poor attenders at antenatal clinics were in abusive relationships. There may be many reasons why these women found it difficult to attend the clinic and the last Report described cases where women had been witheld money for the fare, had been ordered to stay at home by their partner or had no access to the telephone to phone for advice. In most of these cases, outreach midwifery services were not available, as demonstrated by the next case:

> A very young schoolgirl, with a history of non-accidental injury to herself by relatives, failed to keep several appointments and was not followed up by her GP or midwives. She had a history of recurrent urinary tract infections and presented in mid pregnancy with pylonephritis and died shortly afterwards of overwhelming infection.

In this case care was clearly substandard. She was not only a very young mother but was known to be at risk from her family. Social services had also been involved. All these factors independently point to the need for flexible outreach maternity services and the urinary infections she had are a possible indicator of abuse. However her non-attendance was not actively followed up.

**Poor liaison or co-operation between health and social services**

A feature of many of these women was poor co-operation between the health and social services. One case, a very young homeless girl who died under a duvet in a front garden, has already been discussed in Chapters 6 and 14. The following case also highlights the need for closer inter-agency co-operation:

> A sex worker, who died from a malignancy, had numerous social, psychological and medical problems. She was in a physically dependent abusive relationship and her children were subject to a care order. She was also unsupported by her family. She had a past history of poor antenatal attendances. At the start of her next pregnancy she moved to a different part of the country and, although a social service referral was made, she did not receive an appointment, by letter, from her new social service team until several months later. When she failed to attend she was sent a dismissive letter and contact seems to have been lost. In mid pregnancy she developed very distressing symptoms suggestive of a serious pathology but her GP failed to act on them and was also dismissive and disapproving of her lifestyle without seeking to understand why she was in such a situation in the first place. The woman was so concerned about the lack of support from either the health or social services that she moved back to her original place of residence, where she was admitted to hospital and the nature of her illness was finally determined. From this point onwards, her medical care was excellent, although she died, undelivered, a few weeks later, possibly also immunocompromised.

At one level her death could not have been prevented and this case, in the past, would just have been classified as *Coincidental*. However, the lack of care from both the social and health services is stark.

## Recommendations

Recommendations are given at the beginning of this Chapter and are broadly unchanged from those made in the last Report. They are based on the main recommendations from the Department of Health,[16] the Royal College of Obstetricians and Gynaecologists[4] and the Royal College of Midwives.[5] All health professionals who care for pregnant women are strongly urged to read these reports more fully.

## References

1. Bewley S, Friend J, Mezey G, editors. *Violence Against Women*. London: RCOG Press; 1997.
2. Andrews B, Brown GW. Marital violence in the community. *Br J Psychiatry* 1988;153:305–12.
3. Drife J, Lewis G, editors. *Why Mothers Die*. Report of the Confidential Enquiries into Maternal Deaths in the United Kingdom 1993–96. London. The Stationery Office; 1998.

4.  Home Office statistics.

5.  Bacchus L, Bewley S, Mezey G. Domestic violence and pregnancy. *The Obstetrician & Gynaecologist* 2001;3:56–9.

6.  Bacchus L, Bewley S, Mezey G, Haworth A. Domestic violence in pregnancy: does use of a screening instrument increase detection? Unpublished results.

7.  Gazamararian JA, Lazorick A, Spitz AM, Ballard TJ, Saltzman LE, Marks JS. Prevalence of violence against pregnant women. *JAMA* 1996;275:1915–20.

8.  Geilen A, O'Campo PJ, Faden RR, Kass NE, Xue X. Interpersonal conflict and physical violence during the childbearing year. *Soc Sci Med* 1994;39:781-7.

9.  National Children's Home, Action for Children. *The Hidden Victims: Children and Domestic Violence*. London: NCH; 1996.

10. Stark E, Flitcraft A. *Women at Risk*. London: Sage; 1996.

11. Maryland Department of Health. Pregnancy associated homicide. *JAMA* 2001;285:1455–9:1510–11.

12. Royal College of Midwives. *Domestic Abuse in Pregnancy. Position Paper No. 19*. London: Royal College of Midwives; 1997.

13. Heath I. *Domestic Violence: The General Practitioner's Role*. London: Royal College of General Practitioners; 1998.

14. Royal College of Nursing. *Position Paper on Domestic Violence*. London: RCN; 2000.

15. Laurent C. *Domestic Violence: The Role of the Community Nurse*. London: Community Practitioners & Health Visitors Association; 1998.

16. Department of Heath. *Domestic Violence: Resource Manual for Healthcare Professionals*. London: Department of Health; 2000. www.doh.gov.uk/domestic.htm

17. Department of Health. *Working Together to Safeguard Children: A Guide to Inter-Agency Working to Safeguard and Promote the Welfare of Children*. London: Department of Health, Home Office, Department for Education and Employment; 1999. www.doh.gov.uk/domestic.htm

18. Women's Aid. *Health and Domestic Violence Survey 2000*. London: Women's Aid; 2001.

19. Marchant S, Davidson L, Garcia J. Ad, Parson J. Addressing domestic violence through maternity service-policy and practice. *Midwifery* 2001;17:164-70.

# CHAPTER 17
# Midwifery practice

CHRISTINE CARSON on behalf of the Editorial Board

## Midwifery practice: summary of key recommendations

Apart from the specific recommendations given here, midwives should also read the recommendations contained in the rest of this Report or, at very least, the summary of the key recommendations from other Chapters listed at the end of this Chapter. It is also planned to circulate a summary of the key findings and recommendations to all midwives early in 2002.

### Antenatal care

- Midwives should be at the forefront of helping to plan new models of service provision. The planning and delivery of maternity services should focus on regarding each woman as an individual person with different social, physical and emotional needs, as well any specific clinical factors that may affect her pregnancy. Her pregnancy should not be viewed in isolation from other important factors that may influence her health or that of her developing baby.

- Each woman should have a flexible, individual antenatal care plan drawn up at booking, which reflects her own circumstances and needs. This should be reviewed regularly throughout her pregnancy.

- There may be many reasons why women may fail to attend clinic appointments. These women are at higher risk of maternal and fetal complications and death, and regular nonattendance should be personally and actively followed up by the midwife. If the reasons why she felt unable to seek care are ascertained through sympathetic questioning then alternative arrangements should be made that suit the particular circumstances of the woman.

- Targeting care is about developing services that are effective for all women but particularly for those women who would not normally actively seek help and advice. As part of the changes in the delivery of midwifery care, it is crucial that new patterns of antenatal care are developed particularly for those women who are at the greatest risk. In some instances this may require individual antenatal care at home.

- Interpreters should be provided for women who do not speak English. The use of family members, including the use of children as interpreters, should be avoided if at all possible.

## Booking

- At booking, a needs and risk assessment should take place to ensure that every woman has a flexible individual plan for her antenatal care, to be reviewed at each visit, which reflects her own particular requirements for antenatal care.

- With the growing importance of midwifery-led care, it is vital that midwives undertake a full needs assessment at the booking visit, in order to identify women whose past or current medical history may make them unsuitable for this type of care, and that these women be referred for more appropriate care. Conversely, midwives should be prepared to decline taking responsibility for high-risk cases where the involvement of a consultant obstetrician is essential and the reasons for this should be explained to the woman and to the obstetrician.

- The GP booking letter is a referral mechanism and should not be relied upon to provide all the information necessary to plan antenatal care.

- All mothers should have their body mass index calculated at booking as part of the full risk assessment. Further, they should be offered advice about sensible weight reduction, including diet and exercise and referral to a dietician where appropriate. A past history or family history of thromboembolism should be sought and, if present, specialist advice should be obtained.

- Midwives are uniquely placed to provide advice and support on healthy lifestyles, including:

  - diet and exercise

  - smoking, alcohol and substance misuse

  - safety in the home and workplace

  - basic first aid measures, especially for women with existing conditions such as epilepsy

  - the correct use of car seat belts

  - guidance on the warning signs of obstetric complications such as pre-eclampsia.

- All pregnant women should be given advice about the correct use of seat belts as soon as their pregnancy is confirmed:

  - 'Above and below the bump, not over it'

  - Three-point seat belts should be worn throughout pregnancy with the lap strap placed as low as possible beneath the 'bump', lying across the thighs with the diagonal shoulder strap above the bump lying between the breasts. The seat belt should be adjusted to fit as snugly as comfortably possible, and, if necessary, the seat should be adjusted to enable the seat belt to be worn properly.

- Enquiries about previous psychiatric history, its severity, care received and clinical presentation should be made routinely in a systematic and sensitive way at the antenatal booking clinic. Women who have a past history of serious psychiatric disorder, postpartum or non-postpartum, should be referred to a psychiatrist and a management plan should be formulated in light of the high risk of recurrence.

- The term 'postnatal depression' or 'PND' should only be used to describe a nonpsychotic depressive illness of mild to moderate severity, with its onset following delivery. It should not be used as a generic term to describe other mental illnesses. The term 'postnatal depression' or 'PND' in the maternity records diminishes the severity of previous illness and the high risk of recurrence and should not be used unless the illness was minor in nature. Precise details of any previous illness should be sought and recorded in line with the recommendation above.

- All pregnant women should be routinely asked about domestic violence as part of their social history and should have the opportunity to discuss their pregnancy with a midwife, in privacy, without their partner present, at least once during the antenatal period.

## Continuing care

- All providers of maternity services should ensure that there are clear protocols and routes of referral to primary or secondary care when rapid assessment, investigation and treatment are required. This will involve close collaboration with other professionals in both primary and secondary care.

- When referring woman to general practitioners in primary care, midwives should make direct contact with the general practitioner and not ask the woman or her family to do so on her behalf.

- Midwives should have the ability to refer women about whom they are directly concerned to hospital services.

- In order to increase the detection of pre-eclampsia, all mothers should have their urine tested at each antenatal contact after 20 weeks of pregnancy.

## As an individual practitioner

- Midwives must reflect and develop their practice and play an active role in challenging the organisational structure and culture in which they work, to agree policies that reflect the recommendations in this Report.

- Midwives and other health professionals who work with disadvantaged clients need to be able to understand a woman's social and cultural background, act as an advocate for women with medical staff and colleagues, overcome their own personal and social prejudices and practice in a reflective manner.

- Midwives should be prepared to decline taking responsibility for high-risk cases where the involvement of a consultant obstetrician is essential and the reasons for this should be explained to the woman and to the obstetrician.

- Midwives need to fully use existing systems of statutory supervision to ensure continuing professional development and actively demonstrate evidence-based care.

- Continuing professional development should be accepted as the responsibility of the individual practitioner as well as an employer and knowledge and skills should be regularly updated using current research evidence.

## Introduction

This Chapter has, for the first time, been designed to stand alone and provide an overview of the findings of the 1997–99 Confidential Enquiry into Maternal Deaths for midwifery practice. Nevertheless, we urge all midwives to read the Report in its entirety, in order to understand the full impact of the findings on midwifery and obstetric practice. This Chapter includes cross-reference to the other specialised sections. It is planned to issue all midwives with a more comprehensive summary of the key findings in due course.

Together with other Chapters in the Report, this Chapter describes how midwives might effect, directly or indirectly, the safe outcome of pregnancy. It is crucial that the lessons learned from these deaths, and the recommendations drawn up as a consequence, are understood by all midwives, in order that they can continue to develop their professional practice and provide high quality care to all pregnant and recently delivered women.

It is important to note that, while there are areas of concern, midwives have provided exemplary care for many women in this Report. The recommendations should inform the general direction of changes to maternity service-provision but midwives should also take heed of the specific recommendations for individual practice.

Midwives provide the majority of care and are frequently the lead healthcare practitioner for pregnant and recently delivered women. With the increasing emphasis on midwifery-led care, this latter role will continue to expand. Even when midwives are not the lead practitioner, they continue to see most women during their pregnancy, delivery and the postnatal period. Midwives are the professional lead for approximately 70% of births and are involved in the remaining 30%, which are usually higher risk deliveries.[1] Although many women in this Report had higher-risk pregnancies, complications or underlying medical conditions that required specialist obstetric or multidisciplinary care, midwives were also involved in their care. In most cases midwives provided the important continuity, supportive link and point of contact between the woman and a number of different healthcare professionals. In some cases midwives were also the healthcare professional who picked up the early signs of possible complications and referred the woman for appropriate care.

Of the 378 deaths reported to, or identified by, the Enquiry, 106 were classified as *Direct* and 136 as *Indirect* deaths. Twenty-nine were classified as *Coincidental* (*Fortuitous*) and 107 as *Late*. The precise, internationally defined definitions of these categories are given in the Section 'Definitions of Maternal Mortality' at the beginning of this Report. Lessons for midwifery practice, however, can be derived from many of these 378 deaths, irrespective of the category in which they were counted.

All but 21 of the 378 women had had contact with the midwifery services. The 21 who had no contact died before booking or after a miscarriage or termination of pregnancy. A total of eight women had midwifery-led care and a further 42 had joint midwifery/general practitioner-led care. One hundred and ninety women received 'traditional' shared care and 56, who had high-risk pregnancies, were cared for solely in the hospital setting.

The maternal mortality rate for 1997–99, derived from the CEMD data, is 11.4 deaths per 100,000 maternities, a slight decrease from the last triennia. The *Direct* maternal mortality rate, 5.0 deaths per 100,000 maternities, is lower than in any of the other four preceding triennia for which UK data have been collected. However, the *Indirect* maternal mortality rate, 6.4 per 100,000 maternities, is, for the first time, greater than that for *Direct* deaths. Lessons to be learned from *Indirect* causes of death, such as psychiatric illness, heart disease or deaths from underlying medical causes, are just as important as those from *Direct* causes.

Detailed information in relation to substandard care is presented in Chapter 1; Introduction and Key findings. Fifty per cent of *Direct* deaths had major substandard care, in which different treatment may have affected the outcome, and a further 10% were associated with lesser degrees of substandard care, which did not necessarily affect the outcome.

## Overall themes in relation to midwifery practice

From this detailed assessment four key themes emerged:

1. Appropriate provision and targeting of care

2. Professional accountability and responsibility, including advocacy

3. Risk assessment

4. Communication.

These themes are presented here as separate areas for discussion but they are interwoven and share many similarities and common threads.

In addition, this Report contains valuable new information for midwives and other health professionals; for example, in relation to mental illness and thromboprophylaxis. Specific recommendations from the relevant Chapters are summarised later in this Chapter.

## 1. Appropriate provision and targeting of care

Each woman is an individual person with different social, physical and emotional needs as well as specific clinical factors that may affect her pregnancy. Her pregnancy should not be viewed in isolation from other important factors that may influence her health or that of her developing baby.

Midwives have a unique role in providing the majority of antenatal care and are well placed to address health inequalities and health promotion issues. *Making a Difference*[2] suggests that midwives should target vulnerable groups who would not traditionally use the health services. In this triennium, however, midwives appear to have missed many opportunities to do so. Indeed, there were many instances where women appeared to be just slotted in to a rigid antenatal care programme that was inflexible and inappropriate for their specific needs.

## Social exclusion

Although the United Kingdom has low maternal mortality rates compared with developing countries, social deprivation is clearly linked with an increased risk of maternal mortality. This is demonstrated dramatically in Chapter 1 of this Report, where Table 1.16 shows that the risk of maternal death among women from the most disadvantaged groups of society is up to 20 times greater than those women in the two highest social classes. This finding is shared with other developed countries. In the USA, the maternal mortality rate among women living in socially deprived circumstances is ten times higher than the overall US maternal mortality rate.[3] If *Indirect* causes of death such heart disease and suicide had been included in the US data, as they are in the UK, then it is probable that the rates would have been broadly comparable. Social exclusion may be associated with a tendency to delay access to midwifery or health care intervention.

The midwife has a vital role to play, not only in contributing to the health and wellbeing of all mothers and their babies, but also in targeting their care to those mothers most in need. Socio-economic deprivation was a prominent factor in a large number of cases considered by this Report.

Five girls aged 16 years or less and a total of 13 women aged 18 years or less died in this triennium. All but one were severely socially excluded. Four of the five girls aged less than 16 years had been in the care of social services and three of these girls were homeless and living 'rough' at the time of their death. All but one of the deaths in women aged between 16 and 18 years were also characterised by social exclusion. Seven had suffered repeated episodes of domestic violence from within their own family and several of these also had suffered sexual abuse.

All women should have equal access to information and advice, regardless of their social circumstances or how articulate they are. While mothers who live in more deprived circumstances constitute a specific at-risk group, it is important to adopt an individual approach to needs assessment, tailoring the care given to the specific circumstances of each mother. Examples of appropriate targeting of care in specific circumstances are discussed below. Hart *et al.*[4] concluded that midwives who work with disadvantaged clients need to be able to understand a woman's social and cultural background, act as an advocate for women with medical staff and colleagues and overcome their own personal and social prejudices and practise in a reflective manner.

The booking visit presents an opportunity to undertake a complete, holistic needs assessment of the woman. This should include identification of factors relating to social exclusion, including problems such as learning difficulties.

> In a *Late* death discussed in Chapter 15, an obese, unemployed mother whose other children had been adopted, lived in very poor social circumstances. She had been identified as having learning difficulties and was on heparin for an earlier deep vein thrombosis when she became pregnant again. The midwife who took her booking history failed to identify or act on any of the medical or social factors that obviously placed this woman at higher risk and merely told her to make an appointment in four weeks to see the midwife at the surgery. The mother miscarried and subsequently died of pulmonary embolism.

By contrast, the midwifery care in another case of pulmonary embolism was exemplary:

> In this case, counted in Chapter 2; Thromboembolism, a woman with severe learning difficulties booked late in the second trimester. From the moment she booked an individualised plan of care was drawn up and implemented and, with the midwives' encouragement, she then attended all her antenatal appointments and classes. Liaison with social services occurred and the supervisor of midwives was notified in the antenatal period. After a normal delivery she was discharged home and regularly followed up by her midwife. She was anaemic. After a couple of weeks she developed shortness of breath and a slight tachycardia and the midwife properly referred her to the GP. The GP considered the symptoms to be due to her anaemia but she collapsed and died one week later of a pulmonary embolism.

Despite the outcome, it is clear from this case that the midwife had responded appropriately to the individual needs of the mother. In particular, the midwife was instrumental in setting up communication pathways with other outside agencies. Midwives are uniquely placed to have a positive impact, targeting care where it is most needed.

## Poor attenders at antenatal clinic and/or women who booked late

Twenty per cent of the total number of women who died from *Direct* and *Indirect* causes in this Enquiry either booked after twenty weeks of pregnancy or missed more than four or more antenatal visits. While it is not possible to follow up women who are unknown to the service, it was clear in many instances that nonattendance in women who had booked generated a routine appointment by post. It is not known if this was purely an administrative response or whether professionals were involved. Further, it is not clear if this decision was made based on information in the maternity records. Midwives should be aware of their professional responsibility in the protection of the interests of the mother and her baby, ensuring that they are central to the delivery of care.

> In an *Indirect* death, a young schoolgirl with a history of non-accidental injury lived with her mother and stepfather and failed to present for a booked termination of pregnancy. She continued with her pregnancy but after her initial booking visit failed to attend several antenatal appointments. The midwives providing her care knew her past history but they did not follow her up. She was admitted with pyelonephritis in mid-pregnancy and subsequently died.

In this case, non-attendance at antenatal clinic in a young girl with severe social problems was not actively followed up. Targeting care is about developing services that are effective for all women but particularly for those women who would not normally actively seek help and advice. As part of the changes in the delivery of midwifery care, it is crucial that new patterns of antenatal care are developed, particularly for those women who are at the greatest risk. In some instances this may require individual antenatal care at home.

Nearly half of the women who booked after twenty weeks in pregnancy or who were poor attenders at antenatal clinics came from ethnic minority groups. Half of these women did not speak English. In some cases, midwives did go in to the community to follow these women up but in others either no active follow-up was undertaken or letters were sent in English advising the woman to attend her next appointment. There were several instances of such letters not being understood by any family member.

## Ethnicity

Women from ethnic groups other than white were, on average, twice as likely to suffer a maternal death, as shown in Table 1.15 in Chapter 1. Care needs to be taken in interpreting these findings, however, due to the small numbers involved.

Issues to do with late booking and poor attendance in these groups of women are discussed above. There were also many mothers in this triennium whose first language was not English. In all of these groups, language difficulties and lack of knowledge of specific cultural practices may have led to a lack of understanding, which may have contributed to the midwife not being aware of critical signs and symptoms. In some cases midwives asked relatives, who themselves did not speak much English, to contact the GP because the midwife was concerned. The fact that the GP was not subsequently contacted may have been because her instructions were misunderstood or that there was little knowledge of the NHS or, indeed, possibly no one who could make a phone call in English.

In a large number of cases professionals used family members to interpret. There were several difficult cases where children were used inappropriately to interpret intimate personal or social details of the mother, and vital information was withheld. This Report makes a general recommendation about the use of interpreters. Midwives should proactively raise this issue with their trust managers if they are concerned.

Cultural issues also affect other groups. Chapter 1 also shows that a disproportionate number of women from the traditional travelling community were likely to die.

In relation to caring for women from other cultures, midwives and other health professionals should:

- develop a greater awareness of different cultural needs

- request the use of interpreters and/or link workers from within their own organisations

- be at the forefront of developing flexible services for women who are unable, for whatever reason, to regularly attend clinic based antenatal services.

All health care professionals should consider whether there are unrecognised but inherent racial prejudices within their own organisations, in terms of providing an equal service to all service users.

## Domestic violence

Midwives are increasingly recognising the impact of domestic violence on the physical and mental wellbeing of mothers and their families. The Department of Health and the Royal College of Midwives have produced guidelines for the detection and management of domestic violence,[5,6] as have a number of other professional organisations. Domestic violence is of such relevance to this Report that there is now a separate Chapter, Chapter 16, on this subject, which all midwives are strongly urged to read.

In this triennium, 45 (12%) of the women whose deaths were investigated self-reported a history of domestic violence to a healthcare professional. Many women do not admit to being victims of domestic violence due to shame or the fear of reprisal but may do so if questioned in a sensitive manner. From the information made available to this Enquiry, it appeared that no women in this Report had been routinely asked if they had suffered from violence as part of the social history taken at booking, so the figure of 12% is likely to be an underestimate of the prevalence of violence among this group of women.

Current evidence suggests that domestic violence often starts or intensifies during pregnancy. Midwives therefore need to be constantly aware of the possibility, watching for the signs and symptoms suggestive of domestic violence that are discussed in depth in Chapter 16.

Chapter 16 discusses individual cases and it is clear that in some cases midwives provided well-planned and sympathetic care. In one case, the midwife gave the woman at risk her out of hours telephone number. In most cases, however, the case notes clearly gave a past history of assault or indeed stated that the woman had said that she was currently the victim of domestic violence but no action or discussions were recorded. Furthermore, in a few cases when an index of suspicion was raised, the partner was asked about his wife's bruises and the explanation he gave seems to have been accepted without asking the woman herself.

Domestic violence is a difficult issue for healthcare professionals. Many may feel that by opening up the question they may be presented with a situation with which they do not know how to deal and may appear to be offering the woman more support and advice than they believe they can provide. Some midwives will also have experienced violence against themselves. For these reasons, it is important that not only are health professionals, including midwives, trained to understand the importance of confronting these issues but that they are supported by a local network of agencies to whom the woman can be referred for specialised help.

A primigravid woman from an ethnic minority group, who was known to be experiencing severe domestic violence, separated from her husband during pregnancy. She had good support from midwives during the pregnancy and they arranged social service support. Her husband returned to the home after the delivery and her midwives made a further referral to the social worker, whose help she declined. She was murdered a few days later.

Although all the appropriate services seem to have been involved in the antenatal period, there appears to have been a lack of communication in the postnatal period. The midwives reported that all appropriate support had been given but, from the information made available to the Enquiry, they seem to have assumed that by making the referral they had discharged their responsibilities. There also appeared to be a lack of coordination of services, with each professional working in isolation.

All women, whether or not they admit to suffering domestic violence, should have access to information about local services, including the local Women's Aid help line, refuge and the police community safety unit. Midwives should have available a 24-hour help line number that they can give to women at risk of domestic violence.[8] Midwives should consider whether all women should be given this number as part of routine practice.

All health professionals should make themselves aware of the importance of domestic violence in their practice. Chapter 16 of this Report contains recommendations on the identification and management of women who suffer domestic violence.

### Obesity

Obesity is a risk factor for maternal morbidity and mortality from a number of conditions, including thromboembolism and diabetes. Many mothers who died in this triennium were classified as obese although, as there has been a tendency not to weigh mothers routinely in pregnancy, the precise body weights were not always available. All mothers should have their body mass index (BMI) calculated at booking as part of the full risk assessment. Further, they should be offered advice about sensible weight reduction, including diet and exercise and referral to a dietician where appropriate. BMI is defined as the weight (kg) divided by the square of height (m²). An adult BMI greater than 30 would be classified as obese. Midwives should inform mothers who are obese about how to recognise early warning signs of complications. Midwives are also well placed to give advice on healthy eating, diet and exercise.

## 2. Professional accountability and responsibility, including advocacy

The pattern of midwifery care has undergone many changes over the past few years and these changes are set to continue with developments in Government policy and national strategies, such as The NHS Plan[7] and with the new Nurses and Midwives Council taking over from the UKCC and the four National Boards in April 2002.

Midwives must reflect and develop their practice and play an active role in challenging the organisational structure and culture in which they work, to agree policies that reflect the recommendations in this Report. This review will inform midwives, enabling them to work in more effective ways. Midwives are accountable for the care they deliver and should act as an advocate for women, providing a high standard of care in accordance with midwives' rules and code of practice and guidelines for professional practice.[8,9]

One area where a good standard of care was evident was in the care of some women who had cancer in pregnancy. Some midwives excelled in their care of women who were known to be terminally ill. In one case, 'the midwives were unbelievable in the extra care and attention they devoted to this woman'. In another, community midwives visited a mother at home weekly throughout pregnancy and afterwards, when she required care in a hospice.

## Advocacy

Midwives appeared in some cases to miss the opportunity to question the decisions made by other professionals and act as an advocate for the women in their care. The following case discussed in Chapter 3; Hypertensive disease, is an example of this:

> A woman was admitted to hospital, close to term, with severe pre-eclampsia superimposed on essential hypertension. After a failed induction, an emergency caesarean section was performed under general anaesthetic with an estimated blood loss of one to two litres. She was transferred to the recovery area one hour and 40 minutes after delivery. Ten minutes after arrival in the recovery room her blood pressure was recorded as 48/23 mmHg. She remained profoundly hypotensive, with other signs of hypovolaemic shock. Blood was taken for cross matching. While receiving her fourth unit of blood she had a cardiac arrest two hours after reaching the recovery room.

Midwives failed to challenge the decisions made by the junior medical staff in this case. Although the midwives were clearly concerned, they failed to ensure a more senior obstetric and anaesthetic presence when their involvement was required. The on-call anaesthetist had not been made aware of the presence of a woman with severe pre-eclampsia on the delivery suite. The consultant obstetrician was not called and was unaware of the situation. The midwife coordinating the delivery suite did not support the midwives' concerns in that she did not summon senior medical assistance.

## Inappropriate responsibility for care

A number of women, who had features identifying them as high risk at the booking appointment, received shared care suitable only for low-risk women. In some cases, the previous obstetric history did not appear to be part of the planning process when the care was being considered for the current pregnancy:

> A middle-aged woman with an unplanned pregnancy presented at booking with a history of previous caesarean sections for pre-

eclampsia, intrauterine growth restriction and a family history of her mother having worsening pre-eclampsia with each successive pregnancy. Although a consultant obstetrician saw her at a booking appointment, she had the rest of her care provided by the community midwife until the third trimester, after two episodes of proteinuria were documented. When seen by a consultant at the next appointment the fetal growth and blood pressure were normal. She was seen by a midwife two weeks later and had a trace of proteinuria. Four days later, she was admitted as an emergency with symptomatic pre-eclampsia and no fetal heart beat. Soon after admission she had an eclamptic seizure. Ultimately, a large intracerebral haemorrhage was the cause of death.

In this case, there was a failure to appreciate the significance of the past obstetric history and inappropriate low-risk care was given to a woman who was clearly high-risk. Consultant obstetricians and midwives should be aware of the booking history prior to planning the most appropriate antenatal care. The GP booking letter is a referral mechanism and should not be relied upon to provide all the information necessary to plan antenatal care.

Three of the women receiving midwife-led antenatal care were at higher risk and should have been supervised by an obstetrician. One woman had a multiple pregnancy, another was a poorly controlled diabetic and the third, at very high risk of thromboembolism, was in a wheelchair due to an inherited disorder. Conversely, the care appeared excellent for the other cases of midwifery led care, with appropriate transfers for specialist care.

Three further women were receiving joint midwifery/GP-led care and were also higher risk and should not have been cared for in the community.

With the growing importance of midwifery-led care, it is vital that midwives undertake a full needs assessment at the booking visit in order to identify women whose past or current medical history may make them unsuitable for this type of care and who should be referred for more appropriate care. Similarly, midwives should be prepared to decline taking responsibility for high-risk cases where the involvement of a consultant obstetrician is essential and the reasons for this should be explained to the woman and to the obstetrician.

## 3. Risk assessment

The crucial role of the midwife is to perform a continuing risk assessment of the woman, first at booking and then at each point of contact throughout the antenatal, intrapartum and postnatal periods. At booking, this risk assessment includes a detailed review of the woman's personal and family obstetric and medical history with particular reference to significant risk factors, such as thromboembolism and mental illness. Appropriate action should be taken when any deviations from the normal are noted.

The importance of risk assessment at each contact is illustrated by several cases of pre-eclampsia in this Report that may have gone undetected for some time. This may have been due to the woman being seen without a urine specimen being checked and emphasises the need for urinalysis at each antenatal contact after 20 weeks of pregnancy.

Midwives need to be aware of several new findings from this Enquiry when undertaking risk assessments at booking and in the antenatal period.

## Major psychiatric illness

Although not apparent from the figures in this Report, a further study commissioned by the CEMD and discussed in Chapter 1, has found suicide to be the leading cause of maternal death. Chapter 11; Psychiatric causes of death, contains valuable new information and recommendations, many of which are particularly relevant to the provision of midwifery care.

Of great importance to this Enquiry is the risk of recurrence in women with a past history of a previous severe postnatal depression or puerperal psychosis, or of a non pregnancy-related condition such as bipolar illness, schizophrenia or obsessional compulsive disorder. Women with a past history of severe mental illness, be it puerperal or non-puerperal, face a risk of a recurrence of between one in two and one in three following delivery. The risk of recurrence is at its greatest in the first 30 days postpartum. Typically, these illnesses are of rapid onset, escalation of severity and of similar presentation and timing to previous puerperal episodes. This is why we repeat the recommendation made in the last Report that 'a relatively simple procedure should be instituted in every antenatal clinic to identify women at risk of postnatal psychiatric illness and/or self harm'.

In a large percentage of cases clear psychiatric risk factors were present but were not ascertained. Staff, including midwives, often underestimated symptoms of depression or psychosis. For women with a past history of severe mental illness, clear multidisciplinary planning should take place because of the risk of recurrence. This should include referral pathways and criteria for triggering such a referral. There should be a low threshold for seeking intervention where there is a previous personal or family history of mental illness.

The midwife is well placed to identify women at greatest risk of psychiatric illness. This will involve the detection of risk factors at booking, such as a past history of psychosis or depression, whether postnatal or not. The midwife must also be vigilant in looking for signs and symptoms of psychiatric disease developing during pregnancy and the postnatal period. Half of all women who died from psychiatric illness in the postnatal period had a previous history of mental illness. Many of these women appeared to have good social support but frequently the professionals underestimated the severity of acute presentations.

It is clear that the risk assessment for many of these women was cursory, and a relevant history was noted as postnatal depression or PND, without any further enquiry. The women who died suffered from major psychiatric illnesses, not postnatal depression. The term 'PND' should only be used to describe a nonpsychotic depressive illness of mild to moderate severity with its onset following delivery. It should not be used as a generic term to describe other mental illnesses. In this Enquiry, the use of the acronym 'PND' to describe cases of very severe illness complicating previous childbirth may have led to the likely severity of the recurrence being underestimated and to missed opportunities for prevention.

If a woman reports a previous episode of psychiatric illness, it should not be dismissed as 'PND' but enquiry should be made about the severity of the illness, its clinical presentation, the treatment required and the timing of its onset. Most women who have experienced a previous serious postpartum illness will be concerned about future recurrence. Midwives, obstetricians, GPs and psychiatrists must know about the high risk of recurrence and understand that women with early-onset conditions can quickly move from appearing to be merely anxious and depressed to being psychotic and suicidal within a few days. They also need to know that being mentally well in pregnancy does not necessarily reduce the risk of recurrence after delivery. Forewarned is forearmed and, at the very least, a period of skilled monitoring and management plans for early intervention could be instituted.

In nine deaths, where the past history had been recorded in the midwifery notes, it was referred to as 'PND' despite the evidence of previous severe psychiatric illness in relation to childbirth. In no case was there any evidence that the severity of the previous illness, and indeed inpatient care, had been ascertained. The use of the term 'PND' gave the impression that the illness had been less severe than it actually was and no appropriate referral to the psychiatric service or care plans had been made. In one case a past history of a postpartum psychosis was not recorded at all:

> In a *Late* death, a woman died from being hit by a car after absconding from an inpatient psychiatric unit where she was being treated for a postpartum psychosis. She had previously suffered from a postpartum psychosis some years earlier. There was no mention in her antenatal records of her previous psychiatric history and she had midwifery led care and a home delivery. Shortly after this she became psychotic and required inpatient admission during which time she expressed suicidal intentions.

In the absence of a psychiatric report to the CEMD, it is difficult to know whether she had been warned by her previous psychiatrist of the risk of recurrence. Without antenatal detection of this risk it would not possible to take steps to avoid a postpartum recurrence. If her past history had been ascertained, her antenatal and postnatal care could have been planned to involve the relevant health professionals during this high-risk period.

A number of cases involved women in their first pregnancy with a previous history of non-postpartum psychiatric illness. Again the risk of a recurrence or relapse after childbirth appears not to have been recognised either by their psychiatrists or by their midwives. This led to the care being reactive rather than proactive. It seems that the professionals involved in these women's care were taken by surprise by the rapid escalation of symptom severity following the onset of the condition.

## Thromboembolism

Risk factors for thromboembolism were present in 25 of the 31 cases of maternal death discussed in Chapter 2; Thromboembolism. Thirteen women were overweight, five had had a period of bed rest, four had a family history, three had previous thromboembolism and two had undertaken long-haul flights during pregnancy. Some had multiple risk factors. In spite of this multiplicity of risk factors, many of the mothers who died appeared to be treated as low risk. Identified risk factors need to be readily available to all health professionals in the antenatal and postnatal periods. If a woman appears to be at higher risk of thromboembolism she requires referral for medical advice.

Midwives should be aware that pregnancy itself increases the risk of pulmonary embolism, which frequently presents with vague symptoms such as breathlessness. Thirteen women died from pulmonary embolism in the antenatal period. Of these, eight were in the first trimester of pregnancy. Of the 17 postnatal deaths, ten followed a vaginal delivery.

### Planning future care

Allied to the risk assessment discussed above is the need observe relevant care plans that have been made by the medical team during the antenatal period:

> A young woman attended the antenatal clinic regularly. She was a known high-risk patient who had had a retained placenta with a postpartum haemorrhage in her two previous deliveries (the first recorded as a placenta accreta). Delivery was induced over a weekend following admission with a small abruption and, when the placenta was retained, there was midwifery delay in calling the registrar until bleeding was noted. When haemorrhage became profuse there was further delay before the registrar called the consultant. After further delays in proceeding to hysterectomy and obtaining cross-matched blood, cardiac arrest occurred. Ergometrine had been given at delivery, but was not repeated.

In this case, the overall plan for delivery was inadequate and the plans that were made were not communicated effectively. The midwife who conducted the delivery failed to follow the written instructions from medical staff to contact the registrar to attend the delivery. The midwife and her medical colleague appeared not to appreciate the seriousness of this high-risk case. It is crucial to have well documented plans for women at identified higher risk.

## 4. Communication

The importance of communication between the midwives and other health professionals is a recurring theme in this Report, with poor communication being a contributory factor in many cases. In some instances communication with the woman was also poor.

### Communication with other health professionals

In some cases, there was evidence of good communication and multidisciplinary working even though women died. In a case discussed in Chapter 13; Cancer and other tumours, and previously referred to in this Chapter, a woman was diagnosed with cancer in early pregnancy and spent much of her pregnancy in hospital. An excellent summary of the midwifery care demonstrated good planning and communication, delivering a high standard of care. Extra care given by the midwives included liaison with other healthcare teams, staff and family conferences and teaching basic parenting skills to the partner.

The midwife is frequently the professional that will identify factors placing the mother at high risk when taking a booking history. It is essential that the risks identified are communicated effectively to enable the most appropriate care be given.

Midwives working in a primary-care setting appeared to have good communication networks with secondary care and readily referred mothers to maternity hospitals directly. However, referrals to professionals working in primary care were infrequent and were generally conducted via the mother. The midwife should be more proactive where referrals to a woman's general practitioner are deemed to be necessary.

> A moderately obese woman, whose English was very limited, was visited at home by the midwife because she would not attend the clinic. She did not receive any antenatal care for 11 weeks of the pregnancy. During some of this time she went to visit relatives abroad. The next contact was made near term because of intermittent breathlessness and nausea and vomiting for the previous three to four days following her return to Britain. The midwife who visited insisted they must contact the GP if she was still unwell the following day. This woman collapsed and died of a pulmonary embolism three days later, having never contacted her GP.

This case, counted in Chapter 2, demonstrates the difficulty midwives have in making direct referrals within the primary care setting and maintaining their accountability for the care they give a woman. Midwives working in the community feel comfortable referring to the secondary-care maternity services but some do not appear to work in partnership within the primary-care setting and outside agencies. This was particularly evident in terms of communication with other members of the primary healthcare team. If a referral to a GP is thought necessary, midwives should make direct contact with a GP rather than giving the responsibility to the woman.

## Knowing when to refer

In specific instances, midwives appeared reluctant to refer across specialty borders to allied professionals such as community psychiatric nurses, even when there was a serious risk of mental illness. Midwives need to feel comfortable in these horizontal, inter-specialty communications, as well as vertical, hierarchical communication pathways. This may involve overriding the decisions of other health professionals, perhaps by direct referral to other agencies such as accident and emergency departments or consultant led teams. In one case in this Enquiry, a midwife correctly diagnosed and referred a woman with a postpartum thromboembolism which been missed by her GP:

> An obese primigravida was transferred home on the fourth postnatal day after a caesarean section with a haemoglobin of 8.4 g/dl. The next day, she complained to the visiting midwife of not feeling well, with

upper back pain and breathlessness. She also had a pyrexia. The GP was called and visited and the next day the midwife carried out a routine visit. On the sixth postnatal day the mother collapsed at home and died two weeks later of a pulmonary embolism.

The weight in this instance had not been recorded antenatally. The documentation noted she had a low risk for thrombosis. She did not receive any thromboprophylaxis despite her obesity and delivery by caesarean section. The midwife caring for this mother in the community correctly referred the woman to her GP and appeared to be concerned about the possibility of a pulmonary embolism. However, she did not feel able to override the GP when evidently there was no investigation of the woman's symptoms.

Even where the midwife is the lead practitioner, there is a need to work in partnership with other professionals, reflecting their membership of a team. The midwife should feel able to approach senior staff directly, even if this involves bypassing a less experienced doctor:

> A woman with ulcerative colitis who had previously had a colectomy was delivered by caesarean section. She vomited for three days after delivery and was hypotensive for a further three days. Eventually she was diagnosed with an intestinal obstruction after becoming oliguric. She died of multi-organ failure.

The midwives caring for this mother in the first three days of the postnatal period were clearly concerned and called for frequent medical assessment. However, although they were unhappy with the standard of care being given by the junior medical staff, they failed to contact a more senior obstetrician to review the case.

There was evidence that some midwives made appropriate referrals even though the woman died. A case discussed in Chapter 13 describes a mother who was being cared for in a midwifery-led unit and was transferred to consultant care at 24 weeks with non-Hodgkin's lymphoma. The midwives caring for this woman rapidly picked up the fact that there was a problem and referred her for specialist medical opinion.

## Multi-agency working

The midwife is well placed to coordinate partnerships with other professionals and outside agencies. For example, women with problems of substance abuse often appear to default antenatal clinic attendance, while attending the community drug service more regularly.

> A known heroin addict, whose children were being looked after by their grandmother, frequently failed to attend antenatal appointments but did attend a community drugs unit every two weeks for supplies of methadone. In late pregnancy she complained of shortness of breath and weight loss prior to her death from cardiomyopathy.

As discussed in Chapter 11, substance misuse is associated with difficulty in complying with routine services and appointments. Midwives should consider whether they should work in concert with community drug teams and, indeed, plan future services in consultation with the women most likely to use them. In

Glasgow, where service users have been involved in planning their services the uptake and attendance rate is high. Open access to antenatal clinics in conjunction with substance abuse services without the need for making appointments may also improve antenatal attendance.

## Recommendations from other Chapters of specific relevance to midwives

There are a number of recommendations in other Chapters in this Report that may have specific relevance for midwives.

### Thromboembolism (Chapter 2)

- At booking, the BMI should be routinely calculated to identify women whose BMI is over 30 kg/m$^2$. A past history or family history of thromboembolism should be sought and, if present, specialist advice should be obtained.

- Women with other risk factors for thromboemblism (e.g. bed rest, pre-eclampsia, other medical disorders) should be carefully screened and consideration given to thromboprophylaxis.

- All women undergoing caesarean section should receive prophylaxis against venous thromboembolism. Multiple risk factors are often present and the most effective method of prophylaxis, heparin at appropriate doses, should be used.

- Wider use of thromboprophylaxis (not only after caesarean section) and better investigation of classic symptoms (particularly in high-risk women) are urgently recommended.

- Midwives, general practitioners and other medical staff should pay particular attention to women in the puerperium with chest or leg symptoms after vaginal delivery in order to exclude the presence of deep vein thrombosis or potential pulmonary embolism.

### Pre-eclampsia and eclampsia (Chapter 3)

- Pregnant women with a headache of sufficient severity to seek medical advice, or with new epigastric pain, should have their blood pressure measured and urine tested for protein, as a minimum.

- Clear, written, management protocols for severe pre-eclampsia should guide initial and continuing treatment in hospital.

- Automated blood pressure recording systems can systematically underestimate blood pressure in pre-eclampsia, to a serious degree. Blood pressure values should be compared, at the beginning of treatment, with those obtained by conventional mercury sphygmomanometers.

- Magnesium sulphate is the anticonvulsant drug of choice in the treatment of eclampsia.

- Women with moderate to severe pre-eclampsia require a level of clinical observation that may be incompatible with location in a single side room in hospital.

- Women with multiple pregnancies are at increased risk of pre-eclampsia and their antenatal care should reflect that awareness.

---

**Box 17.1  Summary of RCOG Scientific Advisory Committee Advice on preventing thromboembolism in pregnant women travelling by air (See Annex D of Chapter 2)**

| Any gestation and up to six weeks post partum | Short-haul flight (up to four hours) | Long-haul flight (four hours or more) |
|---|---|---|
| No additional risk factors | Calf exercise; move around cabin; avoid dehydration; minimise alcohol and coffee consumption. | Calf exercise; move around cabin; avoid dehydration; minimise alcohol and coffee consumption; well-fitting elastic below-knee compression stockings. |
| Additional risk factors[a] Weight ≥ 100 kg or BMI at booking ≥ 30+ Multiple pregnancy Thrombophilia Past personal or strong family history Medical disorders with increase risk of DVT | Calf exercise; move around cabin; avoid dehydration; minimise alcohol and coffee consumption; well-fitting elastic below-knee compression stockings. | Calf exercise; move around cabin; avoid dehydration; minimise alcohol and coffee consumption; well-fitting elastic below-knee compression stockings; low molecular weight heparin[b] on day of travel (pre-flight) and day after.[c] |

[a]  Women with additional risk factors may need to seek appropriate medical advice. Some, for instance will already be on thromboprophylatic medication
[b]  thromboprophylactic doses are 5000 units dalteparin or 40 mg enoxaparin
[c]  Low-dose aspirin (75 mg per day for three days before travel and on day of travel) is an acceptable alternative in those unable to take low-molecular-weight heparin

---

### Haemorrhage (Chapter 4)

- The speed with which obstetric haemorrhage can become life-threatening emphasises the need for women at known high risk of haemorrhage to be delivered in a hospital with a blood bank on site and appropriate laboratory facilities including haematological advice and therapy.

- Every unit should have a protocol for the management of haemorrhage and this should be reviewed and rehearsed on a regular basis. It should also be included as part of life support training. All members of staff, including those in the blood bank, must know exactly what to do to ensure that large quantities of crossmatched blood can be delivered without delay.

### Sepsis (Chapter 7)

- The onset of life-threatening sepsis at any stage of pregnancy can be insidious and all doctors and midwives must be aware of the symptoms and signs and be prepared to institute immediate treatment to avoid serious consequences.

- A patient with prolonged rupture of the membranes who develops a fever and/or tachycardia should be carefully assessed by senior staff.

- In women with spontaneous rupture of the membranes and not in labour, vaginal assessments should be avoided or kept to a minimum and undertaken with appropriately aseptic precautions.

- There is clear evidence from controlled trials showing the benefits of prophylactic antibiotics for emergency caesarean section. This Report confirms that this policy is still not universally employed.

## Anaesthesia (Chapter 9)

It seems not to be widely appreciated that oxytocin (Syntocinon®) can cause profound, fatal, hypotension, especially in the presence of cardiovascular compromise. Administration should follow the guidance in the *British National Formulary* and other standard formularies. When given as an intravenous bolus the drug should be given slowly in a dose of not more than 5 iu.

## Cardiac disease (Chapter 10)

- Women with severe cardiac disease require multidisciplinary care.

- In women with significant heart disease, delivery must be planned. At the very least, this will involve discussion with the consultant anaesthetist(s) who will be responsible at the time.

- Prepregnancy counselling about the risks of pregnancy should not alienate the woman to such an extent that she does not come for antenatal care if she does become pregnant. These women need the best care that is available throughout pregnancy.

## Psychiatric causes (Chapter 11)

- Protocols for the management of women at risk of relapse or recurrence of a serious mental illness after delivery should be in place in every trust providing maternity services.

- Enquiries about previous psychiatric history, its severity, care received and clinical presentation should be routinely made in a systematic and sensitive way at the booking clinic.

- The term 'postnatal depression' or 'PND' should not be used as a generic term for all types of psychiatric disorder. Details of previous illness should be sought and recorded in line with the recommendations above.

- Women who have a past history of serious psychiatric disorder, whether postpartum or non-postpartum, should be assessed by a psychiatrist in the antenatal period and a management plan instituted with regard to the high risk of recurrence following delivery.

- Women who have suffered from serious mental illness after childbirth or at other times should be counselled about possible recurrence of that illness after further pregnancies.

### Other *Indirect* causes (Chapter 12)

- Women with epilepsy need specific specialist advice in pregnancy. The ideal treatment for pregnant epileptic women, which has already been instigated in some centres, is a dedicated clinic to encompass prepregnancy counselling and attended by an obstetrician, a neurologist/obstetric physician and a specialist midwife or neurological nurse.

- Women with epilepsy should also be made aware of the dangers of bathing in pregnancy. They should be advised to bathe only in shallow water with someone else in the house or, alternatively, to shower.

- All women should be encouraged to have HIV screening at booking.

- Pregnant women appear to be particularly susceptible to infectious diseases. Those who are not improving despite standard treatment should be admitted to hospital.

- The risk to the fetus from poorly treated asthma is much greater than any possible risk to the fetus from steroid drugs. Steroid therapy can and should be continued in pregnancy.

- Pregnancy is not a reason for withholding plain X-ray films of the abdomen, chest X-rays, some computed tomography scans or magnetic resonance imaging from sick women.

### Cancer (Chapter 13)

- Clear and relevant information must be passed from the GP to the antenatal care team at booking concerning any past medical history including previous malignancies and abnormal cervical smears and any relevant family history.

- A clear medical and family history needs to be taken at booking to lower the threshold for the index of suspicion in women who complain of other symptoms during pregnancy.

- When any pregnant woman complains of episodes of vaginal bleeding in pregnancy, other than confirmed causes of haemorrhage, cervical cancer must be excluded by direct observation of the cervix and a cervical smear taken. This should be undertaken irrespective of her past medical history or reports of normal past cervical smears.

- The importance of planned multidisciplinary care for women with cancer and other serious problems cannot be overstressed. Obstetricians, midwives, GPs, oncologists, surgeons, Macmillan nurses and palliative care services need to be involved, in conjunction with the woman and her partner, in planning a course of antenatal care that respects the wishes of the woman and optimise the outcome for the fetus.

- A summary of an excellent midwifery care plan developed for a particular woman in this Report gives a blueprint for others. Apart from providing routine care and support, the midwives' role includes:

- familiarisation visits to the special care baby unit

- support to help the woman come to terms with her condition

- liaison with other health care teams

- provision of information for her and her family

- providing time for rest and privacy

- ensuring the complex set of hand held notes were transferred to all the professionals involved in her care

- teaching her partner parenting skills

- being involved with the first course of post-delivery chemotherapy or treatment.

- Bereavement counselling and access to representatives of religious faiths should be offered on request or when appropriate.

## Domestic violence (Chapter 16)

- All health professionals should make themselves aware of the importance of domestic violence in their practice. They should adopt a non-judgemental and supportive response to women who have experienced physical, psychological or sexual abuse and must be able to give basic information to women about where to get help. They should provide or refer to services that can provide continuing support, whatever decision the woman makes made concerning her future.

- When a woman discloses violence this must be taken seriously. Women who are poor clinic attenders need active outreach services.

- Local trusts and community teams should develop guidelines to identify and provide further support for these women, including developing multi-agency working to enable appropriate referrals or provision of information on sources of further help.

- Information about local sources of help and emergency help lines such as provided by Women's Aid should be displayed in suitable places in antenatal clinic, for example in the women's toilets or printed as a routine at the bottom of hand held maternity notes or cooperation cards.

- Enquiry about violence should be routinely included when taking a social history. Obstetricians and gynaecologists should consider introducing questions about violence during the course of all consultations. In general practice and midwifery, this could be at the booking visit. There are a number of useful documents explaining how this can be achieved, through the use of sensitive questions.

- When routine questioning is introduced, this must be accompanied by the development of local strategies for referral, which should be accompanied by an educational programme for professionals, in consultation with local groups, and preferably delivered by those already working in this area.

- Where the woman is unable to speak English, an interpreter should be provided on at least one occasion, rather than relying on a partner, friend or family member, especially if the index of suspicion is high.

- Every woman should be seen on her own at least once during the antenatal period to enable the disclosure of such information.

## Conclusions

As with previous Reports, there are important lessons for all professionals involved in providing care to women and their babies. This Report should be seen as a contribution to the continuing assessment and development of the role of the midwife. The midwife is at the forefront of the delivery of care and as such is in a position to influence change. The recommendations in this Chapter are intended not only for organisations to inform future policy but also to develop the practice of individual midwives.

The introduction of the consultant midwife in many trusts in the UK will serve to enhance the professional development of the midwife. Allied to this is the role of the midwife as an advocate, crossing health and social care boundaries.

## Assisting with this Enquiry

The case reports completed by midwives for the Confidential Enquiry were frequently disappointing. Midwives often stated merely that 'all appropriate care was given' even though most cases had midwife involvement. If this Enquiry is to continue to improve midwifery practice, midwives must be willing to provide detailed and accurate information about the care they gave. With the introduction of new systems of reporting in the future it is hoped that midwives will provide the information that makes the recommendations made in these Reports as valuable as possible.

## References

1. English National Board for Nursing, Midwifery and Health Visiting. *Report of the Board's Midwifery Practice Audit 1999/2000*. London: ENB; 2001.
2. Department of Health. *Making a Difference: Strengthening the Nursing, Midwifery and Health Visiting Contribution to Health and Healthcare*. London: HMSO; 1999.
3. World Health Organization. *World Health, 51st year. No. 1, Feb–Jan 1998*. IX Geneva: WHO; 1998.
4. Hart A, Lockey R, Henwood F, Pankhurst F, Hall V, Sommerville F. *Researching Professional Education Addressing Inequalities in Health: New Directions in Midwifery Education and Practice. A series from the English National Board for Nursing, Midwifery and Health Visiting*. London: ENB; 2001.
5. Department of Health. *Domestic Violence: A Resource Manual for Health Care Professionals*. London: DoH; 2000.

6. Royal College of Midwives. *Domestic Abuse in Pregnancy. Position Paper No. 19*. London: Royal College of Midwives; 1997.

7. Department of Health. *The NHS Plan A Plan for Investment, A Plan for Reform*. London: DoH; 2000.

8. United Kingdom Central Council for Nursing Midwifery and Health Visiting. *Midwives Rules and Code of Practice*. London: UKCC; 1998.

9. United Kingdom Central Council for Nursing Midwifery and Health Visiting. *Guidelines for Professional Practice*. London: UKCC; 1996.

# CHAPTER 18
# Pathology

HARRY MILLWARD-SADLER on behalf of the Editorial Board

This Chapter is designed to stand alone and to be used by pathologists without the need to read the entire Report.

## The quality of the autopsy

The autopsy is essential in supporting clinical audit and clinical governance and its value has been demonstrated in many studies. Early studies revealed clinical discrepancies in up to 30% of autopsies, with approximately one-third of these being major discrepancies that would have influenced clinical management. Even despite recent improvements in diagnosis, a recent study has found significant clinical discrepancies in approximately 15% of cases.[1] The value of the autopsy in this Enquiry has also been repeatedly demonstrated. Many maternal deaths are both unexpected and dramatic, converting what should be a happy natural event into a tragedy. While no-one should retain organs without consent or take unnecessary or inappropriate histology, a maternal death demands and should command a thorough and detailed pathological investigation with careful clinicopathological correlation. Unfortunately, previous Reports have adversely commented upon the quality of the maternal autopsy when judged against standards defined by the Royal College of Pathologists (1993).[2]

In this Report, the overall standard of the autopsy has improved. Of the 81 *Direct* maternal deaths where an autopsy was performed, 63 (78%) were of adequate standard or better and there have been many examples where careful autopsy investigation and report has significantly aided the review process.

> A young primiparous woman died early in the third trimester in cor pulmonale from idiopathic pulmonary hypertension with the fetus *in utero*. Her mother had died some years earlier from heart disease. Autopsy confirmed marked right ventricular hypertrophy (right ventricle 110 g, left ventricle 138 g). Pulmonary arteries, leg and pelvic veins were carefully dissected and were clear. Histology confirmed grade 6 lesions in the pulmonary arteries, with plexiform lesions and occasional foci of fibrinoid necrosis. There was no evidence of organising thrombus in either the pulmonary arteries or deep calf veins. Post mortem investigations for factor V Leiden were negative. The autopsy report on the mother was traced and confirmed that her mother had died from primary pulmonary hypertension. Tissues were then referred to a specialist centre where the genetic mutation for familial primary pulmonary hypertension was identified.

This overall improvement would have been more marked if the complete documentation from the autopsy had been available. There are many examples where a detailed macroscopic report was made but the histology and/or microbiology, although undertaken, were not provided.

> A very young woman who was in early pregnancy woke up one morning with a right hemiparesis. There was a family history of cardiovascular disease with close relatives dying from a stroke and a myocardial infarct. She deteriorated rapidly and on MRI scan had a large infarct in the region of the middle cerebral artery and a suggestion of dissection of the internal carotid artery within the petrous temporal bone. She died the next day. The autopsy was very thorough and detailed. Thrombus was demonstrated in the middle cerebral artery but there was no apparent underlying arterial pathology in this or in the common carotids. The intrapetrous portion of the internal carotid artery was taken for fixation and decalcification. Embolus could not be excluded because there was thrombus adherent to the aortic leaflet of the mitral valve. The valve was taken for histological examination. Sadly, the results of these further investigations have not been made available to the Enquiry and the differential diagnosis of embolus, primary arterial dissection or idiopathic cerebral thrombosis remains unresolved.

Sadly, other autopsies were technically deficient in one or more ways: no clinical history, inadequate descriptions of organs, no organ weights or no histology. Therefore, for the purposes of this Enquiry, autopsies have been broadly classified as excellent, good, adequate, deficient and appalling. The criteria used are given in Box 18.1.

The essential question to be answered was how well did the autopsy report address the pertinent clinical issues in that patient. While some autopsies did not meet all the RCPath guidelines but adequately identified the causes of death, it was much more common to find that the cause of death was clearly identified from the autopsy, but there was failure to address other clinical problems relating to the case.

Although examples of poor quality could be found from all regions, there was a distinct problem with medico-legal autopsies conducted in a large metropolitan area of the UK; for example, in the case described here:

> An older multigravid patient was admitted towards the end of her pregnancy with severe pre-eclampsia superimposed on essential hypertension. She was given hydralazine, labetalol and nifedipine but, after a second dose of vaginal prostaglandins, she developed fetal distress necessitating emergency caesarean section. At induction of anaesthesia her blood pressure was recorded as 250/160 mmHg and she received magnesium sulphate ($MgSO_4$) in theatre. Although blood loss in theatre was only estimated to be 1.5–2 litres, there was an unexplained delay of nearly two hours between the delivery of the baby and the transfer of the mother to the recovery room. Within a few minutes of arrival in the recovery room her blood pressure was 48/23 mmHg with an unrecordable tachycardia. Blood was then taken for crossmatching and started 30 minutes later. Cardiac arrest occurred two hours later with the patient hypotensive throughout.

> ## Box 18.1 Criteria given by the CEMD to autopsy report
>
> *Excellent*
> A thorough, detailed autopsy report with comprehensive histology and appropriate microbiological, toxicological or other specific directed investigations, with careful exclusion of alternative diagnoses and clarification of a complicated clinical history.
>
> *Good*
> Many of the above features are included but a more straightforward clinical problem with no significant differential diagnoses. Met all the recommendations of the Royal College of Pathologists (RCPath).[2]
>
> *Adequate*
> Established the cause of death but did not necessarily address all the clinical issues. Sometimes there was a lack of supporting evidence because of inadequate documentation. Recommendations of RCPath not necessarily completely fulfilled but deficiencies not apparently affecting the conclusions.
>
> *Deficient*
> Report consistent with clinically suspected cause of death but lacks detail. Lack of supporting investigations, no evidence of clinical correlation or attempt to exclude differential diagnoses. Does not comply with RCPath guidelines in more than one area.
>
> *Appalling*
> All of the 'deficient' criteria but worse. Often the total report including patient details and stated causes of death occupied one side of A4 paper or less. There are discrepancies between the minimally described pathology and the pathological conclusions, there are no supporting investigations and there is no evidence of any knowledge of the clinical problems or of any attempt to exclude differential diagnoses.

The autopsy was conducted in a distant public mortuary, no clinical staff were present and no clinical history was included in the report which, with the external examination, macroscopic findings and conclusions, was less than 300 words long – approximately the length of this vignette. Despite the history of hypertension, the left ventricle was only described as hypertrophied and the kidneys as 'no specific abnormality'. The spleen was not mentioned at all, despite the history of blood loss and hypotension, and there was no detailed attempt to find any source of bleeding in the genital tract or elsewhere. There was no histology so that the evidence of pre-eclampsia, the features of hypertension in the kidneys and the nature of the 'small oval nodules' in the liver was not assessed.

An analysis of the available autopsy reports whose deaths were classified as Direct showed the results given in Table 18.1.

**Table 18.1** Analysis of autopsy reports whose deaths were classified as *Direct*; United Kingdom 1997–99

| Area | Excellent | Good | Adequate | Deficient | Appalling |
|---|---|---|---|---|---|
| London | 0 | 4 | 7 | 2 | 6 |
| Other UK | 13 | 25 | 14 | 9 | 1 |

The reasons for this difference must be multifactorial but it is perhaps of significance that many of the autopsies in the area are performed by visiting pathologists in a non-hospital public mortuary and are directed solely at excluding forensic causes. It is unusual to have any clinical liaison, so that the clinical problems are not addressed and histology is not performed. In some instances, there is such a delay between death and autopsy that histology of tissues is of little value:

> A young primipara had routine antenatal care until 33 weeks of gestation. At that visit 'slight puffiness' was noted but no other features of pre-eclampsia were recorded and she was given a further appointment in three weeks. However, she had seizures at home two weeks later and was dead on arrival at hospital. Autopsy was performed in a distant public mortuary and this was delayed for six days. The report is on one side of A4 paper and comments on atheromatous patent coronary arteries, indurated lungs and bite marks to the tongue. Death was attributed to a pre-eclamptic fit but histology was too autolysed to contribute.

The report failed to address adequately the indurated lungs or the atheromatous arteries and histology was inadequate. Also, it was not clear why there had been such a delay between death and autopsy but it is important that it is as short as possible. Clinicians have a responsibility to report the death to the coroner or to obtain informed consent as quickly as possible and pathologists must endeavour to keep any subsequent delay to a minimum.

## Autopsies by Chapter

### Chapter 2; Thromboembolism

Of the 35 *Direct* deaths attributed to thromboembolism in this Report, several did not have a post mortem and in some further cases no autopsy report was available. Of the remainder, there was an improvement in the quality with 19 acceptable or better and five being deficient. The good reports not only established the cause of death and searched for the source, but also specifically searched for pathological changes that would contribute to understanding other significant episodes in the clinical history.

> A woman from an ethnic minority group died suddenly at home late in her pregnancy after a three- to four-week history of breathlessness. Although visited by the midwife, she and her family were reluctant to involve the general practitioner. The autopsy revealed massive pulmonary embolism with organising thrombus in the left internal iliac vein extending to the common iliac vein. There was no thrombus in the femoral or deep calf veins. Detailed histology of all major organs was undertaken and old organising thromboemboli were found in the lungs as well as the fresh emboli. The heart was referred to a cardiac pathologist because of subendocardial fibrosis in the left ventricular outflow tract. This was attributed to friction from a myxoid mitral valve and the myocyte damage in the right ventricle to

florid catecholamine induced damage. Microbiological cultures of the uterus and spleen were negative and no evidence of thrombophilia was found in a retrieved antemortem sample of blood.

Eight of the 19 acceptable cases have been classified as adequate because the autopsy findings satisfactorily explained the clinical history, even if no histology was taken and the RCPath guidelines were not met.

Sadly, not all cases reached even this standard. Five reports would be considered inadequate or poor even by these relaxed criteria. The most common reason was failure to perform histology on the lungs when there was a clear clinical history suggestive of previous episodes of embolisation that had been misdiagnosed. Six patients had a history of shortness of breath for at least several days preceding the final collapse but in four of these there was no attempt at the autopsy to establish the cause. It is important that an autopsy addresses such clinical audit issues. The following cases are typical examples:

> An older multiparous woman developed shortness of breath late in the first trimester of her pregnancy. This persisted but a month later she was stating that her dyspnoea had improved. She suddenly collapsed and died a week later. At autopsy there was massive pulmonary arterial embolism and thrombi were found in the deep calf veins. There was no attempt to demonstrate older emboli in the pulmonary arteries at autopsy and there was no histology taken of the lungs or of any other organs.

> An overweight parous woman developed thrombophlebitis soon after her pregnancy test proved positive. An older sister was taking warfarin for recurrent deep vein thromboses and pulmonary embolus. At eight weeks of gestation she was referred to the accident and emergency department (A&E) with chest pain, with her GP's diagnosis of pulmonary embolus. After review by the medical registrar, she was allowed home with a diagnosis of musculoskeletal chest pain. Five days later, she represented to the hospital with chest pain and haemoptysis. Pulmonary embolus was diagnosed clinically and she was transferred to a larger centre. There, a V/Q scan was arranged but she collapsed and died on the third day after transfer before this was performed. Massive pulmonary embolism was found at autopsy and an ileofemoral vein thrombosis was identified but there was no attempt either macroscopically or microscopically, to find evidence of previous emboli in the lungs.

Recently, an association between antipsychotic drug therapy and idiopathic venous thromboembolism has been reported.[3] Separating this as a potential cause for pulmonary embolism in pregnancy will be difficult and emphasises the need for meticulous autopsy standards.

> A woman had puerperal psychosis requiring acute psychiatric admission on the fifth day after the birth of another child. She was an inpatient for over two weeks and was successfully treated with risperidone and fluoxetine. Thirteen days after discharge (the 35th postpartum day) she suddenly collapsed and died. Massive

thromboembolism was found at autopsy. The major arteries and veins were described as normal but it is not stated whether the deep calf veins and pelvic veins were examined and no histology was taken.

Clearly, thrombosis in the pelvic veins would have favoured pregnancy in the pathogenesis as might evidence of old organised pulmonary emboli on histology.

## Chapter 3; Hypertensive disorders of pregnancy

There were 15 deaths directly attributed to pregnancy-induced hypertension. Of these, there were ten autopsies of adequate quality or better but there were also three that were substandard. No autopsy was performed or no report was available in the remainder. In the cases coming to autopsy, six died from cerebral haemorrhage or stroke. Of the other cases, two had acute respiratory distress syndrome (ARDS), one had hepatic necrosis with HELLP syndrome, one had postpartum haemorrhage with disseminated intravascular coagulation (DIC) and one had a coincidental viral pneumonia. In two cases, the autopsy was of such poor quality that the mode of death associated with the presumed eclampsia could not be ascertained with confidence.

Clinically severe pre-eclampsia or eclampsia has presented between 26 and 33 weeks of gestation without preceding clinical detection. It is therefore entirely conceivable that fulminating pre-eclampsia, giving rise to unexpected death, may occur *de novo* in the intervals between antenatal assessments. In all autopsies of sudden death in the last trimester of pregnancy, it is critical to exclude pre-eclampsia, even when there is no clinical indication.

> A young primiparous woman had routine antenatal care until 33 weeks of gestation. At that visit 'slight puffiness' was noted but no other features of pre-eclampsia were recorded and she was given a further appointment in three weeks. However, she fitted at home two weeks later and was dead on arrival at hospital. Autopsy was performed in a distant public mortuary and was delayed for six days. The report is on one side of A4 paper and comments on atheromatous patent coronary arteries, indurated lungs and bite marks to the tongue. Death was attributed to a pre-eclamptic fit but histology was too autolysed to contribute.

The poor quality of this autopsy has already been commented on but the case emphasises the need for careful and comprehensive autopsy and histological examination of organs. However, even when pre-eclampsia is being actively treated, death can be due to other causes:

> A primipara with a multiple pregnancy had a caesarean section for suspected (but not confirmed) abruption. On admission, she was noted to be jaundiced and this jaundice, after delivery, became overt and she developed HELLP syndrome. She was transferred to the intensive care unit (ICU) where a further laparotomy was required to drain a retroperitoneal haematoma. She then improved over the next week before rapidly deteriorating with clinical features of septicaemia that did not respond to therapy.

A detailed and thorough autopsy showed multiple foci of necrosis in the myocardium, kidneys and brain with a bile-stained green liver. The lungs were heavy and haemorrhagic with large bloodstained pleural effusions. Histologically, the lungs showed ARDS with pneumonia and there were multiple fungal microabscesses in the brain, kidneys and heart. *Candida albicans* was cultured from the kidney.

> An obese grand multiparous woman with diabetes and chronic hypertension developed superimposed pre-eclampsia and was found dead in her hospital bed one morning. In the days prior to death she had had mild dyspnoea attributed to asthma and her obesity. At autopsy, there was no evidence of any brain pathology and there was no trauma to the tongue to indicate a fit. Extensive histology was undertaken and confirmed the absence of significant pathology in the heart and brain as well as demonstrating the features of pre-eclampsia superimposed on mild chronic hypertensive changes in the kidneys. Surprisingly, the lungs showed evidence of a viral pneumonia with a bronchiolitis; there was no evidence of acute asthma.

The case was reviewed by the local pathology assessor, who confirmed the conclusions. While, ideally, lung cultures should have been performed, it is difficult to identify how the need for this investigation might have been anticipated. However, the assessors believe a diagnosis of sleep apnoea should also be considered: a possibility based on the overall good quality of the autopsy, which excluded some possibilities, and the demonstration of the bronchiolitis in an obese patient.

There is an increasing tendency for death from cerebral haemorrhage not to come to autopsy. Frequently, therefore, the cause of the cerebral haemorrhage – arteriovenous (AV) malformation, berry aneurysm, systemic hypertension or pregnancy-induced hypertension – is not ascertained. Ten deaths in this triennium have been attributed to cerebral haemorrhage or stroke and associated with pre-eclampsia, with three of these being brain stem strokes or haemorrhage. Only five had an autopsy but in one other case there was evidence of an AV malformation in the surgically resected lobe of brain:

> A primiparous woman was admitted at term with mild pre-eclampsia. Planned induction of labour was delayed because the labour ward was busy. She rapidly developed fulminating pre-eclampsia with epigastric pain and bizarre behaviour and, despite hydralazine, had a fit two hours after admission to the delivery suite. Emergency caesarean section was performed and a live but acidotic baby delivered and successfully resuscitated. Within a few hours of delivery, the woman had developed neurological signs and intracranial haemorrhage was diagnosed. She was transferred to a neurological centre where three craniotomies were performed to evacuate the blood and to control the raised intracranial pressure but without success. Histological examination of the resected brain suggested that an AV malformation was present. No autopsy was performed.

While it seems likely that the fulminating eclampsia precipitated bleeding into her AV malformation, autopsy could have provided valuable confirmatory evidence.

**Chapter 4; Haemorrhage**

Postpartum haemorrhage complicates other conditions such as DIC associated with amniotic fluid embolism (AFE), pre-eclampsia and the HELLP syndrome and is discussed in those sections. Of the eight deaths from haemorrhage counted in this Chapter, three were from placenta praevia, three from abruption and two from postpartum haemorrhage where alternative causes could not be identified. No autopsy was done or the report was not available in two of these cases. There were three reports that were adequate or better and three that were deficient or worse. Of the six autopsies, three were patients with placenta praevia, two with an abruption and one with postpartum haemorrhage:

> A consultant performed elective surgery for placenta praevia in a woman who had had previous caesarean sections, but an inexperienced registrar gave the anaesthetic and no special precautions, such as a central line or a second wide-bore cannula, were taken. The estimated blood loss was 6.5 litres and the abdomen had to be reopened within 30 minutes of closure. The woman died before hysterectomy was completed.

The autopsy showed widespread petechial haemorrhages and the lungs were heavy and deeply congested. Death was attributed to DIC complicating severe blood loss but no histology was performed and the possibility of AFE cannot therefore be excluded. No report was available for the resected uterus that had been sent for histopathological examination.

It is important that the sections of uterus, if resected prior to death, are reviewed and the findings incorporated into the autopsy report. Sources of bleeding such as genital trauma and AFE must be carefully excluded as, for instance, AFE can present as post or peripartum haemorrhage.

Two autopsies were so bad that they were non-contributory:

> A registrar performed an elective caesarean section on a patient with known placenta praevia, fibroids and previous uterine surgery. The immediate blood loss was 1200 ml, but bleeding continued and a further five-litre loss occurred at repeat laparotomy for hysterectomy performed by a consultant. Bleeding continued and at splenectomy there was another five-litre loss. There was gradual improvement but two further general anaesthetics were required. The woman finally died of ARDS after proven aspiration during the second of these.

The history was ignored and death was attributed to DIC from placenta praevia. Although the lungs were described as of hard consistency and airless, there was no confirmatory histology and no attempt to demonstrate aspiration. The liver was 'brown and soft in keeping with toxic liver' but was not weighed and, again, no histology was taken.

> A woman with history of postpartum haemorrhage after a previous vaginal delivery was admitted early in the third trimester with pre-eclampsia and a decision to deliver her two weeks later was taken. Although she was known to have an anterior placenta praevia and pre-operative anaemia, a registrar undertook the caesarean section

with a registrar anaesthetist. The placenta was morbidly adherent and there was excessive bleeding. The abdomen was closed but subsequently was reopened for persistent bleeding. Death from hypovolaemic shock occurred during hysterectomy.

The autopsy description was 238 words long, of which, almost half was devoted to the external appearances and the neck tissues. The report mentioned a recently performed hysterectomy but attributed death to DIC from pre-eclampsia. Apart from the heart there were no organ weights and no histology was undertaken.

It has already been identified that obstetric haemorrhage is a difficult diagnostic problem with multiple potential causes and with corresponding difficulties in clinical management. Careful autopsy review can therefore make a significant contribution towards enhancing the quality of clinical practice:

> A woman who was on methadone as treatment for her intravenous drug addiction and who was known to be hepatitis C positive was admitted near term with abdominal pain quickly identified as an abruption. Domestic violence was suspected as the cause of the abruption because she was known to have been at risk and had fresh bruising to the arms, legs and abdomen. Investigations at an earlier admission for abdominal pain had also shown pulmonary hypertension and an anaesthetic assessment concluded that the anaesthetic for her planned caesarean section would require careful preplanning. However, an emergency caesarean had to be performed for fetal distress. A live baby was delivered but cardiac arrest occurred during the anaesthetic. Blood loss was estimated at 1200 ml and fluid replacement was in progress.

A very detailed and thorough autopsy was performed, which included careful description of the external signs of trauma, a detailed account of all organs including the placenta, extensive histology, toxicology and culture of the tricuspid valve. The autopsy confirmed the bruising but was unable to attribute this as a cause of the abruption. It also confirmed that retroplacental haemorrhage had occurred. There was also evidence of right ventricular hypertrophy. The histology confirmed the changes of a chronic hepatitis C infection but the most significant findings were in the lungs, where plexiform lesions of severe pulmonary hypertension were present in association with refractile granulomas of intravenous drug abuse. There was no evidence of AFE. The cause of death was attributed to hypovolaemic shock due to placental abruption.

The *assessors* consider that the blood loss was insufficient to be the sole cause of death and that the pulmonary hypertension was a significant contributory factor. Fortunately, the high quality of the autopsy permits such a retrospective analysis – which would not have been possible with some of the other quoted autopsies. Also, although the *assessors* suspected domestic violence as a possible cause of the abruption, there was no substantial evidence from the autopsy to fully support this concern.

## Chapter 5; Amniotic fluid embolism

This condition has a classical clinical presentation: sudden collapse during labour with cyanosis and rapid onset of DIC, which is so strongly suggestive that in the last triennial Report cases were included in this category that were not confirmed at autopsy. However, in this Report all seven deaths attributed to AFE had been substantiated at autopsy and in contrast to the last triennial report all the autopsy reports were of adequate standard or better. However, because it is rare to encounter an autopsy report where this diagnosis has been carefully excluded from the other causes of massive uterine haemorrhage, the possibility exists that AFE masquerading as intrapartum or postpartum haemorrhage has been missed.

In one case, the fetal squames in the maternal circulation were so numerous that the diagnosis was simply made – but significantly altered the clinical diagnosis:

> A woman was admitted near term with the classic features of an abruption, including intrauterine death. She had a vaginal delivery of a stillborn baby and shortly afterwards passed a litre of blood clot. Clinical and laboratory features of DIC rapidly supervened. Despite major blood transfusion and clinical care involving consultant obstetrician, anaesthetist and haematologist she died in the delivery suite.

The autopsy was thorough and showed congested oedematous lungs with pleural petechiae. There was evidence of placental abruption but there was no evidence of any laceration to the uterus cervix or vagina. Microbiology and toxicology were negative but numerous squames were found in the pulmonary circulation on histology. No special techniques were required for their visualisation.

In another case, AFE was suspected on routine histology but not confirmed by immunocytochemistry:

> A morbidly obese woman with a history of panic attacks had shortness of breath in the first trimester of pregnancy, which was treated as pulmonary embolism with heparin and warfarin. At five months of gestation she was admitted with vaginal bleeding; her international normalised ratio (INR) was 8.3. She was treated with vitamin K and heparin was restarted but she miscarried. Six hours after delivery she complained of chest pain and breathlessness. She was transferred to a medical ward next day, when her INR was 1.9, but she arrested shortly after transfer.

The autopsy was performed 60 hours after death, when skin blistering was noted over the shoulders, upper arms and lower legs. There was gross cardiomegaly with the heart 620 g in weight but, apart from the symmetrical left ventricular hypertrophy, no pathology was found in any of the chambers, valves or coronary arteries. The other major finding was of severe pulmonary oedema and massive (two litres each) bilateral pleural effusions. The pulmonary arteries were patent. Extensive histology and toxicology was undertaken and the opinion of a specialist cardiac pathologist sought. There was no overt cardiac cause of death but numerous platelet thrombi were found in the cardiac and pulmonary vessels together with some possible fetal squames in the lungs. It was therefore tentatively concluded that the cause of death, despite the unusual clinical presentation was DIC from AFE. However, subsequent immunochemistry failed to confirm the presence of fetal squames.

This excellent autopsy, by carefully excluding various alternatives, has prompted a review of the diagnosis. The central *assessors* now believe death could have been from the rare thrombocytopenic complications of heparin administration.[4,5]

Also, the frequency with which fetal squames can be found in the maternal circulation without causing clinical disease is unknown, as is the length of time they remain in the lung capillaries in patients who survive for a period in intensive care before succumbing to their illness.

> A young primigravid woman, recently arrived in the UK, was seen late in pregnancy when intrauterine growth restriction was diagnosed. Fetal distress occurred in labour and an emergency caesarean section was carried out. Soon afterwards, she developed a tachycardia with excessive oozing from the wound, which was re-explored. DIC was diagnosed, she continued to deteriorate and was transferred to ICU. Torrential vaginal bleeding occurred and subtotal hysterectomy was performed. Another laparotomy was required for further bleeding and she then developed renal failure. Despite transfer to a centre for renal dialysis she deteriorated further and died a few days after the caesarean section.

The autopsy was thorough and detailed, demonstrating multi-organ failure from DIC. There was no evidence of AFE on routine staining of the lung histology but, because of the interval between the onset of symptoms and death, a more detailed search for AFE was at first not performed. Subsequently, immunocytochemistry using the cytokeratin markers CAM5.2 and LP34 showed three small foci of squames and a possible lanugo hair.

Modern immunocytochemical techniques are more sensitive than the standard histochemical methods. It is therefore recommended that unless fetal squames are easily found on standard histology, any search for AFE should incorporate probing the maternal lung sections with cytokeratin markers. While CAM5.2 is the most commonly used cytokeratin probe, it is not particularly good at identifying fetal squames and often gives false negative results. LP34 and AE1/2 give stronger marking of fetal squames and a cleaner pulmonary background.

> A woman had a termination of pregnancy at 14 weeks that was apparently performed without complication. After completion of the procedure there was a sudden drop in oxygen saturation with bradycardia. She was transferred to an ICU at another hospital but died a few days later from multiple organ failure. Despite the very unusual clinical presentation in the beginning of the second trimester, AFE was clinically suspected.

A detailed autopsy was performed and many causes, such as uterine perforation, were excluded. The major findings were of heavy rigid lungs consistent with ARDS and infarcts in the kidneys. Extensive histology confirmed ARDS with DIC and numerous microthrombi in all organs. A specific statement is made that there was no evidence of AFE in the lungs but the techniques used histologically for this purpose are not stated; it seems unlikely that immunocytochemistry was employed.

Such findings need to be interpreted against a background of knowledge about the frequency with which fetal squames can be detected in maternal lungs without the clinical syndrome normally associated with AFE. We also need to have information about the survival time of fetal squames in the lung, now that putative clinical cases are surviving.

## Chapter 6; Deaths in early pregnancy

These are most commonly due to ectopic pregnancy but also include other deaths before 24 weeks of gestation. There were 13 deaths from ectopic pregnancy and most are usually due to hypovolaemic shock from massive haemorrhage or DIC supervening after successful resuscitation. The cause of death is therefore usually obvious at autopsy if clinically undiagnosed or apparent if resuscitation has been attempted. Even then, other features may be present that do not directly alter the cause of death but need elucidation.

> An older woman with known alcohol problems, but not known to be pregnant, collapsed after complaining of abdominal pain. The paramedics were unable to resuscitate her and commented on the smell of alcohol. Autopsy showed 1.5 litres of blood in the peritoneal cavity with a 2.5 cm diameter ruptured left fallopian tube at the centre of an ectopic pregnancy. The liver was noted to be fatty. No histology was taken either of the ectopic or the liver and blood alcohol levels were not ascertained.

Some deaths followed attempted treatment and there was one case of an ectopic cervical pregnancy:

> An ectopic cervical pregnancy was diagnosed at 11 weeks and treated by feticide with potassium chloride and methotrexate. The woman was discharged but readmitted with sepsis and evacuation of retained products was attempted. Massive haemorrhage occurred and resulted in hysterectomy. Despite this, death resulted from DIC complicating hypovolaemic shock.

The very thorough and detailed autopsy had a resumé of the clinical events and was consistent with DIC. The surgical histology on the uterus was retrieved and incorporated into the report. This confirmed the presence of retained products in the cervix: histologically, the chorionic villi had almost penetrated the full thickness of the cervix, being within 1 mm of the parametrium. Autopsy histology revealed the microthrombi of DIC and showed widespread non-regional multifocal microscopic infarction in the heart with the formation of contraction bands. No evidence of AFE and no evidence of infection were found.

Adequate documentation of findings is critical and is even more important when conservative treatment for ectopic pregnancies has been attempted.

Deaths from complications of treatment have also occurred. Apart from ectopic pregnancy, there have been three deaths following evacuation of retained products of conception; one of these was for evacuation of a hydatidiform mole, but no autopsy was performed. There are occasions when complications, particularly after abortion, demand a more detailed autopsy. Two deserve comment:

> A known alcoholic woman with a history of fits following alcohol withdrawal had a grand mal seizure the day before a spontaneous

abortion. Evacuation of retained products was performed and she was discharged. She was found dead at home next morning. The autopsy found an enlarged heart, heavy oedematous lungs, pale kidneys and an enlarged bulky uterus weighing 220 g, containing a large amount of fresh blood. The liver was enlarged to approximately twice normal size and showed fatty change. The pancreas was slightly fibrotic. Histology showed some fibrosis and early ischaemic change in the heart, early bronchopneumonia with congestion and oedema in the lungs, severe fatty change in the liver, interstitial nephritis in the kidneys and congested spleen and brain. The cause of death was attributed to uterine haemorrhage from her miscarriage and her alcoholic liver disease. No toxicology or microbiology was undertaken.

The interpretation and conclusions after such a detailed autopsy seem strange and there are clear contradictions within the autopsy and with the clinical events. It is difficult to claim a significant volume of blood loss from the uterus when the organ only weighed 220 g, there was no record of blood loss elsewhere, there had been no fluid replacement and organs, e.g. spleen, were congested. The fatty liver was proposed to have contributed to death by causing abnormal clotting and probable electrolyte disturbance. However, normal electrolytes and clotting were present at the time of the evacuation. It is difficult to determine the scale of the liver disease without formal assessment for the more subtle forms of a steatohepatitis, which may be masked in the presence of such severe fatty change. However, we do know that severe fatty liver is associated with sudden unexpected death even if the mechanisms are speculative. The possibilities of acute alcohol poisoning or drug overdose were not excluded and the role of the interstitial nephritis and the fibrotic pancreas were not explored. It seems unlikely that the latter two would have influenced the sequence of events and been the cause of sudden unexpected death.

A woman had a suction termination of pregnancy at eight weeks, together with insertion of an intrauterine contraceptive device. Death with a diagnosis of thrombotic thrombocytopenic purpura occurred three weeks later. The autopsy findings were considered compatible with the clinical diagnosis. There were petechial haemorrhages with foci of softening in the brain, haemorrhages in the myocardium and soft swollen pale kidneys. The lungs were heavy and congested and the spleen was markedly enlarged though the liver was normal. Although the heart was thought to be of normal size it weighed 486 g. There is no reference to the intrauterine contraceptive device. No specimens were taken for microbiological cultures. Histology confirmed DIC with microinfarcts from platelet thrombi but the more typical fibrin thrombi of thrombotic thrombocytopenic purpura were not identified. Occasional placental structures were still present in the uterus.

Certainly the findings do not disprove the clinical diagnosis but the features are really those of DIC and other causes such as genital tract sepsis have not been completely excluded.

It is necessary to repeat the recommendation from the last Report that it is inadequate not to have taken tissues and swabs for culture and not to have undertaken extensive histology in such cases.

## Chapter 7; Genital tract sepsis

There were 14 deaths from genital tract sepsis, five following miscarriage. Only one of the deaths in women who had delivered was post surgical. Sepsis was a major factor in some deaths discussed in other Chapters. This includes a patient dying of peritonitis from bowel perforated during a laparoscopy for an ectopic pregnancy.

There were no cases of necrotising fasciitis in the period under review.

Death was due to streptococcal septicaemia in five cases and to coliforms in four, but the organism was unknown in five. Because of the speed with which streptococcal septicaemia progresses, a high index of clinical suspicion, rapid laboratory responses and vigorous therapy are needed to combat it. There is often no evidence that the primary route of infection is through the genital tract and other symptoms such as diarrhoea and vomiting may be dominant and misleading. These features therefore demand a careful and thorough autopsy.

> An older woman was admitted at 30 weeks of gestation with a history of sore throat, diarrhoea and vomiting, with abdominal pain of short duration. She collapsed on arrival and the fetal heart rate dropped to 40 bpm. Emergency caesarean for presumed abruption delivered a live baby but there was no evidence of abruption. The diagnosis of septic shock rapidly became apparent and she was started on multiple antibiotics following microbiological advice. She was transferred to an ICU at a tertiary centre under the care of an infectious diseases physician but died next day. Group A streptococci were cultured from the placenta.

Autopsy showed widespread petechial haemorrhages and bleeding into the peritoneal cavity but there was no obvious source of sepsis in the genital tract or elsewhere. Externally, the body showed a purplish red diffuse discolouration of the skin with several small cutaneous haemorrhages as well as numerous petechiae. No cultures were taken and no histology was performed.

> A woman from an ethnic minority group was admitted moribund in the third trimester after a short illness. Septic shock was diagnosed and resuscitation started but she arrested shortly after admission. Cultures of blood and vagina grew Group A beta-haemolytic streptococci. At autopsy, there were numerous haemorrhages into all tissues and the uterus was a dark red colour. Again, the skin showed an intense lividity and there was no obvious source of infection. Culture of a variety of organs produced a heavy growth of streptococci from the placenta but not from the amniotic fluid. Extensive histology confirmed the widespread DIC with microthrombi in most organs.

The skin lividity described in these two cases seems to be a typical autopsy feature of streptococcal septicaemia, although it is not consistently present ante mortem. When present, it should initiate the taking of samples from different organs, e.g.

vagina, uterine cavity, placenta, amniotic fluid, spleen, lungs, larynx, for microbiological culture. It is unknown how many of these streptococcal septicaemias originate from the genital tract and how many are from sore throats or other loci. There was a delay of four days between death and autopsy in both these cases so that autolysis was present. However, if the autopsy is conducted within 36 hours of death then a striking feature is the haemolytic staining of intimal surfaces throughout the body and the premature autolytic changes on histology.

There was one unusual case of toxic shock syndrome due to mixed infection including Group C streptococci.

Classic cases of ascending genital tract infection do still occur but the organisms are varied:

> An older woman from an ethnic minority group had an *Escherischia coli* urinary tract infection treated in early pregnancy. At 24 weeks, she was seen with a five-day history of passing offensive fluid associated with abdominal pain and a temperature. This was also diagnosed as an *E. coli* urinary infection sensitive to the administered antibiotic. She was discharged the following day but readmitted a day later with spontaneous rupture of her membranes. Steroids were started and she was transferred, apyrexial, to a tertiary centre with neonatal ICU facilities. Steroids were continued. A few days after transfer she became pyrexial, blood cultures were taken and she was transferred to the labour ward. A stillborn baby was delivered a few hours later but the placenta was retained. This required manual removal under general anaesthesia but afterwards she could not be extubated because of her hypoxic state. She was transferred to an ICU where hysterectomy was performed two days later to eliminate a source of infection. She survived there for four weeks before succumbing from multi-organ failure.

The autopsy was sound but the findings were those of multi-organ failure. However, histology of the placenta showed a chorioamnionitis and infection in the uterine wall, which emphasises the necessity of reviewing all previously resected tissues in compiling a report.

Sadly, in other cases of sepsis, the poor quality of the autopsy has significantly hampered review of the circumstances leading to death:

> An older woman had an amniocentesis following a high risk result for Down syndrome. She was readmitted that day with right iliac fossa pain and next day had pyrexia and miscarried. Evacuation of retained products was performed but she arrested during the procedure. Gram-negative rods were isolated from the placental tissues. The patient died several days later but in the interim had received 50 units of blood and 74 units of blood products. Autopsy showed widespread ischaemic lesions in the digits and blistering and ulcers on the skin. There were the features of ARDS in the lungs and numerous petechial haemorrhages in all organs. No histology and no cultures were taken.

Despite all the evidence for DIC complicating septicaemia and the failure to perform any histology or demonstrate an alternative cause, the cause of death was given as AFE. The *assessors* cannot accept this conclusion.

> A woman with Ehlers Danlos syndrome and chronic alcoholism was admitted at 32 weeks of gestation with abdominal pain, hypotension and a productive cough. Abruption was suspected and an emergency Caesarean section was performed. During the procedure, the haematologists reported that the blood film suggested severe sepsis. She deteriorated rapidly with DIC and had to be transferred to a teaching hospital because of a lack of ICU beds. She died on arrival.

Despite dying in a teaching hospital the autopsy was not performed for another six days. The gross findings revealed very heavy oedematous lungs but did not identify any definite cause of death. No locus of infection was identified but the spleen, at 102 g, was unremarkable. Nonetheless, death was attributed to septicaemia. No cultures were attempted though the results after the six-day delay would have been of dubious value. Histology was limited but the lungs were only congested. There was 'no evidence' of AFE but the techniques used to exclude this diagnosis are not given. The delay in conducting this autopsy has adversely affected review of the diagnosis and therefore the relevance of the given care.

## Chapter 8; Genital tract trauma and other *Direct* deaths

There were two cases of haemorrhage leading to DIC following genital trauma. In both, there was adequate documentation of the trauma. Curiously, in the one case, macroscopic pathology was described but the histology was documented as normal. For instance, the kidneys had mottled cortical surfaces and the swollen brain was consistent with the history of DIC, brain damage and convulsions. Both brain and renal histology showed 'no significant abnormality'. It is difficult to have confidence that other conditions such as AFE were satisfactorily excluded.

In cases of genital trauma, it is important to provide a detailed description of the injuries, to identify the site of the placenta and to exclude amniotic fluid embolus.

There were six deaths from liver disease of which four were due to acute fatty liver, one to acute hepatic necrosis of unknown cause and one to haemoperitoneum from a ruptured subcapsular liver haematoma. There was no autopsy in two of the cases diagnosed as acute fatty liver: all the autopsies in the other cases of liver disease were of very high standard. One case is highlighted because of the very early stage of pregnancy at which it occurred:

> A young primagravida was found dead in bed at approximately 24 weeks of gestation. She had had headaches, nausea and vomiting for two weeks prior to death following her last normal antenatal review and died two days before she could get an appointment with her GP. Gross fatty liver was the major finding at autopsy and severe diffuse microvesicular fatty change was confirmed on histology. There was no significant abnormality in any of the other sampled organs and extensive toxicological, microbiological, and virological studies were all negative.

Fatty liver of pregnancy almost invariably occurs in the last trimester of pregnancy and the rare occurrences in the second trimester have been the subject of case reports even in the last few years. The earliest recorded case was at 22 weeks of gestation. Nonetheless, in this instance it is difficult to find any alternative diagnosis given the documented findings and the meticulous way that other diagnoses were excluded.

One other case deserves mention in this Chapter, as the differential diagnosis was of ruptured caecum secondary to caesarean section:

> A woman had a multiple pregnancy successfully delivered by elective caesarean section. Her puerperium was normal until day five, when she developed increasing abdominal distension and then became acutely unwell. Conservative treatment for paralytic ileus failed and laparotomy was performed. Faecal peritonitis from a ruptured caecum was found and right hemicolectomy with ileostomy and mucus fistula colostomy performed. She was transferred to ICU but died the next day.

Autopsy was careful and thorough demonstrating DIC from sepsis. There were hard scybala in the left colon and review of the resected caecum showed mucosal ulcers as well as the perforation. The pathologist concluded that death was due to perforation of the caecum from pseudo-obstruction of the large bowel (Ogilvie's syndrome). Acute colonic pseudo-obstruction can complicate surgery and presents with abdominal distension after a mean of 3.5 postoperative days.[6] It can also occur after caesarean section.[7] The assessors had to consider whether the perforation was directly due to surgical trauma at the caesarean section. This is thought to be unlikely as, in this case, presentation was on day five and the surgically resected caecum showed other mucosal ulceration as well as the perforation. The case, therefore, is considered to be a rare type of *Direct* maternal death.

## Chapter 9; Anaesthetic deaths

The pathology of an anaesthetic death is usually one of careful exclusion: aspiration of gastric contents is perhaps one of the most positive findings to be made. It is much more difficult to determine the cause of death by exclusion and, of necessity, this must entail a particularly careful and thorough autopsy. It is therefore very disappointing to find an autopsy that was of such poor quality that no cause of death could be formally ascertained from an independent inquiry:

> The mother was in labour under spinal anaesthesia that was subarachnoid rather than the intended epidural. When caesarean section was necessary, the anaesthetic was topped up but the spinal block was higher than expected. She developed hypotension and bradycardia that was appropriately treated but her blood pressure had only increased to 80 mmHg systolic when the baby was born apnoeic and pulseless. As the paediatrician had not arrived, the anaesthetist intubated and resuscitated the baby. By the time this had been achieved, the mother was bleeding and the obstetrician requested oxytocin to improve the uterine tone. Cardiac arrest rapidly followed and resuscitation was unsuccessful.

Separate pathological review of the autopsy for the independent inquiry concluded that the autopsy was not of the standard recommended for the investigation of maternal deaths. Specific attention was drawn to the lack of organ weights apart from heart and brain; despite, for instance gross pulmonary oedema, the lack of microbiological studies (which was considered to be a major omission) and the inadequate histological investigation. The reviewer was able to retrieve blocks of lung specifically to stain for AFE and these were negative. The conclusion was that it was impossible confidently to define or exclude a cause of death from the report and this Enquiry was deprived of valuable negative information.

The anaesthetic *assessors* consider that a combination of the cardiovascular effects of a high spinal block and the large dose of administered oxytocin could be sufficient to precipitate cardiac arrest. This diagnosis, however, is dependent upon satisfactory exclusion of other causes, which should have been provided from the autopsy.

## Chapter 10; Cardiac deaths

### Congenital

There were ten deaths associated with congenital cardiac anomalies and one *Late* death. Two deaths were due to pulmonary hypertension complicating Eisenmenger's syndrome but no autopsies were performed.

There were four cases of primary pulmonary hypertension: the available autopsy reports are of a very good standard:

> A young primiparous woman died, undelivered, early in her third trimester in cor pulmonale from idiopathic pulmonary hypertension. Her mother had died a few years earlier from heart disease.

Autopsy confirmed marked right ventricular hypertrophy (right ventricle 110 g, left ventricle 138 g). Pulmonary arteries, leg and pelvic veins were carefully dissected and were clear. Histology confirmed grade 6 lesions in the pulmonary arteries with plexiform lesions and occasional foci of fibrinoid necrosis. There was no evidence of organising thrombus in either the pulmonary arteries or deep calf veins. Postmortem investigations for factor V Leiden were negative. The autopsy report on the mother was traced and confirmed that her mother had died from primary pulmonary hypertension. Tissues were then referred to a specialist centre where the genetic mutation for familial primary pulmonary hypertension was identified.

> A primigravid woman had had a congenital atrial septal defect (ASD) repaired but it subsequently reopened and pulmonary hypertension developed necessitating further repair. She was reviewed regularly through the antenatal period but early in the third trimester had some 'funny turns' including a fit. She was delivered, by caesarean section, just before term, after spontaneous rupture of her membranes. She had a cardiac arrest just after the placenta was delivered and resuscitation was unsuccessful.

There was a thorough and detailed autopsy where the major macroscopic abnormality was in the heart. This was dilated with right ventricular hypertrophy but the ventricles were not separately weighed. The ASD had been closed with a patch and there was no communication between the atria. Histology was taken from many organs. The lungs showed grade 5 pulmonary hypertensive changes with no evidence of embolism or AFE. Subsequently a cardiac pathologist examined the heart and confirmed the right ventricular hypertrophy and the severe pulmonary hypertension. The cause of death was attributed to primary pulmonary hypertension but on review is probably secondary to the ASD prior to its repair.

### Endocarditis

There were two cases of endocarditis. One was in a patient with a bicuspid aortic valve and the other occurred in a patient with a long-standing patch repair of an aortic coarctation. In addition, there was a *Late* case of an acute endocarditis without underlying valve pathology:

> A grande multiparous woman had had an aortic coarctation repaired many years earlier. She was a heavy smoker with poor social circumstances. In mid-trimester she presented with central chest pain, breathlessness and a continuous heart murmur on the left sternal edge. Endocarditis was diagnosed but no blood cultures were ever positive. She was treated with antibiotics and valve replacement was deferred until the baby was more mature. A caesarean section had to be done two weeks later and was immediately followed by open-heart surgery for mitral and aortic valve replacement and excision of vegetations on the tricuspid valve. Postoperatively she developed DIC and died within 12 hours of the operation.

The autopsy was detailed with careful description of the valve replacements and the repaired tricuspid valve. There was no evidence of residual endocarditis and no source of infection was found. Detailed histology was taken but the report on this is not available, nor is the histology of the resected heart valves. It is not known whether microbiological samples were taken.

## Acquired heart disease

### Myocardial infarction

There were five deaths related to myocardial infarction/ischaemic heart disease. There was no autopsy in one and no report on the autopsy in a second. Heavy smoking in women in their thirties again emerges as a key risk factor in three of the cases and one was an insulin-dependent diabetic. Details of a positive family history were present in one case. Three cases were sudden and unexpected. In the three available reports, the coronary thrombus was histologically confirmed in two. One autopsy report was of very poor quality:

> An older woman died suddenly at home a few weeks after a normal vaginal delivery. Clinical details are brief as her partner destroyed her hand-held records. No clinical history was given in the autopsy report, which was exceedingly brief: half of the 200 words used were devoted to the external appearances and the head and neck. Apart from the heart, there were no organ weights. Fresh blood clot occluded the

anterior descending branch of the coronary artery but there is no description of the underlying vessel wall. No histology was taken.

The autopsy failed to meet even the most relaxed interpretation of the standards set by the RCPath.

### Cardiomyopathy

There were seven deaths attributed to puerperal cardiomyopathy.

> In one case, a woman was admitted just before term with a one-week history of increasing breathlessness. An echocardiogram showed a dilated cardiomyopathy and she was transferred to a tertiary centre, where an elective caesarean section was performed. There was no significant change in the postpartum echocardiogram but clinically she improved and was discharged home to be with her baby. Five days later, she felt unwell and shortly afterwards her husband found her unconscious. Resuscitation was unsuccessful.

The features of a dilated cardiomyopathy were present at autopsy with the heart weighing 706 g and showing subendocardial fibrosis. The heart and the histology were reviewed by cardiac pathologists and confirmed as a dilated puerperal cardiomyopathy.

There were another eight cases of other forms of cardiomyopathy or myocarditis. The pathology and aetiology of these conditions are poorly understood. They are therefore difficult to categorise, even after a well-conducted autopsy:

> A younger multiparous woman suddenly collapsed a few days after a normal full-term vaginal delivery. She survived four days in ICU, during which time an enlarged heart consistent with hypertrophic cardiomyopathy was found on echocardiogram.

Autopsy showed an enlarged heart (570 g) with a concentrically hypertrophied left ventricle and diffuse endocardial thickening. There was no localised subaortic endocardial pathology and the valves and coronary arteries were normal. The kidneys were normal with no evidence of hypertensive changes and no other pathological cause of hypertension could be found. Histology of the heart confirmed the myocyte hypertrophy, without the characteristic disarray found in hypertrophic cardiomyopathy, and was referred for expert cardiac pathological opinion. It was confirmed that the findings were atypical and could not be categorised as puerperal, dilated or hypertrophic cardiomyopathy, or as a myocarditis. A category of pseudohypertrophic cardiomyopathy was suggested, as this would not have the familial implications for the relatives. Nonetheless a simple echocardiographic analysis of the left ventricular shape and size was advised for first-degree relatives.

With this variation in pathology, it can be difficult to differentiate puerperal from other types of cardiomyopathy, which themselves can be difficult to classify. It is disappointing, therefore, when an opportunity to investigate death attributed clinically to a cardiomyopathy is not taken.

> An older grandmultiparous woman had two admissions for chest pain and palpitations early in pregnancy before presenting again with the same complaints a third time, which quickly progressed to cardiac

arrest. She had a history of episodes of cardiac failure in her previous recent pregnancies. These had been diagnosed as due to a dilated cardiomyopathy. Two sisters also had 'cardiomyopathy' and her mother had died of 'palpitations'.

The autopsy was confined to an external examination of the body only. A full autopsy should have been undertaken and the nature of the cardiomyopathy established, and any other undiagnosed pathology identified.

Other cases may have been inappropriately classified as cardiomyopathy following autopsy:

> A grossly obese woman was admitted near term with a history of increasing shortness of breath over the previous two days. A presumptive diagnosis of pulmonary embolism was not substantiated on investigation. She also had hypertension and proteinuria. Two days after admission she became dizzy and unwell with a tachycardia. Her symptoms persisted over the next few days and a consultant nephrologist review attributed her proteinuria to pregnancy. A caesarean section was planned for an unstable lie but she arrested at the start of anaesthesia.

The autopsy revealed a dilated hypertrophied heart weighing 510 g with mild right ventricular hypertrophy (85 g). There was no evidence in the report of subaortic stenosis or of other macroscopic left ventricular abnormality. The coronary arteries were normal. There were no pulmonary emboli in the oedematous lungs. A 6-cm diameter carcinoma was found in the lower pole of the left kidney. The remainder of the genitourinary tract was normal: the uterus showed the anticipated changes following caesarean section. No histology was taken and the cause of death was attributed to a cardiomyopathy. This autopsy was inadequate because extensive histology was needed but not performed. The heart pathology and the renal cell carcinoma should have been histologically confirmed. The possibility of secondary hypertension from the renal carcinoma should have been investigated and the changes of pre-eclampsia should have been evaluated. It is difficult to accept a diagnosis of cardiomyopathy in the absence of these further investigations.

> A known multiparous drug addict booked late. Previously, her drug addiction had resulted in gangrene of the fingertips and a radial artery thrombosis. She was first seen after 20 weeks of gestation, when she was complaining of breathlessness, but then failed to attend her clinic appointments for another three months. At this stage, she was still complaining of breathlessness. Shortly afterwards, she was admitted in a collapsed state, peripherally shut down, cyanosed and hypotensive. Cardiac arrest occurred.

An extensive and detailed autopsy included histology, microbiology and toxicology. The heart was dilated and weighed 350 g; the ventricles were not separately weighed. The myocardium appeared focally pale but otherwise no significant pathology was found. Elsewhere, there were haemorrhages into the mesentery and the liver showed a nutmeg pattern of intense congestion. Toxicology found therapeutic levels of methadone in the blood and mixed organisms were present in the blood cultures. Sepsis was considered possible from these findings. However, the histology showed a florid foreign body giant cell reaction to doubly refractile material in and around vessels in the lungs and similar changes were present in the heart and liver. The granulomas had produced focal scarring and foci of necrosis in the heart. Death was given as cardiac failure due to pregnancy associated cardiomyopathy. While the hyperdynamic changes in pregnancy were a major determinant in the timing of this death, the underlying pathology is that of right ventricular strain from the granulomatous scarring in the lungs further exacerbated by the granulomatous myocarditis.

### Aneurysms

In this triennium, five deaths were due to dissecting aneurysms of the aorta. There was one other death from a ruptured mesenteric artery aneurysm and one *Late* death from a ruptured splenic aneurysm. The diagnosis of dissecting aortic aneurysm was made clinically in three cases but in one only preterminally and confirmed at autopsy. Autopsy established the cause of death and its source in the remaining cases:

> A woman was four months pregnant when she complained of severe abdominal pain at work. On arrival at hospital she was shocked and resuscitation was commenced. Investigations quickly revealed evidence of an aortic dissection and thoracotomy with cardiac bypass was commenced approximately two hours after admission. The dissection was confirmed and involved the coronary arteries: it was not possible to wean her off by-pass.

The autopsy was thorough and sound. No features of Marfan syndrome could be identified. The aortic dissection started 2–3 cm above the root extended back around the origin of the left coronary artery and gave origin to extensive haemomediastinum. Histology was consistent with heart failure in all tissues and there was no evidence of cystic medial necrosis either in the root of the aorta or in the abdominal aorta.

In only one case were the features of Marfan syndrome present:

> A young woman, with a close relative with Marfan syndrome who had died from ruptured aortic aneurysm, was admitted with severe back pain at term. Computed tomography (CT) scans demonstrated aortic root dissection and emergency laparotomy with delivery of a live baby was performed. Two days later, she had further episodes of severe chest pain and had a cardiac arrest.

Marfanoid features were confirmed at autopsy, as was a 20-cm dissection in the wall of the aorta starting in a tear 8 cm from the aortic valve. There had been extensive haemorrhage into the mediastinum. Histology confirmed the cystic medial necrosis.

### Other cardiac deaths

As might be expected, there are a variety of conditions under this heading, including three deaths attributed to cardiac arrhythmia in the absence of other pathology.

One of these cases was a woman with a past history of palpitations investigated some years earlier and diagnosed as mitral valve prolapse. She was found dead at home at 32 weeks of gestation. The autopsy showed a normal heart and valves and was very detailed, with extensive negative microbiology and toxicology. The histology was also very detailed and comprehensive. The only abnormality was chronic thyroiditis but an antenatal sample of blood was retrieved; analysis showed normal thyroid function tests.

The report can be criticised only from failure to have the heart examined by a specialist cardiac pathologist but, given the otherwise excellent quality of the report, the diagnosis of sudden cardiac arrhythmia seems sound.

This contrasts sharply with another case:

A woman with morbid obesity and known to suffer from Wolff-Parkinson-White syndrome died a few weeks postpartum. During her pregnancy she had developed gestational diabetes and there had been several multiprofessional meetings to plan her antenatal care and the delivery.

The heart weighed over 500 g at autopsy, the liver over 4 kg and the spleen over 600 g. The kidneys showed features of shock, with pale cortices, and death was due to heart failure from left ventricular hypertrophy. It is regrettable that after so much professional effort that there was no histology or more detailed investigation of the heart and other organs to complete the investigation.

Other causes include a strange case of idiopathic myocardial fibrosis and one of eosinophilic myocarditis:

A multiparous mild asthmatic had a normal pregnancy and vaginal delivery. After discharge she became depressed and moclobemide was prescribed. After almost four weeks of treatment, the drug was changed to fluoxetine because the patient had developed a rash. However, a further rash developed within a week. After 11 days of fluoxetine she was complaining of shortness of breath followed within a few days by diarrhoea and vomiting. No abnormal signs could be found on examination but she spent the next week in bed before suddenly collapsing. Paramedics identified a cardiac arrest but, despite resuscitation, she was asystolic on arrival at hospital.

The autopsy was thorough and detailed with heavy oedematous lungs, pleural effusions and inflamed airways. The heart was of normal size but the myocardium was pale and showed a mottled yellow discolouration throughout both ventricles. Histologically, there was a marked dense eosinophilic infiltrate in the myocardium with many small foci of necrosis. There was no evidence of a vasculitis in any of the many organs examined, although a patchy perivascular infiltrate in the lungs and kidneys also included many eosinophils. There was no generalised eosinophilia. These are the findings of an eosinophilic myocarditis, which has been described in pregnancy.[8] Despite this, it is usually associated with atopic conditions or drug reactions and is therefore considered *Indirect*, especially as the symptoms started in the postnatal period.

## Chapter 12; Other *Indirect* deaths

These cover a miscellany of diseases and, in many cases, the relationship and interaction of the disease with pregnancy is uncertain.

### Cerebral haemorrhage/thrombosis

There were 11 deaths from subarachnoid haemorrhage from ruptured berry aneurysm. Details were very sparse in these cases. The lesion was demonstrated by angiography in five and at autopsy in three. These three were the only cases to have an autopsy. It is perhaps significant that, in all three, there was sudden collapse and death before admission to hospital and investigation could be achieved. No histology was taken in any of the three cases, so ancillary factors were not excluded. Perhaps more surprisingly, in one case, toxicology was not taken:

> A cocaine addict was on a rehabilitation programme when she suddenly collapsed and died in the street. She was in her third trimester but had defaulted her last antenatal clinic appointment.

The autopsy was very detailed and identified a ruptured berry aneurysm 0.3 cm in diameter on the anterior communicating artery. There was no histology or toxicology. The quality of the autopsy was marred slightly by failure to search for features of eclampsia histologically and by failure to check for recent cocaine abuse. Subarachnoid haemorrhage can occur up to six hours after taking cocaine and the aneurysms are both smaller (5 mm versus 11mm) and rupture at an earlier age in cocaine users (33 years versus 52 years).[9]

There were five cases of intracerebral haemorrhage, three of which occurred in the antenatal period and two after delivery. Despite detailed autopsies, no cause or contributing factors could be found. Three cases of dural sinus thrombosis occurred. All were in the postpartum period: one complicated congenital hydrocephalus at two weeks and one was nine days postpartum in a patient with a strong family history of thrombophilia. All autopsies were very good.

> An older woman had had an abruption late in the second trimester. Approximately one week later she was admitted with unsteadiness and headache. A CT scan showed cerebellar lesions interpreted as infarction. She was discharged after six days, only to be readmitted three days later with drowsiness and right-sided weakness. A further CT scan showed a left frontoparietal haematoma with a sagittal sinus thrombosis. She continued to deteriorate and she died a few days later. Investigations for thrombophilia were all negative.

There was a comprehensive and detailed autopsy, with specialist neuropathological referral and supporting histology and microbiology. No source of infection was found. The sagittal sinus thrombosis was confirmed with extension into the internal jugular vein as well as many of the tributaries of the sinus. In addition, there was a thrombosis of the right vertebral artery, extending from its subclavian artery origin to the vertebrobasilar confluence. This appeared to have been the cause of the original infarcts in the brain stem and cerebellum.

### Epilepsy

In this triennium, there were nine deaths attributed to epilepsy but only eight of these were known epileptics on drug maintenance therapy. Of the eight, two deaths occurred in the first trimester, four in the second, one in the third and one in the postpartum period. All these eight deaths occurred suddenly at home. Although, in epileptic deaths, the evidence is largely negative by exclusion of other causes, in two alternative causes of death could not be excluded. In one there was the possibility of a sudden cardiac arrhythmia. In the other, differentiation from a diabetic death was adversely affected by a poor autopsy report:

> An epileptic woman also had poorly controlled diabetes with several complications including nephropathy with heavy proteinuria, neuropathy and retinopathy. She was found dead at home in the first trimester of pregnancy.

The autopsy was inadequate, being very brief, ignored most of the clinical problems and even some of the macroscopic pathology with no histology taken from any tissue. Death was attributed to hypoglycaemic fitting but a postmortem blood sugar was greater than 2 mmol, which makes this diagnosis very unlikely. Given the very poor quality of the report, no alternative cause of death can sensibly be considered.

Obviously, the role of the autopsy is crucial in establishing the cause of death in these patients. It is an essential part of the autopsy to exclude other causes of fits, such as eclampsia, and to establish the therapeutic drug levels in the body at the time of death. While epilepsy is controlled by the clinical response to therapy without reference to drug blood levels, knowledge of these levels at autopsy can identify failure to comply with therapy or changes in therapeutic concentrations induced by the pregnant state.

> A poorly controlled epileptic had been much improved by the addition of lamotrigine to her valproate medication. When she became pregnant, a neurologist recommended tapering her valproate and increasing her lamotrigine because of fears about valproate teratogenicity. Her next outpatient appointment was three months later but, 12 weeks into her pregnancy, she was found dead in her bath.

The autopsy was consistent with death from epilepsy and no other pathological conditions were present. No histology was taken and no drug levels were measured. Although the cause of death is undoubtedly accurate, in the absence of postmortem toxicology we do not know whether there was compliance with the altered drug regimens. It is conceivable that she had prematurely tailed off the valproate because of the risks to her fetus.

Three epileptic deaths, including the one described above, were associated with drowning in the bath, although one of these was in bizarre circumstances:

> An epileptic woman was last seen alive one evening when preparing to bathe her newborn baby. She was later found dead with her face in the baby bath, which contained 2 inches of water. Frothy oedema fluid was exuding from the nose; there was postmortem livido to the face and numerous petechiae to the eyes, forehead and neck. There were no visible signs of external trauma and the tongue was not bruised. The major abnormality internally was the congested oedematous lungs. Extensive histology was non-contributory and toxicology showed

therapeutic levels of drugs: the carbemazepine level was just below the therapeutic range. A few weeks before delivery her blood levels of carbemazepine had been in the high therapeutic range, suggesting that a change in her drug regimen had occurred.

Drug levels were only assayed in four cases but, as in the above case, were of value in assessing the clinical management.

## Asthma

Five deaths were attributed to asthma in this triennium: a further two *Late* deaths from asthma are also recorded. Of these, five autopsy reports are available for review and in one case no autopsy was performed but would have been of value. Three of the autopsies were high standard with supporting histology: a minor criticism would be the failure to search for a precipitating upper respiratory tract infection. One autopsy was inadequate and one failed to resolve the clinical problems:

> A woman from an ethnic minority group had severe asthma that had previously necessitated hospital admissions. At her booking, she had been assessed as high risk because of her asthma and a previous caesarean section. At six months of gestation she suddenly complained of shortness of breath, collapsed and had a cardiac arrest at home. When admitted to A&E, resuscitation and a perimortem classical caesarean section were attempted, without success, but intestinal petechiae were noted. There was no evidence of an abruption.

The autopsy findings were those of congestion of organs and oedema of the lungs. Extensive histology, independently reviewed, confirmed these findings and demonstrated platelet thrombi in lung capillaries. No fetal squames and no mucus plugging of airways were found. There was no toxicology or microbiology performed.

This death is classified as being due to asthma because of the preceding clinical history, the absence of alternative diagnoses and because in many confirmed deaths from asthma the autopsy findings may be minimal. No mucus plugging was found at autopsy but it is possible that the resuscitation could have removed this evidence. Unfortunately, there is no histological description of the small airways. Because of the petechiae at caesarean section, DIC was clinically suspected and the thrombi in lung capillaries could be supportive evidence. The petechiae were not described in the organs at autopsy even though skin petechiae were noted.

## Infections

There were 13 deaths from infections that may be regarded as opportunistic and two have been assessed as being the probable consequence of HIV infection. In other instances, the fulminating infection may have been the result of the pregnancy. Such examples would include two deaths from influenzal pneumonia, one death from tuberculosis and the second known case in pregnancy of a streptococcal gastritis.

> A young woman had a normal antenatal period apart from a mild refractory anaemia. She had a spontaneous labour but three weeks

postpartum she complained of a headache and the GP was called. He in turn arranged for a domiciliary visit: the consultant physician diagnosed a tension headache. Three days later she collapsed and was admitted. CT scan showed a large tumour in the right frontal lobe and, although brain-stem dead, she was transferred to a neurological centre where the diagnosis was confirmed.

There was a very detailed autopsy that revealed a large tumour centred on the right caudate nucleus with herniation of the uncus and the cerebellar tonsil as well as infarction of the pons. Elsewhere in the body there was generalised lymphadenopathy and there was a white necrotic tumour 1.5 cm in diameter in the apex of the right lung. There were also areas of thickening in the wall of the ascending colon and in the ileum where there was associated mucosal ulceration. The cause of death was given as brain-stem infarction due to a malignant tumour. Histology showed caseating tuberculosis in the brain, ileum and lymph nodes and the case was referred for public health contact tracing and assessment.

It is difficult to explain the rapid progression in this patient without incriminating the diminished immune status of pregnancy as a contributing factor.

When the maternal death is sudden with no clinical explanation, the diagnosis rests entirely on the post mortem examination:

> Late in her pregnancy, which had been uneventful throughout, a primigravida with no history of previous illness was found lying dead in her home. From the circumstances her death had been sudden. A thorough autopsy revealed only a very abnormal gastric mucosa, which histology showed to be typical of acute phlegmonous gastritis. This is an extremely rare condition with a high mortality caused by an acute haemolytic streptococcal gastritis with septicaemia. Fortunately, the pathologist had submitted a large number of samples for bacteriological examination. Both beta and alpha haemolytic streptococci together with *Strep. pneumoniae* were isolated from multiple sites. This allowed the consultant bacteriologist and the consultant pathologist to each provide thoughtful comments on the case and to substantiate their diagnosis. The regional assessors accepted that their careful investigations were convincing, despite the lack of any supportive clinical history. A literature search found one other similar case, in Denmark, of fatal acute phlegmonous gastritis in pregnancy, also late in pregnancy.[10]

When the disease disclosed is so unexpected and rare, the pathologist has to be able to justify its validity. This can only be done if the autopsy has been exhaustive, well-documented and all relevant investigations undertaken. These criteria were met in both of these most unusual cases and illustrate the positive contribution of an autopsy to assessing the circumstances giving rise to a maternal death.

## Tumours and miscellaneous causes of death

### Tumours
The full range of tumour-related deaths is separately considered, in Chapter 13, for the first time in this triennial Report. There were 52 deaths from malignant

tumours: 28 of these have been classified as *Indirect* or *Late Indirect*, as there was evidence that the pregnant status interfered with diagnosis or subsequent clinical management. There are very few cases where there was evidence that the pregnancy directly altered the biological behaviour of the tumour. As identified in Chapter 13, a full spectrum of malignant tumours has been reported with no unusually frequent cancer, given the age profile of the cases.

In many instances no autopsy was done but histology had established the diagnosis:

> A woman who booked at 15 weeks of gestation was regularly seen in clinic. At 31 weeks of gestation, abnormal liver function tests with pruritis were diagnosed as cholestasis of pregnancy. Placenta praevia was diagnosed the following week and she was admitted shortly afterwards. After two episodes of antepartum haemorrhage she underwent a successful caesarean section and was discharged on the sixth postpartum day. She was readmitted with ascites a month after delivery. Investigations showed liver metastases and a supraclavicular lymph node was biopsied. This showed a poorly differentiated adenocarcinoma with a tubular and cribriform pattern. Immuno-cytochemistry was negative for both oestrogen receptor status and for serum CA125 levels. The patient died a few months after delivery: no autopsy was done and the primary site was never established.

Breast, stomach and pancreas seem to be lead candidates: ovary can probably be excluded because of the negative serum CA125. In retrospect the abnormal liver function tests at 31 weeks of gestation were a manifestation of her carcinomatosis.

### Phaeochromocytoma

There were no deaths from phaeochromocytoma in this triennium but the condition must always be considered in the differential diagnosis of fulminating pre-eclampsia and in cerebral haemorrhages.

### Other causes

There were two deaths from peritonitis complicating intestinal obstruction from adhesions. Symptoms were present but not investigated with abdominal X-rays because of the patient's pregnant status. Both were diagnosed at autopsy, although one report is sketchy and poor in quality.

As might be expected, there are a variety of deaths from other rare causes and some of these are exotic. One patient died from acute gestational hyperlipidaemic pancreatitis but unfortunately the pathology has not been available for review. Acute pancreatitis was the probable cause of death in another patient:

> A patient with long history of alcohol abuse booked in early pregnancy and was then admitted at three months of gestation with severe vomiting of five days duration. Ultrasound scan showed a missed abortion that was evacuated but she continued to deteriorate and had marked electrolyte disturbances. She died shortly after admission in multi-organ failure.

The autopsy included review of the clinical history and was quite detailed, with supporting histology but no microbiology. The cause of death was given as acute hepatic failure from fatty liver. This is surprising, given that the fatty change without cirrhosis was confirmed histologically and because there was a very careful description of chronic pancreatitis with a large (5-cm diameter) pancreatic pseudocyst filled with green sludge. It is considered more probable that this was multi-organ failure from alcohol-induced pancreatitis and that the interpretation of the vomiting as hyperemesis places this death in the *Indirect* category.

One patient died suddenly on an acute psychiatric ward, having been admitted for suspected puerperal psychosis:

> A young woman had a vaginal delivery at term after induction because of proteinuria, hypertension (130/90 mmHg) and generalised oedema. The following day she seemed confused but she clinically responded to lorazepam and thioridazine and was discharged next day. She was readmitted two days later with symptoms of 'hearing voices', diagnosed as probable postpartum psychosis. She was found dead in bed a few days after admission.

No cause of death could be ascertained from the comprehensive and detailed autopsy. Toxicology was taken but was negative and there was extensive histological sampling. No histological abnormalities were found in any of the organs apart from the brain. Multiple areas of brain were sampled and showed severe damage in the thalamus where there was diffuse bilateral neuronal loss as well as marked reactive gliosis. Expert neuropathological opinions were sought and prion diseases were excluded by immunocytochemistry. The conclusions were that the gliosis preceded the birth of the baby and had been present for some time. The changes were considered to be a consequence of hypoxic damage but the cause was not identified. The final diagnosis was 'diffuse cerebral gliosis'.

The cause of death is considered unascertained. The small vessel damage of pre-eclampsia was not found but this possible cause cannot be completely excluded. It is of note that without such extensive brain sampling the cause of death might have been attributed to a cardiac arrhythmia.

> An obese woman who had a history of postnatal depression had a normal pregnancy and spontaneous vaginal delivery at term. Postnatal depression again occurred and she was treated with haloperidol. Shortly after this, she had to be admitted to a psychiatric ward when she had stiffness, fever and breathing difficulties. Clinically malignant neuroleptic syndrome due to haloperidol was suspected. She recovered after a brief spell in ICU, where she had been intubated, and was transferred to a medical ward where she suddenly collapsed and died.

Autopsy revealed a large (490 g) heart with left ventricular hypertrophy and petechial haemorrhages on the epicardium. There were bloodstained effusions in the pericardial and pleural cavities, the lungs were heavy and congested and there was some blood in the cerebellopontine region. Blood was present in the stomach and small bowel but not the large bowel: three superficial mucosal tears were identified in the gastric antrum. The liver and spleen were congested. The death was attributed to gastric haemorrhage from an adverse drug reaction. No histology was taken.

It is difficult to believe that sudden death without warning can occur from three superficial mucosal tears. In other circumstances, there is usually time for patients to be resuscitated from well-defined causes of massive haemorrhage such as bleeding oesophageal varices. Also there was no evidence of hypovolaemia – the liver and spleen were congested. There was no attempt to assess the cardiac pathology nor was there any attempt to establish the cause of the cerebellopontine bleeding or the petechiae. This cannot be considered to be an adequate autopsy and it is difficult to assess care when the cause of death has not been accurately defined.

### Chapter 14; *Coincidental* deaths

While the medical causes of many of these deaths are not directly relevant to the Enquiry, it is important that the survey is comprehensive. These cases often also identify important public health issues and social exclusion. Even when death is classified as *Coincidental*, useful information relevant to pregnancy may be available for analysis. There are several deaths from road traffic accidents in this Report and many of these are from acceleration/deceleration injuries. It is often not known whether or not a seat belt was being worn and whether some of the injuries, particularly to the large gravid uterus, were seat belt associated or not. In one case, there was clear evidence that the seat belt was not in the recommended position. Only a lap belt was used and the fetus was forced through both uterus and diaphragm into the chest.

The assessors have also noted reports of domestic violence in some clinical histories, which are described in Chapter 16. Even when not affecting the cause of death, it is felt important to identify the problem so that help and support can be offered to the mother.

As the circumstances of these *Coincidental* deaths are so varied, it is difficult to formulate precise recommendations except to re-emphasise the importance of the RCPath guidelines[2] in the conducting and reporting of autopsies. For this Report, however, we would recommend that the information on the use of seat belts and any evidence of domestic violence be recorded as accurately as possible in the autopsy report.

**This Chapter has been seen and discussed with Elizabeth Gray FRCPath, Philip Roberts FRCP FRCPath and Nigel Kirkham MD FRCPath.**

# References

1. Sonderegger-Iseli K, Burger S, Muntwyler J, Salomon F. Diagnostic errors in three medical eras: a necropsy study. *Lancet* 2000:355:2027–31.
2. Royal College of Pathologists. *Guidelines for Post Mortem Reports*. London: RCPath; 1993.
3. Zornberg GL, Jick H. Antipsychotic drug use and risk of first-time idiopathic venous thromboembolism: a case–control study. *Lancet* 2000:356:1219–23.
4. Meyres D, Ayalou H, Virag I, Weisbort Y, Zakut H. Heparin induced thrombocytopenia and recurrent thrombosis in pregnancy. A case report. *J Reprod Med* 1986:31:993–6.

5. Warkentin TE, Sikov WM, Lilleycrap DP. Multicentric warfarin-induced skin necrosis complicating heparin-induced thrombocytopenia. *Am J Hematol* 1999:62:44–8.

6. Clarke HD, Berry DJ, Larson DR. Acute pseudo-obstruction of the colon as a postoperative complication of hip arthroplasty. *J Bone Joint Surg Am* 1997;79:1642–7.

7. Tang PT, Collopy BT, Somerville M. Ogilvie syndrome with caecal perforation in the post-caesarean patient. *Aust N Z J Obstet Gynaecol* 1995:35:104–6.

8. Sagesaka T, Liang SG, Morioka H, Watanabe T, Kaibara M, Dobha N. Acute myocarditis with eosinophilia presenting as asymmetric hypertrophy during pregnancy. *J Obstet Gynaecol Res* 1997:23:147–51.

9. Fessler RD, Esshaki CM, Stankewitz RC, Johnson RR, Diaz FG. The neurovascular complications of cocaine. *Surg Neurol* 1997:47:339–45.

10. Anaes S, Pedersen SN, Theilade P. Phlegmonous gastritis in pregnancy: a case with fatal outcome. *Ugeskr Laeger* 1993:155:1806–7.

## ANNEX A to Chapter 18
## The maternal death autopsy: recommendations for pathologists

The following *abbreviated* guide to the requirements for a maternal death autopsy should be regarded as supplementing and not replacing the Guidelines issued by the Royal College of Pathologists.[1] If in doubt, advice and help should be sought from the local CEMD regional pathology assessor: the current list of assessors can be found at the end of this Report.

## In general

- Maternal deaths are still under-reported and pathologists performing autopsies on women who are pregnant or are known have been pregnant within a year of their death should contact their local director of public health or the lead clinician to check that the case has been reported.

- Clinical information for the Enquiry is sometimes incomplete and pathologists should provide a review of the clinical history in autopsy reports including height and weight of the woman.

- Review all organs or tissues that had been resected/examined prior to death, e.g. placenta, uterus.

## Specific disorders

- Check and note existence of local guidelines for the management of hypertensive disorders of pregnancy.

- Identify fluid balance; minimum histology of lungs, liver, kidney, brain, placental site; exclude previous hypertension.

### Thromboembolus

- Identify any local risk-factor protocol, note family history, test for thrombophilia where appropriate, significance of chest symptoms and heparin prophylaxis.

- Describe the nature and distribution of emboli; site of origin; evidence of previous episodes and histology.

### Haemorrhage: ante and postpartum haemorrhage

- **Macroscopic**: identify the site and severity of bleeding; location of placenta and detail genital tract trauma.

- **Histology**: placental histology; search for disseminated intravascular coagulation; exclude amniotic fluid embolism; review other tissues resected.

### Early pregnancy

*Ectopic pregnancies*
- Diagnostic awareness, ultrasound monitoring and diagnosis.

- Location and size of ectopic, estimate blood loss and review other tissues resected.

*Terminations of pregnancy*
- Sites and locations of bowel perforations and culture of tissues.

### Amniotic fluid embolism

- **Macroscopic**: detailed examination of genital tract for trauma.

- **Histology**: detailed histology of both lungs; immunocytochemistry for cytokeratins using LP34 or AE1/2 rather than Cam5.2 if in doubt.

- Women dying after labour, of causes other than suspected amniotic fluid embolism, should have their lungs examined for amniotic squames to check whether amniotic fluid can enter the circulation without a fatal outcome.

### Hyperemesis

- Exclude acute Wernicke's encephalopathy.

### Epilepsy

- **Macroscopic**: exclude specific brain pathology and establish anticonvulsant drug levels.

- **Histology**: exclude eclampsia as cause of fits.

### Cardiac deaths

- **Macroscopic**: full description of heart and weigh/measure ventricles separately.

- **Histology**: both ventricles: assess conducting system, seek cardiac pathology opinion if in doubt.

### Aneurysms

- **Macroscopic**: nature and site of aneurysm.

- **Histology**: distribution of arterial pathology.

## Reference

1. Royal College of Pathologists. *Guidelines for Post Mortem Reports*. London: RCPath; 1993.

# CHAPTER 19

# Intensive care

SHEILA M WILLATTS on behalf of the Editorial Board

## Intensive care: key points

- In over 31% of deaths in this Report there was a recorded need for intensive care. The reasons for intensive or high-dependency care range from a short period of attempted resuscitation to several weeks' intensive care and organ support.

- In some cases death occurred before admission to an intensive care unit (ICU), either because of lack of availability of beds or because of the distance between the maternity unit and intensive care facilities.

- Regardless of the original diagnosis, the quality of the intensive care may determine the outcome.

- Currently, when scrutinising death certificates, it is difficult to identify women who are or have been pregnant during an intensive care episode.

## Intensive care: key recommendations

- Women at known higher risk of complications should not be delivered in maternity hospitals separate from acute hospital facilities. Clear and workable arrangements should be in place between all maternity units and their local intensive care unit to enable rapid transfer of any woman who suddenly requires intensive care.

- Arrangements for the transfer of critically ill obstetric patients should be improved. There were several occasions where delay in transfer occurred, due to lack of either staff or a suitable transport vehicle.

- Early communication of anticipated problems and review of the patient by a critical care clinician would prevent delay in admission in many cases. This applies particularly in cases identified to be at increased risk such as those with HELLP, which can deteriorate rapidly, as shown in this Report.

- The recent recommendations in the Department of Health of England's report *Comprehensive Critical Care*[1] should be considered in respect of the increased availability of intensive care and outreach services for pregnant or recently delivered women.

- As maternal mortality is low in developed countries, the development of a severe morbidity–mortality ratio would be useful in helping to evaluate the effects of new treatments or management guidelines.

- Information systems should be developed to enable the easier identification of pregnant or recently delivered women who require intensive care.

## Summary

In this triennium, there were 119 maternal deaths for which there had been a recorded need for intensive care. These are shown in Table 19.1. Of these, 53% of *Direct* deaths and 35% of *Indirect* deaths had required intensive care. The relevant section of the Enquiry form is not complete in every case, so it is likely that the number of cases is actually higher than this. The reasons that intensive or high-dependency care is required have not changed in this triennium.

**Table 19.1** Maternal deaths admitted to an intensive care unit (ICU) by cause of death; United Kingdom 1997–99

| Principal disorder | Admitted to ICU (n) | Total cases (n) | Cases admitted to ICU (%) | Duration of stay (days) |
|---|---|---|---|---|
| *Direct:* | | | | |
| Thromboembolism | 12 | 35 | 34 | 0.1–90 |
| Hypertensive diseases of pregnancy | 11 | 15 | 73 | 0.5–13.0 |
| Haemorrhage | 3 | 7 | 43 | 0.1–32 |
| Amniotic Fluid Embolism | 5 | 8 | 63 | 0.1–2.0 |
| Early pregnancy | 7 | 18 | 39 | 0.2–6.0 |
| Sepsis | 10 | 13 | 77 | 0.3–16 |
| Other | 6 | 7 | 86 | 1.0–17.0 |
| Anaesthetic | 2 | 3 | 66 | 1.0–39.0 |
| Total *Direct* | 56 | 106 | 53 | |
| *Indirect:* | | | | |
| Cardiac | 17 | 35 | 48 | 0.2–12.0 |
| Psychiatric | 3 | 15 | 20 | 2.0–14.0 |
| Other | 28 | 86 | 33 | 2.0–34.0 |
| Total *Indirect* | 48 | 136 | 35 | |
| *Coincidental* | 3 | 29 | 10 | 4.0–6.0 |
| *Late* | 9 | 107 | 8 | 1.0–45.0 |
| Total | 116 | 378 | 31 | |

The reasons for admission range from a short period of attempted resuscitation to up to 90 days' intensive care and organ support for patients with hypoxic encephalopathy or multiple organ failure. In one instance, three months of intensive care was provided after brain damage had occurred:

> A patient collapsed in early pregnancy due to a pulmonary embolus. She was resuscitated and transferred from one hospital to another for lack of an intensive care bed. She was left on a ventilator, initially, to allow pregnancy to reach maturity, but subsequently could be managed on an acute medical ward when spontaneous respiration was re-established. She subsequently became febrile and vaginal delivery occurred, but two hours after delivery she collapsed and died.

In some cases, death occurred before admission to an ICU, either because of lack of availability of beds, which seems to be a continuing and possibly increasing problem, or because of the distance between isolated maternity units and general hospital facilities. Some services are only available in very specialised units, such as those managing liver failure and those providing extracorporeal membrane oxygenation (ECMO) for acute respiratory distress syndrome (ARDS). In these circumstances, transport of a critically ill patient requires a very skilled team.

Sepsis is still a significant cause of maternal mortality but is also common after patients are admitted to an ICU and often precipitates multiple organ failure:

> A patient who was discharged home a few days after delivery was readmitted two weeks later with fever, pelvic pain and bleeding. She was cyanosed with a systolic blood pressure of only 40 mmHg. Septic shock was diagnosed and she was resuscitated and given intravenous antibiotics. Group C beta-haemolytic Streptococcus was grown from her vagina but blood cultures were sterile. Respiratory, cardiac and renal support were required. Disseminated intravascular coagulopathy (DIC) led to vascular injury of the extremities. This patient was not transferred to an ICU until 24 hours after admission, by which time aggressive inotropic support was required to supplement her fluid management. However, she rapidly deteriorated, despite ventilation and invasive monitoring, and developed multiple organ failure by the third day. Haemofiltration was started, with slight improvement over the next 24–48 hours but then barotrauma required insertion of chest drains, peripheral gangrene set in and eventually she sustained a cardiac arrest from which she could not be resuscitated.

The following case, counted in Chapter 9; Anaesthesia, demonstrates that, regardless of the cause of the original problem, overall management and specific events may be a greater determinant of outcome than the primary disorder:

> The patient, of high parity and a smoker, bled at delivery. There was difficulty with transfusion because of antibodies and she had a significant postpartum haemorrhage (PPH). During examination under anaesthesia, she developed bronchospasm and pulmonary oedema. Fluid overload was suspected, as a large volume of Gelofusine® (Braun) had been given. She was transferred to the ICU, where she developed a coagulopathy. Although bronchospasm improved, oxygenation remained a problem. Chest X-ray showed pulmonary oedema, so frusemide was given and ventilatory support was escalated. She became stable over the next few days but, a few days after delivery, she became oliguric despite cardiovascular stability. She was transferred to a regional centre for renal support. Tracheostomy was performed to expedite weaning off the ventilator but problems of bleeding from the tracheostomy site developed, although she continued to wean from ventilation. A few days later she became acutely hypoxic and a suction catheter could not be passed through the tracheostomy tube. Fibre-optic bronchoscopy suggested a suboptimal position of the tracheostomy. Ventilatory support was reintroduced, formal revision of the tracheostomy was suggested and she returned to theatre next day for this purpose. A size-8

endotracheal tube was passed but did not bypass the tracheostomy stoma sufficiently to ventilate the patient. A smaller tube was passed but did not result in satisfactory ventilation so a size-8 was again attempted but there was no chest movement nor $CO_2$ elimination. Hypoxia and hypotension required adrenaline. All attempts to obtain access to the trachea failed. Tracheobronchial fistula was suspected, the cardiothoracic surgeons were contacted but despite all attempts at providing a secure airway she remained severely hypoxic and died. At autopsy, the soft tissues around the tracheostomy site were haemorrhagic with a 1-cm tear in the right main bronchus and copious blood in the airways in addition to changes of ARDS.

The cause of death in this patient was airway obstruction due to problems with the position of the tracheostomy. There is evidence that her lung injury was improving, in that she was weaning from ventilation. The originating factor for her death was PPH and subsequent development of ARDS but all this could have been reversible in the absence of the airway problem.

A further case, counted in Chapter 15 as a *Late Direct* death, relates to failure of postoperative management:

The mother, who spoke no English, sustained a massive PPH from multiple vaginal tears and subsequently developed a vescicovaginal fistula after a hysterectomy, which was repaired many months later. After this operation she was over-transfused and developed dilutional hyponatraemia as a result of receiving five litres of dextrose/saline overnight (to force a diuresis in the presence of oliguria). She had a fit on the ward followed by a cardiorespiratory arrest and was intubated and ventilated. No intensive-care bed was available on site so she was transferred to another hospital for intensive care and died a few days later without recovering consciousness. Prior to her collapse her plasma sodium was 122 mmol/l$^{-1}$ and potassium 2.5 mmol/l$^{-1}$.

There are no records of her intensive care management and it is not clear why diuretics were not given. There is no information about her pituitary from the autopsy and the possibility of Sheehan's syndrome developing as a result of her original PPH remains. In any event, her fluid balance was grossly mismanaged. This case also illustrates the difficulties that arise when an intensive-care bed is not readily available.

## Recent reviews of maternal mortality and morbidity associated with intensive care

Since the last triennial Report, there have been a number of publications relating to maternal death. Maternal mortality in France has been shown to be higher than in comparable countries, resulting in a study on all obstetric patients treated in ICU in three French regions for one year.[2] The frequency of critical illness was estimated at 310 per 100,000 live births. Hypertensive disease was the most frequent diagnosis (26%) and haemorrhage accounted for 20%. The authors concluded that the relationship between critical illness, maternal mortality and the delivery of health care deserved further in depth study. A similar review from China[3] over an eight-year period reported the outcome of critically ill obstetric patients using the Acute Physiology And Chronic HEalth (APACHE II) scoring system. Obstetric admission to an ICU during the study period represented 0.12% of all deliveries during the period of study. Massive PPH accounted for 53% of admissions. The maternal mortality rate was 5.1 deaths per 100,000 total births. Applying the APACHE II scoring system to predict outcome showed that these obstetric patients had a better outcome than predicted.

An Italian study[4] reviewed the causes for transfer of obstetric patients to an ICU. Twenty eight patients required transfer for three major reasons; worsening of pre-existing pathology, deterioration of diseases related to pregnancy and complications of delivery. Seven of these patients died, all following cardiovascular complications.

A study in South Africa[5] identified nearly five times as many 'near-misses' (defined as acute organ system dysfunction, which, if not treated appropriately, could result in death) as cases of maternal death. This extent of morbidity helps to define the intensive care needs of obstetric patients as almost all near-misses will require some intensive care.

A 14-year review from Canada of women who required transfer for critical care found an incidence of 0.7 per 1000 pregnancies.[6] A total of 55 patients required 280 days in a critical care environment. There were two maternal deaths (2.6 per 100 000 live births).

Maternal outcome in severe pregnancy-related liver disease has been reviewed in one large liver unit in the United Kingdom.[7] Over a ten-year period, 46 women developed hepatic dysfunction sufficiently severe to require admission to the liver failure unit; 70% had acute fatty liver of pregnancy and 15% had HELLP syndrome. One patient had pre-eclamptic liver rupture requiring transplantation. Infectious complications occurred in 53% of patients with acute fatty liver of pregnancy and 29% of those with HELLP. Major abdominal bleeding occurred in a quarter of these patients often requiring laparotomy. In this series, four patients with acute fatty liver of pregnancy died but there were no maternal deaths associated with HELLP.

The outcome for patients with pulmonary vascular disease in pregnancy remains poor. A recent analysis[8] found a maternal mortality of 36% in 73 patients with Eisenmenger's syndrome, 30% in 27 patients with primary pulmonary hypertension and 56% in 25 patients with secondary vascular pulmonary hypertension, all deaths occurring within 35 days of delivery. Maternal prognosis depends upon intensive surveillance in the postpartum period.

A recent analysis of obstetric admissions from the Intensive Care National Audit and Research Centre (ICNARC) case-mix programme database was presented to the Intensive Care Society in July 2000.[9] Cases were identified between December 1995 and March 1999 from 91 units and a total of 46,587 ICU admissions. Obstetric admissions were those with a primary or secondary obstetric reason for admission or with pregnancy identified as a condition relevant to the admission. Obstetric admissions by these criteria constituted 0.8% (*n*=393) of all ICU admissions (of which, 53.9% as a primary reason, 24.7% as a secondary reason, and 21.4% as another relevant condition). The 393 admissions were classified as in Table 19. 2.

**Table 19.2**   Obstetric admissions (ICNARC 2000)[9]

| Diagnosis | Admissions[a] | |
|---|---|---|
| | (n) | (%) |
| Haemorrhage | 138 | 35.1 |
| Peri and postpartum | 97 | 24.7 |
| Ectopic pregnancy | 25 | 6.4 |
| Antepartum haemorrhage | 16 | 4.1 |
| Vascular | 112 | 28.5 |
| Pre-eclampsia | 67 | 17.1 |
| HELLP | 41 | 10.4 |
| Amniotic fluid embolus | 3 | 0.8 |
| Intrauterine death | 24 | 6.1 |
| Infection | 15 | 3.8 |
| Septic abortion | 6 | 1.5 |
| Infected retained products of conception | 5 | 1.3 |
| Pelvic infection or abscess | 3 | 0.8 |
| Amnionitis | 1 | 0.8 |
| Trauma, perforation or rupture | 10 | 2.5 |
| Overactivity (ovarian) | 3 | 0.8 |
| Other | 91 | 23.2 |

[a] n = 342

The overall hospital mortality for these admissions was 3% but a number (n=13, 3.3%) had severe comorbidities (n=4, 1.2% very severe cardiovascular disease). The median length of stay in intensive care was one day and in hospital ten days.

The authors state that the present difficulties in identifying pregnant women during an intensive care episode through NHS information systems require a solution. This conclusion has also been reached by the authors of this Enquiry, mainly in order to identify deaths that occur outside maternity units which are not always reported leading to an underestimation in the number of deaths.

A recent study from the South East Thames NHS Region[10] reported the estimation of severe maternal morbidity by developing clinically based definitions for severe haemorrhage, eclampsia, severe pre-eclampsia, HELLP syndrome, severe sepsis and uterine rupture. Thromboembolic disease, a leading cause of maternal death in this country, was excluded because of the difficulty of diagnosis in non-fatal cases. There were 48,865 deliveries in 19 maternity units and six neighbouring hospitals between 1 March 1997 and 28 February 1998, the study period. There were 588 cases of severe obstetric morbidity (12 per 1000 deliveries) and five maternal deaths due to the conditions studied. Disease specific morbidity was 6.7 per 1000 deliveries for severe haemorrhage, 3.9 for severe pre-eclampsia, 0.2 for eclampsia, 0.5 for HELLP syndrome, 0.4 for severe sepsis and 0.2 for uterine rupture. Age greater than 34 years, non-white ethnic group, past or current hypertension, previous PPH, delivery by emergency caesarean section, antenatal admission to hospital, multiple pregnancy, social exclusion and taking either iron or antidepressants at booking were independently associated with morbidity. Maternal mortality is low in developed countries, so the development of a severe morbidity–mortality ratio might be more useful to evaluate the effect of new treatments or management guidelines. Risk adjustment will be required to account for differences in risk profile between maternity units.[11]

A further retrospective cohort study of 51,576 women delivered at a university teaching hospital found 50 patients who required transfer for intensive care (0.97/1000) with three maternal deaths (5.8/100 000). The main indications for transfer were hypertensive disease (32%), haemorrhage (24%) and maternal cardiac disease (24%).[12] The perinatal mortality rate was 14%. Thirty-two of the 50 women conserved their fertility. Transfer to intensive care in this study was the criterion for near-miss morbidity.

These reports help to evaluate the risk of pregnancy and facilitate discussion on the adequacy of critical care facilities for those at risk.

A recurring theme in this enquiry is the problem for junior doctors in particular, in recognising patient deterioration at an early stage where pre-emptive treatment is likely to be effective. A number of systems exist for early identification of patients at risk, with accompanying training schemes and outreach systems to treat at risk patients early. Examples include the (modified) early warning system ([M]EWS), the ALERT course and the patient at risk team.

The studies discussed here and mechanisms for early intervention provide support for ensuring adequate critical care facilities, including transfer services, for pregnant and postpartum patients, whose outcome from critical illness is, overall, better than predicted.

## References

1.  Department of Health. *Comprehensive Critical Care*. London: DoH; May 2000.
2.  Bouvier-Colle MH, Ancel PY, Varnoux N, Salanave B, Fernandez H, Papiernik E, Breat G. Intensive care of pregnant women. Characteristics of patients and health management structure. *J Gynecol Obstet Biol Reprod (Paris)* 1997;26:47–56.
3.  Tang LC, Kwok AC, Wong AY, Lee YY, Sun KO, So AP. Critical care in obstetric patients; an eight year review. *Chin Med J* 1997;110:936–41.
4.  Bastianelli C, Valente A, Farris M, Lucantoni V, Lippa A, Primiero FM. Causes for transfer of obstetric patients to an intensive care unit. *Minerva Ginecol* 1997;49:443–6.
5.  Mantel GD, Buchmann E, Rees H, Pattinson RC. Severe acute maternal morbidity: a pilot study of a definition of near-miss. *Br J Obstet Gynaecol* 1998;105:985–90.
6.  Baskett TF, Sternadel J. Maternal intensive care and near-miss mortality in obstetrics. *Br J Obstet Gynaecol* 1998;105:981–4.
7.  Pereira SP, O'Donohue J, Wendon J, Williams R. Maternal and perinatal outcome in severe pregnancy-related liver disease. *Hepatology* 1997;26:1258–62.

8. Weiss BM, Zemp l, Seifert B, Hess OM. Outcome of pulmonary vascular disease in pregnancy: a systematic overview from 1978 through 1996. *J Am Coll Cardiol* 1998;31:1650–7.

9. Rowan K, Goldfrad C. Obstetric Admissions to the Case Mix Programme. Presentation to the Intensive Care Society; 2000.

10. Waterstone N, Bewley S, Wolfe C. Incidence and predictors of severe obstetric morbidity: case-control study. *BMJ* 2001;322:1089–93.

11. Murphy DJ. Commentary: Obstetric morbidity data and the need to evaluate thromboembolic disease. *BMJ* 2001; 322:1093–4.

12. Murphy DJ, Charlett P. Cohort study of near-miss maternal mortality and subsequent reproductive outcome. *Eur J Obstet Gynaecol Reprod Biol* 2001;3935:1–6.

# CHAPTER 20

# Caesarean section

MARION H HALL on behalf of the Editorial Board

Case fatality rates for elective or emergency surgery of any kind are always an amalgamation of the risk associated with the disorder for which the surgery is indicated and the risk associated with the procedure itself (including anaesthesia and pre- and postoperative care). These risks can be disaggregated only where trial evidence is available comparing different interventions. Hardly any such evidence is available in respect of caesarean section. Nevertheless, since CEMD is a population-based study with large numbers, data are presented here so that women, midwives and obstetricians will know that although caesarean section is major abdominal surgery, it is associated with a very low case fatality rate, as is instrumental delivery and, indeed, spontaneous vaginal delivery. Interpretation of the differences in rates is complex.

Of the 378 maternal deaths counted in this Report, 120 women had a caesarean section. The case fatality rate for vaginal birth is significantly less than for caesarean section and other forms of operative delivery. Among *Direct* deaths, the case fatality rate was lower for elective than for emergency caesarean section, although there was very little difference among *Indirect* deaths.

Of the 276 deaths that occurred at more than 24 weeks of gestation, 24 women died undelivered, leaving 252 who did deliver. Of those, 120 (44.6 %) were delivered by caesarean section, considerably more than the average rate of 21.3% as found in the Royal College of Obstetricians and Gynaecologists' National Sentinel Caesarean Section Audit, which took place over a three-month period in 20001.[1] However, of the deaths among delivered women, 29 were classified as *Coincidental (Fortuitous)* and 107 as *Late* and not in any way related to pregnancy or delivery. Thus, these deaths are excluded from further consideration here.

Of the remaining deaths among women who delivered, 69 were *Direct*, of whom 40 (57.8 %) had a caesarean section and 87 were *Indirect*, of whom 51 (58.6 %) had a caesarean section. These are shown in Table 20.1 and classified by the RCOG system shown in Box 20.1. However, in two of the *Direct* deaths, the caesarean section was postmortem and in another four it was perimortem. Similarly, among the *Indirect* deaths, three were carried out postmortem and another nine perimortem. None of these deaths is considered further, since those operations carried out postmortem could not have caused the mother's death and where caesarean section was carried out perimortem, the mother was already undergoing resuscitation and very likely to die.

Determination of the case fatality rates for the different types of delivery required detailed assessment of the timing and indication for intervention. All the deaths were categorised using the four-point classification adopted by the Royal College of Obstetricians and Gynaecologists,[2] given in Box 20.1, and the results are shown in Table 20.2.

**Table 20.1**  Maternal deaths following caesarean section; United Kingdom 1997–99

| Class of section[a] | Type of maternal death | | | |
|---|---|---|---|---|
| | *Direct* | *Indirect* | *Fortuitous* | *Late* |
| Emergency | 14 | 9 | 0 | 0 |
| Urgent | 14 | 14 | 2 | 6 |
| Scheduled | 1 | 3 | 0 | 0 |
| Elective | 5 | 13 | 3 | 14 |
| Perimortem | 4 | 9 | 2 | 0 |
| Postmortem | 2 | 3 | 2 | 0 |
| Total | 40 | 51 | 9 | 20 |

[a] Definitions of caesarean section adopted by the RCOG[2]

Box 20.1  Definitions of caesarean section adopted by the Royal College of Obstetricians and Gynaecologists[2]

| Type | Definition |
|---|---|
| Emergency | Immediate threat to life of woman or fetus |
| Urgent | Maternal or fetal compromise which is not immediately life-threatening |
| Scheduled | Needing early delivery but no maternal or fetal compromise |
| Elective[a] | At a time to suit the patient and the maternity team |
| Perimortem | Carried out *in extremis* while the mother is undergoing active resuscitation either to save the fetus or the mother |
| Postmortem | Carried out after the mother has died in order to try to save the fetus |

[a] All of these cases had a medical indication for caesarean section

**Table 20.2**  Caesarean section by cause of death; *Direct* deaths, United Kingdom 1997–99

| Cause | *(n)* | Total (Peri or post mortem) |
|---|---|---|
| 2  Thrombosis[a] | 11 | 4 |
| 3  Hypertensive disease | 12 | |
| 4  Haemorrhage | 4 | |
| 5  Amniotic fluid embolism | 4 | 2 |
| 7  Sepsis | 6 | |
| 8  Trauma/other | 1 | |
| 9  Anaesthesia | 2 | |

[a] includes cerebral thrombosis

## *Direct* deaths

Using Hospital Episode Statistics (HES) data, it has been possible to the estimate the overall number of caesarean sections that took place in the United Kingdom between 1997 and 1999 in each of the four RCOG categories.[2] Estimated case fatality rates and relative risk ratios for the different types of caesarean section are shown for *Direct* deaths in Table 20.3.

**Table 20.3** Estimated case fatality rates per million maternities and relative risk by type of delivery for *Direct* deaths; United Kingdom 1997–99

| Type of delivery | Total[a] (n) | Delivered *Direct* deaths (n) | Death rate per million | Relative risk | 95% Confidence interval |
|---|---|---|---|---|---|
| All maternities | 2,124 | 63 | | | |
| Vaginal deliveries | 1,710 | 29 | 16.9 | 1.0 | |
| All caesarean sections | 413[b] | 34 | 82.3 | 4.9 | 2.96–7.97 |
| Emergency | 69 | 14 | 202.9 | 12.0 | 6.32–22.65 |
| Urgent | 137 | 14 | 102.2 | 6.0 | 3.18–11.40 |
| Scheduled | 78 | 1 | 12.8 | 0.8 | 0.10–5.55 |
| Elective | 130 | 5 | 38.5 | 2.3 | 0.88–5.86 |

[a] In 1000s; [b] estimated number of caesarean sections does not add up directly due to rounding

The case fatality rate for *Direct* deaths following caesarean section, as derived from the NHS activity data for all caesarean sections, was around five times greater than for vaginal delivery, and for emergency caesarean sections was 12 times as great. Even for elective caesarean sections the rate was twice that for vaginal delivery, but this was not statistically significant.

However, as shown in Table 20.4, instrumental vaginal delivery also appears to be associated with greater risk and this should be borne in mind when considering the risks associated with emergency and urgent caesarean section.

**Table 20.4** Estimated case fatality rates per million maternities and relative risk by different types of vaginal delivery for *Direct* deaths; United Kingdom 1997–99

| Type of delivery | Total[a] (n) | Delivered *Direct* deaths (n) | Death rate per million | Relative risk | 95% Confidence interval |
|---|---|---|---|---|---|
| Spontaneous vaginal deliveries | 1463 | 19 | 12.9 | 1.0 | |
| Assisted or instrumental delivery | 247 | 10 | 40.5 | 3.1 | 1.29–7.05 |

[a] In 1000s

Since these are observational data, it can not be concluded that caesarean section is necessarily more dangerous than vaginal birth. The extra deaths from caesarean section may be due to an antecedent condition, such as placenta praevia or pre-eclampsia, which predisposed to both the decision to perform caesarean section and to the death of the woman. It is not possible to determine the proportion of the increased risk that is attributable to antecedent conditions and what (if any) to the procedure itself. Nevertheless, there were several cases in which caesarean section, although done in good faith for reasonable indications, may well have contributed to the fatal outcome; for example, four cases of thromboembolism, two cases of cerebral thrombosis, three cases of haemorrhage and two cases of intestinal obstruction.

Previous caesarean section scars may occasionally cause serious problems at or after subsequent delivery, both by making it less likely that vaginal delivery will occur, and by causing morbidity;[3] there were several examples among the deaths, e.g. placenta accreta.

Although sufficient detail was not always available, an analysis was done of whether the indication for caesarean section was primarily maternal or fetal (giving maternal indications priority if both were involved) and is shown in Table 20.5. Maternal and fetal welfare may sometimes be in conflict but, among *Direct* deaths, it is clear that the majority of the indications are maternal, suggesting that the mothers were at risk prior to the procedure.

**Table 20.5** Indication for caesarean section by type of section for *Direct* deaths; United Kingdom 1997–99

| Type | Indication for surgery | | |
| --- | --- | --- | --- |
| | Fetal (*n*) | Maternal (*n*) | Not determined (*n*) |
| Emergency | 4 | 9 | 1 |
| Urgent | 3 | 8 | 3 |
| Scheduled | 1 | 0 | 0 |
| Elective | 1 | 4 | 0 |
| Total | 9 | 21 | 4 |

## *Indirect* deaths

Table 20.6 shows the estimated case fatality rates and relative risks for *Indirect* deaths by the four categories of caesarean section. Table 20.7 shows the estimated case fatality rates and relative risk for *Indirect* deaths by different types of vaginal delivery.

**Table 20.6** Estimated case fatality rates per million maternities and relative risk by type of delivery for *Indirect* deaths; United Kingdom 1997–99

| Type of delivery | Total[a] (*n*) | Delivered *Direct* deaths (*n*) | Death rate per million | Relative risk | 95% Confidence intervals |
| --- | --- | --- | --- | --- | --- |
| All maternities | 2,124 | 75 | | | |
| Vaginal deliveries | 1,710 | 36 | 21.1 | 1.0 | |
| All caesarean sections | 413[b] | 39 | 94.4 | 4.5 | 2.85-7.06 |
| Emergency | 69 | 9 | 130.4 | 6.2 | 2.99-12.86 |
| Urgent | 137 | 14 | 102.2 | 4.8 | 2.62-9.00 |
| Scheduled | 78 | 3 | 38.5 | 1.8 | 0.56-5.93 |
| Elective | 130 | 13 | 100.0 | 4.7 | 2.52-8.96 |

[a] In 1000s; [b] estimated number of caesarean sections does not add up directly due to rounding

**Table 20.7** Estimated case fatality rates per million maternities and relative risk by different types of vaginal delivery for *Indirect* deaths; United Kingdom 1997–99

| Type of delivery | Total[a] (*n*) | Delivered *Direct* deaths (*n*) | Death rate per million | Relative risk | 95% Confidence interval |
|---|---|---|---|---|---|
| Spontaneous vaginal deliveries | 1,463 | 28 | 19.1 | 1.0 | |
| Assisted or instrumental delivery | 247 | 8 | 32.4 | 1.7 | 1.07-5.13 |

[a] In 1000s

The relative risk associated with all caesarean sections is very similar to that for *Direct* deaths (about five times greater than for vaginal delivery). In contrast to *Direct* deaths, the relative risk of *Indirect* death associated with elective caesarean section compared with vaginal delivery is greater, but there is very little difference between the relative risks for elective and emergency/urgent caesarean section. There may often be good indications for caesarean section relating to the woman's medical condition, but it should not be assumed that it will always be safer for the mother. The indications for surgery were predominantly maternal (73 %) and the operation was deemed to be relevant to the death in only 29 % of cases.

## Comment

There is no trial evidence of any overall benefit to the mother of caesarean section. There is now trial evidence of benefit from caesarean section to the fetus in breech presentation[4] but this was as yet unpublished during 1997–99 and could not have informed practice. Evidence from the Confidential Enquiry is difficult to interpret since there is no way of knowing how many identical or similar scenarios may have had better outcomes. The use of a control group (as in Waterstone's study of severe obstetric morbidity[5]) only partially solved the problem since it is possible to control only for factors that are known or believed to confer risk.

The relative risks of deaths associated with elective and emergency caesarean section compared with vaginal birth are similar to those in the previous triennium,[6] though improved for elective/scheduled caesarean section among *Direct* deaths. This may be because caesarean section is now being performed with less strong medical indications, thus diluting the denominators.

There are very few incontrovertible indications for caesarean section (e.g. placenta praevia, transverse lie, cord prolapse, uterine rupture). When deciding upon caesarean section for the more arbitrary indications, such as previous section, dystocia and fetal distress, careful consideration should be given to the possible risk of increasing maternal mortality and problems in future reproduction. Both the mother and the obstetrician need to be aware of this, but it must be clear also that the absolute risk involved is very small. There is no evidence as to whether mortality would be reduced or increased by performing an elective caesarean section on those women thought likely to have an emergency caesarean section. The sensitivity and specificity of current methods of prediction is so poor that a policy of increasing elective caesarean section rates cannot be recommended.

## References

1. Royal College of Obstetricians and Gynaecologists Clinical Effectiveness Support Unit. *The National Sentinel Caesarean Section Audit Report.* London: RCOG Press; 2001.

2. Lucas DN, Yentis SM, Kinsella SM, Holdcroft A, May AE, Wee M, Robinson PN. Urgency of caesarean section: a new classification. *J R Soc Med* 2000;93:346–50.

3 Rageth JC, Grossenbacher H. Delivery after previous Caesarean: a risk evaluation. Swiss working group on Obstetric and Gyanecologic Institutions. *Obstet Gynaecol* 1999;33:332–7.

4 Hannah ME, Hannah WJ, Hewson SA, Hodnett ED, Saigal S, Willan AR for the Term Breech Trial Collaboration Group. Planned caesarean section versus planned vaginal birth for breech presentation at term: a randomised multicentre trial. *Lancet* 2000;356;1375–83.

5 Waterstone M, Bewley S, Wolfe C. Incidence and predictors of severe obstetric morbidity: case–control study. *BMJ* 2001;322:1089–94.

6 Hall MH, Bewley S. Maternal mortality and mode of delivery. *Lancet* 1999;354:776.

CHAPTER 21

# Near misses and severe maternal morbidity

MARION H HALL on behalf of the Editorial Board

As maternal mortality rates, at least in developed countries, are now so low, it becomes difficult to formulate guidelines on very small numbers. Also, with no control group, there is a risk of seeming wise after the event. Scrutiny of near misses, that is women who were at serious risk of death but survived, may be useful for several reasons:

- larger numbers of cases are available for scrutiny, allowing more robust conclusions on risk factors and substandard care

- larger numbers could permit more contemporaneous reporting

- lessons to be learned from the management of cases who survived may be at least as useful as from those who died

- near-miss cases could also be seen as controls for deaths

- if the requirement for total confidentiality is modified it may be possible to interview survivors, to help in determining both risk factors and substandard care

- requirements for intensive care unit (ICU) beds can be estimated

- ratios such as that of deaths to near-misses can be calculated and could be compared between areas or over time; this concept is illustrated in Figure 21.1 (adapted from Mantel et al.[1]).

A comparative analysis of several recent near-miss reports is shown in Table 21.1. In this table, the near-miss rate per 1000 maternities varies from three to 12 in the prospective, more recent, studies. The lower rate from Nova Scotia includes historical data from an era when ICU care was used less than it is now. The death–near-miss ratio varies from 1:5 in Pretoria to 1:118 in London. The Pretoria study is not population-based (it includes referrals) and is in a setting with higher overall rates of morbidity and mortality. In any event, these differences cannot be interpreted without attention to the characteristics of the studies, which are shown in Table 21. 2.

Two of the studies[3,4] included only women admitted to ICU. In the Scottish study,[2] however, only 28% of the cases went to ICU (many obstetric units can provide high-dependency care). Every case admitted to ICU was included even if system-based criteria were not met. One study[5] specifically excluded thromboembolism, which was included in others, either by clinical criteria[3,4] or by the system-based criteria[1,2]. It is clear that most of the variation in the rates and ratios described is due to different inclusion criteria, with the very high rate of near-miss in London[5] being due to a much lower threshold being used for the case definition (e.g. 1500 ml blood loss compared with 2500 ml in Pretoria[1] and Scotland[2]). A drop in haemoglobin was also used in the London study,[5] but anaemia is hardly ever life-threatening.

**Table 21.1**   Summary of recently published data on surveys of near misses/severe maternal morbidity

| Location of study | Reference | Study period (years) | Deliveries (n) | Near-misses (n) | Near misses (per 000) | Deaths (per 000) | Death to near-miss (ratio) |
|---|---|---|---|---|---|---|---|
| Pretoria, SA | 1 | 1996–97 | 13,429 | 147 | 10.9 | 2.2[a] | 1:5 |
| Scotland | 2 | 2000 | 23,166 | 68 | 3.3 | 0.12[b] | 1:27 |
| France | 3 | 1995 | 140,322 | 435 | 3.1 | 0.16[a] | 1:19 |
| Nova Scotia (Canada) | 4 | 1980–93 | 76,119 | 55 | 0.72 | 0.03[a] | 1:24 |
| London | 5 | 1997–98 | 48,865 | 588 | 12.0 | 0.10[a] | 1:11 |

[a] includes only deaths occurring to women included in the study
[b] estimated from published figures for UK 1994-6 for *Direct* and *Indirect* Deaths

**Table 21.2**   Summary of the characteristics of recent near-miss reports

| Characteristic | Location of study | | | | |
|---|---|---|---|---|---|
| | Pretoria[1] | Scotland[2] | France[3] | Nova Scotia[4] | London[5] |
| Population-based | No, referrals also | Yes | Yes | Yes | Yes |
| Research or routine? | Routine | Routine | Research | Research | Research |
| Prospective? | Yes | Yes | Yes | No | Yes |
| Inclusion criteria | System + ICU | System + ICU | ICU | ICU | Clinical |
| Severity Score | No | No | Yes | No | No |
| Thrombosis included | ? | ? | Yes | Yes | No |
| Controls? | No | No | No | No | Yes |
| Sub-standard care assessed? | Yes | No | No | No | No |

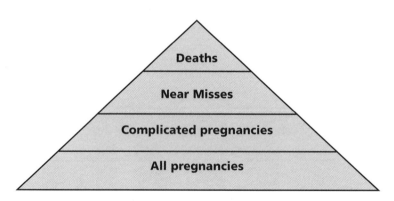

**A high death to near-miss ratio might reflect poor care or a high threshold for categorisation as a near-miss**

**Figure 21.1**   Relationship between death and near-miss in an obstetric population (not in proportion) (adapted from Mantel *et al.*[1])

All of the studies defined their criteria clearly, but there is no scientific basis for choosing a high or a low threshold. Admission to ICU alone is easy to identify from an administrative point of view but is subject to the major flaw that it is likely to occur more frequently when and where provision is plentiful than when it is not.

Only one of the above studies[1] made any assessment of whether care was or was not substandard. If this were to be attempted in the United Kingdom (using standards similar to those used in the assessment of maternal deaths) it would be essential to use inclusion criteria with a high threshold, so as to have manageable numbers and to make the near-misses comparable to the deaths. Using existing risk-management structures, a pilot study is underway in Scotland (of which reference 2 is an interim report) that adopts a modification of the inclusion criteria described by Mantel *et al.*[1] (i.e all cases with failure or severe dysfunction of any major system and all cases admitted to ICU). This pilot study will allow accurate estimation of the annual numbers of near misses and of ICU bed requirements.

Further work is required to make the assessment of substandard care more scientific and of how to incorporate it into current risk-management protocols.

**This Chapter has been seen and commented on by Dr Gillian C Penney FRCOG.**

# References

1. Mantel GD, Buchmann E, Rees H, Pattinson RC. Severe acute maternal morbidity: a pilot study of a definition for a near-miss. *Br J Obstet Gynaecol* 1998;105:985–90.
2. Penney GC, Hall MH on behalf of the Scottish assessors for the Confidential Enquires into Maternal Deaths (unpublished data).
3. Bouvier-Colle MH ,Salanave B, Ancel PY et al. Obstetric Patients treated in Intensive Care Units and Maternal Mortality. *Eur J Obstet Gynecol Reprod Biol* 1996;65:121–5.
4. Baskett TF Sternadel J. Maternal Intensive care and near-miss mortality in obstetrics *Br J Obstet Gynaecol* 1998;105:981–4.
5. Waterstone M, Bewley S, Wolfe C. Incidence and predictors of severe obstetric morbidity: case-control study. *BMJ* 2001;322:1089–94.

# Appendices

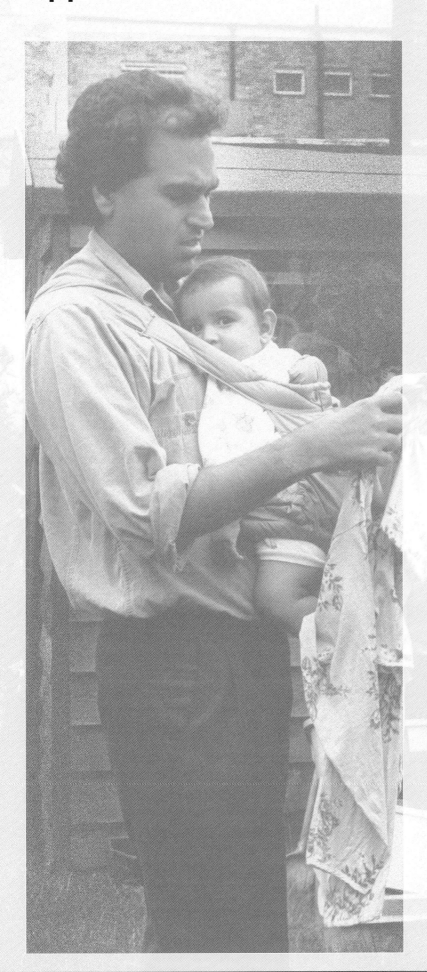

APPENDIX 1

# Trends in reproductive epidemiology and women's health

BEVERLEY BOTTING on behalf of the Editorial Board

## Introduction

The purpose of this Appendix is to provide statistics that place in context the data on maternal deaths given earlier in this Report. Changes in the population at risk could change the number of deaths expected if rates remain at the same level. This Appendix provides an overview of trends in reproductive epidemiology by discussing conceptions, terminations of pregnancy, embryonic deaths (miscarriages) and births. It discusses the fertility of women in different age groups and at different parities, and presents relevant information about problems around the time of delivery. The Appendix also discusses other aspects of women's health highlighted in this Report. In particular, a section is devoted to statistics on obesity and on smoking in pregnancy.

## Maternal deaths identified by the Registrars General

As described in Chapter 1, the numbers of *Direct* and *Indirect* deaths identified by the Enquiry always exceeds those identified from an examination of the cause of death given on death certificates. The Office for National Statistics (ONS) death certificates are examined to select deaths where there is a mention anywhere on the certificate of a pregnancy-related condition, such as eclampsia. Women who die while pregnant but where no mention is made of the pregnancy on the certificate will not be identified this way. In Scotland, however, there is a box on the death certificate that can be ticked to identify that the woman was pregnant or had recently given birth.

In 1997–99, 142 deaths in the UK were identified from death registrations as having a pregnancy-related condition mentioned on their death certificate (Table A1.1) This represented a rate of 3.9 per million women aged 15–44 years and contributed 0.6% of all deaths in the age group (Table A1.2). The Enquiry identified 106 *Direct* maternal deaths and 136 *Indirect* maternal deaths, suggesting that only 59% of maternal deaths mention the pregnancy at death registration. This problem will be rectified in part by the new procedures described elsewhere in this Report, which link female deaths to recent birth registrations. This will help identify additional women who die shortly after giving birth.

**Table A1.1** *Direct* and *Indirect* maternal deaths and mortality rates per 100,000 maternities reported to Registrars General and to the CEMD; United Kingdom 1985–99

| Triennium | Maternal deaths known to Registrars General | | Direct deaths known to Enquiry | | Indirect deaths known to Enquiry | | Total known to Enquiry | | Total maternities |
|---|---|---|---|---|---|---|---|---|---|
| | (n) | Rate | (n) | Rate | (n) | Rate | (n) | Rate | (n) |
| 1985–87 | 156 | 6.9 | 137 | 6.0 | 86 | 3.8 | 223 | 9.9 | 2,268,766 |
| 1988–90 | 172 | 7.3 | 145 | 6.2 | 93 | 4.0 | 238 | 10.1 | 2,347,529 |
| 1991–93 | 150 | 6.5[a] | 128 | 5.5 | 100 | 4.3 | 228 | 9.8 | 2,317,328 |
| 1994–96 | 175 | 8.0[b] | 134 | 6.1 | 134 | 6.1 | 268 | 12.2 | 2,197,640 |
| 1997–99 | 142 | 6.7[c] | 106 | 5.0 | 136 | 6.4 | 242 | 11.4 | 2,123,614 |

[a] Final ONS revised figures for 1991–93: the rate available at the time for the publication of the 1991–93 Report was 6.0; [b] England and Wales figures for 1994 now include underlying cause and mentions (ICD9 630–676); [c] the rate for 1994–96 in the previous report was 7.4

**Table A1.2** Mortality rates per million in the female population ages 15–44 years; all causes and maternal deaths; United Kingdom 1979–99

| Triennium | All causes Rate | Maternal deaths Rate | Deaths in age group due to maternal causes (%) |
|---|---|---|---|
| 1979–81 | 697.2 | 6.7 | 1.0 |
| 1982–84 | 641.6 | 5.0 | 0.8 |
| 1985–87 | 622.3 | 4.2 | 0.7 |
| 1988–90 | 624.9 | 4.6 | 0.7 |
| 1991–93 | 607.7[a] | 4.1 | 0.7 |
| 1994–96 | 606.7 | 4.8 | 0.8 |
| 1997–99 | 599.2 | 3.9 | 0.6 |

[a] England and Wales figures for 1994 now include underlying cause and mentions (ICD9 630–676)

# Overall trends in reproductive epidemiology

## Maternities and estimated pregnancies

Maternities are pregnancies that result in a live birth at any gestation or a stillbirth occurring at 24 weeks of completed gestation or later. Statistics on these outcomes can be given with great confidence, since they are required by law to be registered. It is impossible to know the exact number of pregnancies that occurred during this or any preceding triennium, however, since not all pregnancies result in a registrable live or stillbirth. Other outcomes of a pregnancy can be a legal termination (which is also registrable by law), an embryonic death or an ectopic pregnancy.

## Estimated pregnancies

The combination of the number of maternities, together with legal terminations, hospital admissions for embryonic death (at less than 24 weeks of gestation) and

APPENDIX 1 | 331

Trends in reproductive epidemiology and women's health

ectopic pregnancies, with an adjustment to allow for the period of gestation and maternal ages at conception, provides an estimate of the number of pregnancies, is shown in Table A1.3. The resulting total, however, is still clearly an underestimate of the actual number of pregnancies, since these figures do not include other pregnancies that miscarry early, those where the woman is not admitted to hospital or, indeed those where the woman herself may not even know she is pregnant. Data in earlier Reports were given for England and Wales only and these are included for comparison.

**Table A1.3** Estimated pregnancies (in thousands); England & Wales 1976–93 and United Kingdom 1991–99

| Triennium | Maternities (n) | Legal abortions (n) | Spontaneous abortions (n) | Ectopic pregnancies (n) | Total estimated pregnancies (n) |
|---|---|---|---|---|---|
| *England and Wales* | | | | | |
| 1976–78 | 1,781.3 | 316.4 | 158.3[a] | 11.6 | 2,267.6 |
| 1979–81 | 1,910.9 | 378.1 | 134.3[b] | 12.1 | 2,435.4 |
| 1982–84 | 1,905.8 | 392.3 | 113.6[b] | 14.4 | 2,426.1 |
| 1985–87 | 1,987.9 | 444.9 | n/a | n/a | 2,432.8 |
| 1988–90 | 2,073.2 | 512.7 | 277.2[b] | 24.8 | 2,887.9 |
| 1991–93 | 2,046.2 | 485.7 | 233.8[b] | 27.0 | 2,792.7 |
| | | | | | |
| *United Kingdom* | | | | | |
| 1991–93 | 2,317.3 | 525.6 | 266.4[b] | 30.2 | 3,139.5 |
| 1994–96 | 2,197.6 | 519.1 | 164.7[b] | 33.5 | 2,914.9 |
| 1997–99 | 2,123.6 | 564.1 | 153.6[b] | 31.9 | 2,873.3 |
| | | | | | |
| Percentage | 73.9 | 19.6 | 5.3 | 1.1 | 100.0 |

[a] ICD (8th revision) 640–645; [b] ICD (9th revision) 634–638; n/a = not available

Sources: ONS Birth statistics Series FM1; ONS Abortion statistics Series AB; Department of Health: Hospital Episodes Statistics; Welsh Office: Hospital Activity Analysis; Scottish Morbidity Records (SMR) 1 Inpatients and Daycases Acute; Scottish Morbidity Records (SMR) 2 Inpatients and Daycases Maternity; DHSS Northern Ireland

Using these sources of data, ONS estimated that 74% of pregnancies in the United Kingdom between 1997 and 1999 led to a maternity resulting in one or more registrable live or stillbirths. A further 20% of pregnancies were legally terminated under the 1967 Abortion Act. The remaining 6% of known pregnancies were admitted to hospital following an embryonic death or an ectopic pregnancy. Embryonic deaths that resulted in a day stay or that were not admitted to hospital are not included in these data. The striking changes in the estimated number of embryonic deaths and ectopic pregnancies between 1982–84 and 1988–90 are most likely to be due to the different ways the data were collected during these triennia and the different sampling and grossing up procedures used. There appears to be no obvious change in clinical patterns over this period that could have contributed to this increase in number.

## Trends in legal abortion

Some women die following legal (and in the past, illegal) abortion. Since the introduction of legal abortion in 1968, following the Abortion Act 1967 in England, Wales and Scotland, and up to the end of 1999, over 4.4 million legal terminations of pregnancy have been carried out for residents of Great Britain. The Abortion Act 1967 does not apply to Northern Ireland, where only a small number of legal terminations are performed each year on medical grounds under the case law that applied in England and Wales before the Abortion Act 1967. However, some women having legal terminations in Great Britain, of which there were 4,583 in 1997–99, gave a usual address in Northern Ireland.

Table A.4 shows both the number of legal abortions in Great Britain and the rate per 1,000 women aged 15–44 years for each of the most recent four triennia. Figure A1.1 shows the legal abortion rate for each individual year over the period 1970 to 1999. From 1990 to 1995, the rate of abortion to women aged 15–44 years decreased continually. This trend reversed in 1996, however, when the rate increased. The peak rate was in 1998, at 15.7 per 1,000 women aged 15–44 years, being slightly higher than the previous peak of 15.3 in 1990. This was due, at least in part, to a 'pill' scare in September 1995.[1] In this current Report, the deaths of three women following legal abortion were investigated.

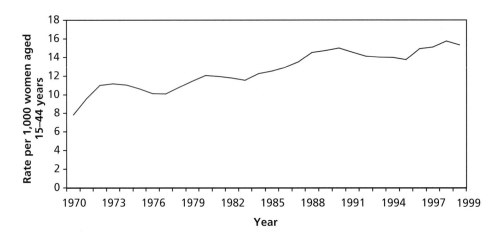

**Figure A1.1** Legal abortions in Great Britain to women resident in the United Kingdom; 1970–99

Following the introduction of legal abortion, the number of maternal deaths following illegal abortions fell sharply. In 1970–72 (the first full triennium during which legal abortion was available) there were 37 reported deaths from illegal abortion, falling to one in 1979–81. No maternal deaths from illegal abortion have been reported since, including for this triennium.

## Birth rates and general fertility trends

Birth rates and fertility trends are important in the context of this Enquiry, as changes in patterns of childbearing may affect the number of maternal deaths. Since the England and Wales Enquiry started in 1952, joined by Scotland and Northern Ireland in 1985, 39 million births have been registered in the United Kingdom. The total number of births and the fertility rate for each triennium since 1976–78 are given in Table A1.5. Figure A1.2 shows the general fertility rate (births per 1,000 women aged 15-44) over the period 1952–99.

**Table A1.4** Legal abortions in Great Britain to women resident in United Kingdom; 1988–99

| Triennium | Abortions[a] (n) | Women aged 15–44 years Rate per 1,000 |
|---|---|---|
| 1989–90 | 551.1 | 14.7 |
| 1991–93 | 525.6 | 14.2 |
| 1994–96 | 519.1 | 14.2 |
| 1997–99 | 564.1 | 15.4 |

[a] In 1000s

Sources: England and Wales: ONS Abortion statistics Series AB; Scotland: Information and Statistics Division

**Table A1.5** Births (live and still) and fertility rate; United Kingdom 1976–99

| Triennium | Total births[a] | Fertility rate[b] |
|---|---|---|
| 1976–78 | 2,038.3 | 60.9 |
| 1979–81 | 2,235.2 | 64.2 |
| 1982–84 | 2,182.5 | 60.7 |
| 1985–85 | 2,292.9 | 61.9 |
| 1988–90 | 2,374.0 | 63.4 |
| 1991–93 | 2,346.8 | 63.4 |
| 1994–96 | 2,227.5 | 60.9 |
| 1997–99 | 2,155.3 | 58.8 |

[a] In 1000s; [b] Rate per 1000 women aged 15–44 years

Sources: England and Wales: ONS Birth statistics series FM1; Scotland: Registrar General's Annual Report series; Northern Ireland: Registrar General's Annual Report series

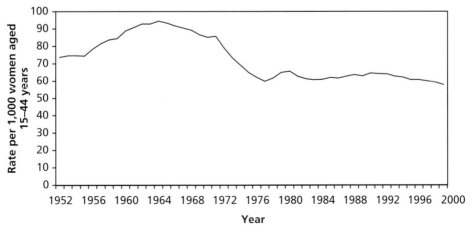

Figure A1.2 General fertility rate; United Kingdom 1952–99

As can be seen in Figure A.2, fertility increased from 1952 until it peaked in 1964 at 94 births per 1,000 women. This was followed by a steady decrease in the general fertility rate until 1977 when it reached a minimum of 59 births per 1,000 women. The rate then fluctuated but, between 1982 and 1990, there was a small but sustained increase, reaching 64 per 1,000 in 1990. The rate for the three years covered by this Report fell to 59, the lowest rate in any triennium since the Enquiry began.

The small fluctuations in fertility rates since 1977 conceal wider medical and social changes affecting reproductive epidemiology. Reduced perinatal and infant mortality means that more babies are surviving into childhood. An increasing proportion of births occur outside marriage and there are changing patterns in the age at which women have children.

### Maternities by age and parity

The pattern of fertility in terms of maternal age and age at first birth has changed over recent years. Women are, on average, older at childbirth, in part due to older ages at marriages. On the other hand, figures for parity remain constant. These changes can make an important contribution to maternal mortality because the risk of maternal mortality becomes higher with increasing age and parity.

Between 1986 and 1999 fertility rates increased considerably among women in their thirties and forties. In contrast, rates fell among women in their twenties. The late twenties were the peak childbearing years, with fertility rates substantially above those for all other age groups. This pattern has changed in the last triennium, with 30% of births occurring in both age groups 25–29 and 30–34.

As a result of a special exercise undertaken in England and Wales, shown in Table A1.6, it is possible to estimate separately, using survey data, the changes in the age and parity distribution of live births in England and Wales for each triennium between 1988–90 and 1997–99. More women are delaying childbearing: in 1988–90, 49% of women having their first child were aged under 25 years, whereas by 1997-99 only 38% were aged under 25 years. Similar data are not routinely available for Scotland and Northern Ireland.

### Maternities by marital status

One of the most striking trends in recent years has been the dramatic increase in both the number and proportion of all births occurring outside marriage. By 1999, 39% of births in the United Kingdom were outside marriage. Nevertheless, this increase has been concentrated in births outside marriage registered by both parents, usually giving the same address. During the period 1980 to 1999, the proportion of all births that occurred outside marriage and were registered by the mother alone remained at 6–8%. The proportion of births outside marriage in England and Scotland were similar (39% and 41%, respectively). In Wales, the proportion of births outside marriage has been increasing faster than for the other countries, reaching 46% in 1999. The proportion of births outside marriage in Northern Ireland (30%), was less than in Great Britain, although the rate of increase over the previous decade was similar, as shown in Figure A1.3.

Fertility rates in the four constituent countries of the United Kingdom follow the same pattern but those for Northern Ireland always remain higher than for the other countries. This is due, at least in part, to women having, on average, more children. In 1997–99, 33% of births within marriage in Northern Ireland were the woman's third or higher order birth, compared with 23% of births in England and Wales.

**Table A1.6**  Percentage distribution of all live births by parity and age at first birth; England and Wales 1988–99

|  | 1988–90 (%) | 1991–93 (%) | 1994–96 (%) | 1997–99 (%) |
|---|---|---|---|---|
| *Parity* | | | | |
| 0 | 41 | 40 | 40 | 41 |
| 1 | 34 | 34 | 34 | 33 |
| 2 | 16 | 17 | 18 | 18 |
| 3 | 6 | 6 | 6 | 6 |
| 4 | 3 | 3 | 3 | 2 |
| Total | 100 | 100 | 100 | 100 |
| | | | | |
| *Maternal age (years)* | | | | |
| < 20 | 8 | 7 | 7 | 8 |
| 20–24 | 27 | 24 | 20 | 18 |
| 25–29 | 35 | 35 | 34 | 30 |
| 30–34 | 21 | 24 | 28 | 30 |
| 35–39 | 7 | 8 | 10 | 12 |
| 40+ | 1 | 1 | 2 | 2 |
| Total | 100 | 100 | 100 | 100 |
| | | | | |
| *Maternal age (years) at first birth* | | | | |
| < 20 | 16 | 15 | 14 | 16 |
| 20–24 | 33 | 29 | 25 | 22 |
| 25–29 | 33 | 34 | 33 | 30 |
| 30–34 | 14 | 17 | 21 | 24 |
| 35+ | 4 | 5 | 7 | 8 |
| Total | 100 | 100 | 100 | 100 |

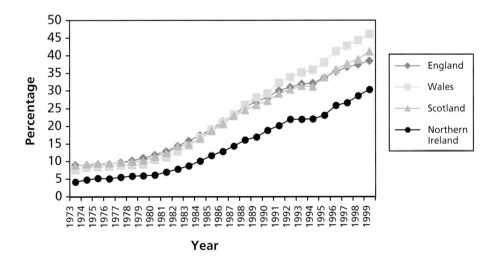

**Figure A1.3** Proportion of births outside marriage, countries of the United Kingdom; 1973–99

*Maternities by ethnic origin*

Since 1994, ethnic origin has been collected on the Enquiry notification forms. Therefore, to place these data in context it would be ideal to compare with the proportion of maternities by the mother's ethnic origin. Unfortunately, however, ethnic origin is not collected at birth registration. Instead, the parent's countries of birth are recorded. This is becoming a less reliable proxy for ethnic origin, as increasing proportions of women from different ethnic groups were born in the United Kingdom. Ethnic origin is collected by the Hospital Episode Statistics (HES) but this information is incomplete in many areas, so is not of sufficient quality for analysis. For comparisons with the data recorded for this Enquiry, therefore, we analysed the population of all women aged 15–44 years by their ethnic group. Ethnic origin was asked for the first time in the 1991 Census of Great Britain and can be estimated from the Labour Force Survey. Table A1.7 shows the female population of Great Britain in 1999 in the childbearing ages by ethnic group. In 1999, 3% of all women aged 15–44 years considered themselves of Black ethnic origin (including Mixed), 2% Indian and 1% Pakistani. These are the same proportions as in 1996. In total, 8% of women in these age groups considered they belong to an minority ethnic group, a slight increase on the 7% in 1996.

**Table A1.7**  Female population of Great Britain (in 1,000s) by ethnic group and age: 1999

| Ethnic Group | Total | | Age (years) | | | | |
|---|---|---|---|---|---|---|---|
| | 15–44 (*n*) | % | 15–19 (*n*) | 20–24 (*n*) | 25–29 (*n*) | 30–34 (*n*) | 35–44 (*n*) |
| Black: | | | | | | | |
|    Caribbean | 130 | 14 | 13 | 14 | 16 | 29 | 57 |
|    African | 110 | 12 | 15 | 14 | 15 | 27 | 39 |
|    Other(non-mixed) | 36 | 4 | **6** | **5** | **6** | **10** | **10** |
|    Mixed | 35 | 4 | **8** | **8** | **7** | **7** | **5** |
| Indian | 232 | 24 | 36 | 37 | 42 | 40 | 78 |
| Pakistani | 158 | 16 | **29** | 34 | **29** | **28** | 37 |
| Bangladeshi | 56 | 6 | **13** | **13** | **10** | **9** | **11** |
| Chinese | 42 | 4 | **3** | **8** | **6** | **11** | **15** |
| Other: | | | | | | | |
|    Asian (non-mixed) | 66 | 7 | **6** | **8** | **12** | **12** | **27** |
|    Non-mixed | 44 | 5 | **6** | **6** | **5** | **8** | 20 |
|    Mixed | 48 | 5 | **10** | **9** | **8** | **9** | **12** |
| All minority ethnic groups | 959 | 8 | 146 | 156 | 156 | 190 | 312 |
| White | 10,825 | 92 | 1,578 | 1,482 | 1,819 | 2,069 | 3,876 |
| Total females | 11,785 | 100 | 1,724 | 1,638 | 1,975 | 2,260 | 4,188 |

[a] In 100s

Source: Labour Force Survey (Average of 1999 Spring, Summer, Autumn and Winter quarters)

WARNING: The population estimates above are based on a sample survey and are consequently subject to sampling error. Estimates based on very small sample numbers, i.e. where the standard error of the estimate exceeds 20% of the estimate itself, appear in bold and should not be used in any analysis – they are provided solely as an approximate indication only

Note: The percentages for the individual minority ethnic groups represent the proportional breakdown of All Minority Ethnic Groups total of 8%

*Maternities by multiplicity*

One of the major changes in birth rates in the past two decades has been the increase in multiple births, especially triplet and higher-order births. In the United Kingdom, the number of twins increased from 6,697 in 1978 to 9,891 in 1998. The number of triplet and higher-order births increased over the same period from 80 to 331. Much of this increase has been a result of increasing use of *in vitro* fertilisation (IVF) and other assisted conception techniques. In the period 1 April 1998 to 31 March 1999 there were 1,891 twin and 264 clinical pregnancies confirmed following IVF.[2]

## Mode of delivery

The proportion of deliveries by caesarean section, whether elective or emergency, has been increasing steadily. The level was 3% in the 1950s and rose to about 10% in the early 1980s. It then rose from 11% in 1989–90 to about 15% in 1994–95.[3] In 1997–98 in England, over 18% of deliveries were by caesarean section; more than half of these were emergency caesareans.[4] The recent National Sentinel Caesarean Section Audit[5] in the UK in 2000 gives an overall rate of 21.3. A similar proportion of caesarean sections was seen in Northern Ireland and in Scotland. This trend is important in the context of this Enquiry, since complications of a caesarean section may lead to a maternal death. An increase in the proportion of deliveries by caesarean means that more women are at risk of these complications.

The mode of delivery is highly related to both parity and age. In 1994–95 in England, 5% of deliveries to women aged under 25 years were elective caesareans, compared with 8% of those aged 25–34 years and 13% of those aged 35 years or over. Within these age groups, however, primiparous women were less likely than other women to have an elective caesarean (Table A1.8). The same pattern of increasing proportions with age was also seen in the proportion of women whose delivery was by emergency caesarean. In contrast, however, emergency caesarean rates were higher for primiparous women in each age group.

**Table A1.8**  Percentage of singleton deliveries by caesarean section by parity and age; England 1994–95

| Age (years) | | Caesarean | |
|---|---|---|---|
| | | Elective (%) | Emergency (%) |
| All ages | Total | 7 | 9 |
| | 0 | 5 | 12 |
| | 1+ | 9 | 6 |
| Under 25 | Total | 5 | 7 |
| | 0 | 4 | 9 |
| | 1+ | 6 | 5 |
| 25–34 | Total | 8 | 9 |
| | 0 | 5 | 14 |
| | 1+ | 9 | 5 |
| 35 and over | Total | 13 | 12 |
| | 0 | 11 | 21 |
| | 1+ | 13 | 8 |
| Source: | Hospital Episode Statistics | | |

## Complications during delivery

Hypertensive disorders and oedema during pregnancy were recorded as an antenatal complication in 7% of deliveries in England in 1997–98.[4] Labour was induced in over half of all cases where hypertension was recorded as having complicated pregnancy.

Twenty per cent of women had an epidural before or during delivery, 4% had a general anaesthetic and 7% a spinal anaesthetic. There have been major changes in anaesthetic use for women who had caesarean sections. In 1989–90, over 50% of women having an elective caesarean section had a general anaesthetic; by 1997–98 the proportion had fallen to under 20%. In 1989–90, over 30% had an epidural but the proportion fell to 10% in 1997–98. To balance these reductions, the proportion with a spinal anaesthetic rose from 11% to 55% and a further 5% of women in 1997–98 had both epidural and spinal anaesthetic.

Postpartum haemorrhage was reported in 5% of deliveries.

# Other aspects of women's health

## Obesity

The body mass index (BMI) is the most widely used measure of obesity. It is defined as weight (kg) divided by the square of height ($m^2$). Adults with a BMI between 25 and 30, inclusive, are described as overweight and those with a BMI over 30 as obese. In 1996, in England the mean BMI for women aged 16–64 years was 25.8 $kg/m^2$; 17% of women aged 16–64 years were obese.[6] Between 1993 and 1996, the mean BMI increased and the prevalence of obesity increased by 1.6% for women in this age group (Figure A1.4). The increase was greater in women aged 25–34 years and 55 years and over than those in the other age groups.

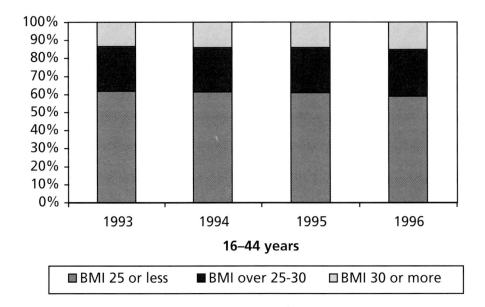

**Figure A1.4** Women's body mass index (BMI) by age; England 1993–96

## Blood pressure

Raised blood pressure is a risk factor for both coronary heart disease and stroke. Various initiatives have been suggested to reduce the mean systolic blood pressure, including promoting healthy eating, sensible drinking and the reduction of obesity. Table A1.9 shows that in 1996 4% of obese women were hypertensive compared to 1% of women with a BMI below 30. A further 4% of obese women were not hypertensive but were taking medication affecting blood pressure, compared with 1% of other women.

**Table A1.9**   Blood pressure level of females aged 16–44 years by body mass index (BMI) and age, 1996

| Blood pressure level[a] | BMI | | | | Total |
| --- | --- | --- | --- | --- | --- |
| | 20 or under | Over 20–25 | Over 25–30 | Over 30 | |
| Normotensive untreated | 98 | 99 | 98 | 92 | 97 |
| Normotensive treated[b] | 0 | 1 | 1 | 4 | 1 |
| Hypertensive treated | 0 | 0 | 0 | 1 | 0 |
| Hypertensive untreated | 1 | 1 | 1 | 3 | 1 |

[a] Informants were considered hypertensive if their systolic blood pressure was 160 mmHg or over or their diastolic blood pressure was 95 mmHg or over or they were taking medicine affecting blood pressure; [b] 'treated' means taking medication affecting blood pressure

Source: Health Survey for England, 1996

## Smoking

Women's cigarette smoking in 1996 in England was about half a percentage point higher than in the previous three years. This suggests that the long-term downward trend in cigarette smoking among women has halted. There is evidence, however, those women do reduce their levels of smoking when they are pregnant. In England in 1995, a survey of women who had recently given birth[7] showed that, although 35% of these women smoked before pregnancy, only 23% continued to smoke during pregnancy. Figure A1.5 show that this reduction in the prevalence of smoking during pregnancy was seen in all age groups, although the overall prevalence of smoking was highest for the youngest mothers and reduced at higher ages.[7]

## Contraceptive pill usage

The proportion of women using contraceptive pills remained steady since the mid 1980s. However, the number of women attending clinics using contraceptive pills as their primary method of birth control and the number of prescriptions for the pill issued by GPs, both fell following the 1995 'pill scare' and have not since regained the levels observed in 1995 and earlier years.[8]

In Great Britain during the period covered by this Enquiry, it is estimated that one-quarter of all women aged 16–49 years used the contraceptive pill. This proportion varied for different age groups as seen in Table A1.10, from just 50%

of women aged 20–24 years to 4% of women aged 45–49 years. Using these data from the General Household Survey, there was a statistically significant decrease between 1995 and 1998, from 29% to 24%, in the percentage of women aged 30–34 years claiming to use the pill as their usual form of contraception. In the other age groups, none of the changes between 1995 and 1998 was statistically significant. In the past, there have been suggestions that the contraceptive pill carried a relatively higher risk of thrombosis. The most recent warning about possible risks of this form of contraception was during the period covered by the previous Enquiry. On 18 October 1995, the Committee on Safety of Medicines issued a warning that seven brands of the contraceptive pill carried such a risk. There were concerns that this scare would result in an increase in unplanned pregnancies. There was a rise in conception rates, which coincided with the timing of the announcement about the safety of contraceptive pills, and so it seems likely that the pill scare had an upward effect on conceptions.[1]

**Table A1.10** Trends in use of the pill as a usual method of contraception in women aged 16–49 years, by age; Great Britain 1986–98

| Age (years) | 1986 (%) | 1989 (%) | 1991 (%) | 1993 (%) | 1995 (%) | 1998 (%) |
|---|---|---|---|---|---|---|
| 16–17 | 20 | 19 | 16 | 20 | 25 | 17 |
| 18–19 | 42 | 39 | 46 | 42 | 37 | 41 |
| 20–24 | 55 | 48 | 48 | 50 | 49 | 52 |
| 25–29 | 38 | 36 | 42 | 44 | 41 | 41 |
| 30–34 | 21 | 22 | 25 | 29 | 29 | 24 |
| 35–39 | 8 | 12 | 11 | 16 | 20 | 18 |
| 40–44 | 4 | 4 | 4 | 7 | 9 | 9 |
| 45–49 | 1 | 3 | 2 | 4 | 3 | 4 |
| | | | | | | |
| Total 16–49 | 23 | 22 | 23 | 25 | 25 | 24 |

Source: Living in Britain 1998 General Household Survey

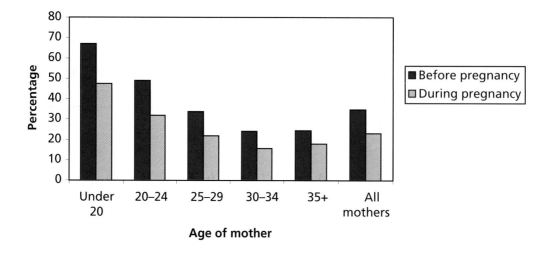

**Figure A1.5** Prevalence of smoking before and during pregnancy; England 1995

## Health of travellers

The term 'travellers' is taken here to refer to both 'new travellers' and traditional travellers. New travellers are people from the settled community and who, for various reasons, have decided to adopt a nomadic lifestyle similar to that of traditional travellers. Traditional travellers are not a homogeneous group. In the United Kingdom, they mainly comprise English and Welsh Romanichal or Romany Gypsies, Irish travellers and Scottish travellers.[9] Estimating the number of travellers is difficult because of their nomadic lifestyle. There are no national morbidity statistics on these groups and very little information on their health status. United Kingdom studies have, however, shown higher proportion of babies with low birthweight and a higher rate of asthma.[10,11] A 1999 study[12] showed that the health status of Gypsy travellers was significantly poorer than in the lowest socio-economic United Kingdom population group but was not so markedly different from a matched, socially deprived resident group.

## Health of ethnic populations

The Health Survey for England in 1999 focused on the health of minority ethnic groups.[13] For women, Black Caribbean and South Asian groups were 20–45% more likely to report limiting long-standing illness than women in the general population. Pakistani and Bangladeshi women were more than five times as likely as the general population to have diabetes and Indian women were almost three times as likely. Black Caribbean and Pakistani women were over 20% more likely than the general population to have high blood pressure. Black Caribbean and Pakistani women were 60% more likely to be classified as obese than women in the general population, while Bangladeshi women were 40% and Chinese women 80% less likely to be obese. Irish women (33%) were more likely to smoke cigarettes than women in the general population (27%), while prevalence among Black Caribbean women was similar (25%). Among women in other groups, cigarette smoking was very low, ranging from 1% of Bangladeshi women to 9% of Chinese women.

# References

1. Wood R, Botting B, Dunnell K, Trends in conceptions before and after the 1995 pill scare. *Popul Trends* 1997;89.
2. Human Fertilisation and Embryology Authority. *Annual Report 1999*. London: HFEA; 2000.
3. NHS Maternity Statistics, England:1989–90 to 1994–95, Department of Health Statistical Bulletin, December 1997.
4. NHS Maternity Statistics, England:1995–96 to 1997–98, Department of Health Statistical Bulletin, June 2001.
5. Royal College of Obstetricians and Gynaecologists Clinical Effectiveness Support Group. *National Sentinel Caesarean Section Audit Report*. London: RCOG Press; 2001.
6. Prescott-Clarke P, Primatesta P, editors. *Health Survey for England 1996*. London: HMSO; 1998.

7. Foster K, Lader D, Cheeseborough S. *Infant feeding survey 1995*. London: HMSO; 1997.

8. NHS Contraceptive Services, England: 1999–2000, Department of Health Statistical Bulletin, October 2000.

9. Cleemput PV. Health care needs of travellers, *Arch Dis Child* 2000;82:32–7.

10. Crout L. *Traveller Health Care Project. Facilitating Access to the NHS*. Walsall: Walsall Health Authority; 1987.

11. Anderson E. Health concerns and needs of traveller families. *Health Visitor* 1997;70:148–50.

12. Cleemput PV, Parry G. Health status of Gypsy travellers. *J Public Health Med* 2001;23:129–34.

13. Erens R, Primatesta P, Prior G, editors. *Health Survey for England – the Health of Minority Ethnic Groups* 1999. London: TSO; 2001.

APPENDIX 2

# Method of enquiry

## Historical background

This is the fifth Report to cover the whole of the United Kingdom. The English and Welsh Reports were published at three-yearly intervals from 1952 until 1984. The Reports for Scotland were published at different intervals from 1965 to 1985, the last covering both maternal and perinatal deaths. Northern Ireland Reports were started in 1956 and were published four-yearly until 1967; because of the small number of maternal deaths the next report covered ten years from 1968 to 1977 and the last Report covered the seven-year period 1978 to 1984. The relatively small number of deaths in Scotland and Northern Ireland led to the decision of the four Chief Medical Officers to change to a combined United Kingdom Report after 1984. This decision also ensured maintenance of confidentiality. Separate figures for England and Wales, previously included to facilitate comparison with earlier Reports, will, for the most part, no longer be given.

## England and Wales

The responsibility for initiating an enquiry into a maternal death rests with the director of public health (DPH) of the district in which the woman was usually resident. If the case can be identified from death certificate data, the Director of the Enquiry notifies the DPH, together with the appropriate forms (MDR[UK]1)to be completed. In about 40% of cases the death is not coded as pregnancy-related on the death certificate and the DPH and/or Director of the Enquiry are notified directly by one or more of the health professionals concerned. The DPH completes the first part of the form, which is then sent to obstetricians, anaesthetists, pathologists, general practitioners, midwives and any other professionals who were concerned with the care of the woman.

When all available information about the death has been collected, the DPH forwards the form to the appropriate assessor in obstetrics, who in turn reviews the case and seeks further assessments from the other professional assessors. Anaesthetic assessors review all cases where there had been involvement of an anaesthetist and midwifery assessors where the involvement of a midwife may have affected the outcome. In addition, every possible attempt is made to obtain full details of any autopsy or pathological investigations, which are then reviewed by the appropriate pathology assessors. The assessors add their comments and opinions regarding the cause or causes of death.

The completed form is returned to the medical co-ordinators, acting on behalf of the Chief Medical Officers of the Department of Health or for Wales, as appropriate. The central assessors in obstetrics and gynaecology, midwifery, anaesthetics, pathology, psychiatry and general medicine then review, as required, all available recorded facts about each case and assess the many factors that may have led to death.

Statistical data are supplied by the Office for National Statistics (ONS).

## Scotland

In Scotland, the system of enquiry is broadly similar except that a single panel of assessors covers more than one health board. A single assessor representing each of anaesthetics, pathology and midwifery comments on all cases. The panel of assessors meets twice a year (in April and October) to assess and classify each case.

The Scottish Programme for Clinical Effectiveness in Reproductive Health (SPCERH) administers the Enquiry on behalf of the Chief Medical Officer. The Programme office receives copies of the death certificates of all relevant deaths from the General Registrar's Office (Scotland) and then sends an enquiry form to the DPH of the health board of residence of the woman concerned. The enquiry form used is MDR(UK)1. As in England and Wales, the DPH takes responsibility for organising completion of the form by all professional staff involved in caring for the woman. When this is achieved, it is passed to the appropriate obstetric assessor, who determines whether further data are required before the case is submitted for discussion and classification to the full panel of assessors. In cases where an anaesthetic had been given, an autopsy or pathological investigation undertaken or where there were significant midwifery issues, the obstetric assessor passes the form to the assessors from relevant disciplines for their further comments. The form is then returned to the SPCERH medical coordinator, who retains it from that time until it has been fully considered, classified and used for preparation of the Report. As for the other countries, at all times each form is held under conditions of strict confidentiality and is anonymised before being provided to UK assessors compiling the Report.

Additional information is obtained from statistics collected and analysed by the Information and Statistics Division of the Scottish Health Service Common Services Agency. This is available from routine hospital discharge data collected by general and maternity hospitals. The coverage by Form SMR2, the maternal discharge summary, is now almost universal at 98% of registered births. General practitioners and hospital and community medical and midwifery staff assist in ensuring that deaths occurring at home are included in the Enquiry.

## Northern Ireland

Maternal deaths are reported to the DPH of the health and social services board in which the woman was resident. The DPH is responsible for organising completion of the maternal death form MDR(UK)1, by those involved in the care of the patient. On completion, forms are sent to the medical coordinator at the Department of Health, Social Services, and Public Safety. The medical coordinator, acting on behalf of the Chief Medical Officer, forwards the form, accompanied by an autopsy report, when one has been conducted, to the obstetric assessor who coordinates the input of the pathological, anaesthetic and midwifery assessor as appropriate. A single panel of assessors deals with all cases. The assessors are asked to consider the report and to provide their comments regarding the cause of death. The obstetric assessor returns the completed form to the medical co-ordinator. The form is anonymised and forwarded to the central CEMD coordinator.

## Central assessment

The central assessors review each case thoroughly, taking into account the case history, the results of pathological investigations and findings at autopsy given in the CEMD report form before allotting the case to be counted in a specific Chapter in the Report. Their assessment occasionally varies with the underlying cause of death as given on the death certificate and classified by the Registrars General using the International Classification of Diseases, Injuries and Causes of Death, ninth revision (ICD9). This is because, although the death may have been coded for multiple-organ failure as the terminal event, it could have been precipitated by an obstetric cause, such as septicaemia from an infected caesarean section. Although each maternal death reported to this Enquiry is only counted and assigned to one Chapter, it may also be referred to in other Chapters; thus, a death assigned to hypertensive disorder of pregnancy, in which haemorrhage and anaesthesia also played a part, may be discussed in all three Chapters.

## Authors

Chapters are initially drafted by individual central assessors and then discussed in detail by the whole panel before the Report is finalised. Other acknowledged professionals who have a particular and expert interest in specific diseases or areas of practice may be asked to review and comment on the recommendations prior to publication.

## Confidentiality

Strict confidentiality is observed at all stages of the Enquiry and identifying features are erased from all forms. After preparation of the Report and before publication, all the already anonymised maternal death report forms, related documents and files are destroyed.

346

## APPENDIX 3

# Enquiries into maternal deaths during the 20th century

## ALISON MACFARLANE

Enquiries into maternal deaths in the United Kingdom took their current form in the 1950s and 1960s but the methods used were developed over a much longer period. Studies of maternal mortality date back at least to the end of the eighteenth century, when Robert Gordon investigated an outbreak of puerperal fever in Aberdeen and identified its contagious nature.[1,2]

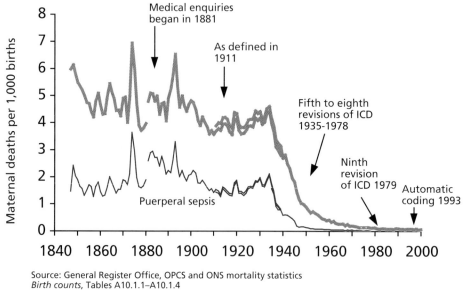

Source: General Register Office, OPCS and ONS mortality statistics
*Birth counts*, Tables A10.1.1–A10.1.4

**Figure A3.1** Maternal mortality, England and Wales 1847–2000

Debates about the nature of puerperal fever and its contribution to the high maternal mortality rates observed in the 'lying-in hospitals' set up by charities continued throughout the 19th century. Statistics were compiled for these hospitals and compared with those for the population as a whole derived from death registration. Supporters of the lying-in institutions took the view that maternal deaths were under-reported in the general population. Their critics acknowledged that under-ascertainment was a problem but felt that it was unlikely to be sufficient to explain the differences between the rates fluctuating from just below four to nearly seven per thousand live births reported in the Registrar General's population statistics shown in Figure A3.1 and rates ranging from ten to over 49 deaths per thousand live births reported from lying-in hospitals.[3,4]

## The early years of the twentieth century

In his Milroy lectures on *Deaths in Childbed, a Preventable Mortality*, given to the Royal College of Physicians in 1904, William Williams reviewed trends and variations in maternal mortality in the population and discussed the high mortality rates in 'lying-in' hospitals.[5] His second lecture described the aetiology and bacteriology of puerperal fever and used series of individual cases to illustrate how it spread. In his last lecture, he discussed the implementation of the Midwives Act 1902, which had come into force the previous year and gave his views on ways in which improving midwives' training could prevent maternal deaths.

The first report of a national enquiry into maternal deaths in England and Wales was published in 1915 by the Local Government Board, the government department whose responsibilities included public health. Entitled *Maternal Mortality in Connection with Childbearing and its Relation to Infant Mortality*,[6] it was undertaken to complement a series of four reports on infant and child welfare.[7–10]

The publication of the report coincided with the implementation of the Notification of Births (Extension) Act 1915. This required birth attendants and parents to notify births to local authorities which were given funds to provide maternal and child welfare schemes or make grants to voluntary organisations to do so.[11] The schemes included home visiting by health visitors and maternal and child welfare centres offering antenatal and postnatal care. This legislation came about in response to political campaigns, notably from the Women's Cooperative Guild, whose book, *Maternity, Letters from Working Women*, gave first hand accounts of women's experiences of motherhood at this period.[12]

In his introduction to the report, Arthur Newsholme, Medical Officer to the Board, referred to the very excessive mortality still associated with childbearing in some parts of the country and set out the aims of the enquiry:

> 'The present report is intended to draw attention to this unnecessary mortality from childbearing, to stimulate further local inquiry on the subject, and to encourage measures which will make the occurrence of illness and disability due to childbearing a much rarer event than at present. The attainment of these ends is important as much in the interest of the child as of its mother'.[6]

The Local Government Board's report drew heavily on birth and death registration statistics provided by the General Register Office, along with aggregated data from other sources. The first part reviewed national trends in births and infant mortality and the second looked at trends and geographical variations in maternal mortality. It showed that mortality rates attributed to puerperal fever were similar throughout the country, while those attributed to other causes of maternal death were more variable. Rates were much lower in London than in the provinces. Some deprived areas had high rates but other similar areas did not.

Possible reasons for this were explored in the third section which concluded that 'general experience, apart from statistical evidence, appears to point to differences in availability of skilled assistance when needed in pregnancy, and at and after childbirth'.[6] The fourth and last section described steps being taken under the new legislation and possible further action. It closed with contributions from two medical officers to the board. Janet Lane-Claypon discussed the impact of the maternity grant, introduced under the 1911 National Insurance Act, on midwives' fees and calls for medical assistance. Her colleague, Isabella Cameron, attempted to use the limited data available to compare infant and maternal mortality in selected hospitals and at home at a time when puerperal sepsis still contributed substantially to the high mortality in hospitals.

## Enquiries into individual maternal deaths in the 1920s and 1930s

Unlike infant mortality and adult mortality in general, maternal mortality remained at a high level up to the mid 1930s, as Figure A3.1 shows. It was therefore a cause for great public concern, which prompted a series of official investigations. These used a range of methods, including analyses of aggregated mortality data, enquiries into individual deaths and studies focusing on areas with high mortality.

The first enquiry into individual maternal deaths was set up in 1917 in Aberdeen by Matthew Hay, the Medical Officer of Health.[13] Local registrars of births and deaths were asked to forward to the Medical Officer of Health a return showing deaths of women within four weeks after childbirth or during pregnancy. Steps were then taken to obtain information about home conditions, the woman's health during the antenatal period and whether she had received antenatal care, details of the birth and her previous obstetric history from the midwife or health visitor working in the district.

A preliminary report, based on data from these enquiries, was sent to the Scottish Departmental Committee on Puerperal Mortality and Morbidity in 1923. In reviewing the subject of maternal mortality and looking into individual case histories, the Committee's report, published in 1924, concluded that 'puerperal mortality is but a section of a much wider group of causes of puerperal morbidity'.[14] It felt that, while environmental factors were important, the solution lay in the improvement and extension of the maternity services and giving particular attention to puerperal sepsis.

A fuller analysis of individual deaths in Aberdeen, based on a detailed analysis of records of 252 maternal deaths between 1918 and 1927, was published by the Scottish Board of Health in 1928.[13] It included a special census of births in Aberdeen in 1924, so that mortality rates could be calculated by age of mother, parity, occupation, financial circumstances degree of overcrowding of housing and other factors.

In England and Wales, enquiries were led by the Maternal and Child Welfare Division of the Ministry of Health, formed in 1919 when government departments were reorganised after the First World War. The Division was headed by Janet Campbell, 'assisted by a staff of women doctors, nurses and midwives'.[15] The Welsh and Scottish Boards of Health were set up in the same year and included maternal death enquiries among their responsibilities for maternal and child welfare in their countries.

After producing short reports, in which she looked critically at the teaching of obstetrics and the training of midwives and made recommendations for improvement,[16,17] Janet Campbell went on to a wider review of maternal mortality. Using aggregated data, she found that the geographical differences were similar to those observed ten years earlier. Like the authors of the Local Government Board report and the Scottish report, she concluded that access to skilled maternity care should be a top priority.[18] She proposed looking into individual maternal deaths but her next report, *The Protection of Motherhood*, published in 1927, reviewed the ways in which maternity services were developing. It set out proposals for a complete maternity service in which the work of midwives and doctors in private practice would be complemented by local authority services.[19]

Public pressure for action increased when a voluntary maternal mortality committee was set up in 1927. Led by May Tennant, an infant welfare campaigner and Gertrude Tuckwell, a labour movement activist, the committee encompassed all shades of political opinion and a wide range of voluntary groups, including the Women's Cooperative Guild and the National Birthday Trust.[20] Responding to this in 1928, the Ministry of Health appointed the Departmental Committee on Maternal Mortality and Morbidity 'to advise upon the application to maternal mortality and morbidity of the medical and surgical knowledge at present available, and to enquire into the needs and direction of further research work'.[21]

To inform the Committee's work, an enquiry into individual maternal deaths was set up in England and Wales. Medical Officers of Health were invited to obtain information about every maternal death in their area and send confidential reports to the Ministry. The reports were then scrutinised and classified by two medical examiners, GF Gibberd and Arnold Walker. They were asked to subdivide deaths into those directly due to childbearing, over a third of which were attributed to puerperal sepsis, and those not primarily due to pregnancy. The purpose was to look for 'the primary avoidable factor'.[21]

Reports on 5805 deaths, analysed in two series, were included in the Committee's interim and final reports published in 1930[21] and 1932.[22] The Committee recommended that the enquiries should continue on a routine basis. The Ministry of Health therefore sent out a circular asking medical officers of health to continue sending reports to the Department of Health on a revised and shortened form 97 MCW.[23] The two medical examiners continued their work of assessing the reports. Summary statements were included in the *Chief Medical Officer's Annual Report* from 1932 to 1953. Similar systems continued in Wales, Scotland and Northern Ireland.

As well as reporting the results of the confidential enquiries, the Committee's reports ranged more widely. The *Interim Report* discussed abortion in relation to maternal mortality, antenatal care, the use of anaesthetics and analgesics in obstetric practice and medical education in obstetrics before setting out its ideas for a national maternity service.[21] These were developed further in the *Final Report*, which included descriptions of the maternity services of the Netherlands, Denmark and Sweden.[22] It also included a statistical memorandum from the Registrar General. Other chapters focussed on areas with high maternal mortality, which were investigated in a separate report by Janet Campbell, Isabella Cameron and Dilys Jones,[24] and on maternal morbidity.

Both reports discussed detailed accounts of puerperal sepsis and measures to be used to prevent it. These included both antiseptic and aseptic technique and optimising the size and layout of hospitals.[21,22] The *Final Report* also reviewed research in progress. This included bacteriological research about the nature of the streptococcus in which the leading figures were Leonard Colebrook, a member of the Committee and his sister Dora, both of whom were members of the Medical Research Council's scientific staff.[25]

In Scotland, the enquiry method developed in Aberdeen was used at a national level. As well as recording particulars about 2,527 maternal deaths that occurred from 1927 to 1932, data were also collected about all the 39,205 births occurring in a six month period, so that comparisons could be made between the two groups of women.[26] This approach, involving the use of appropriate comparison or control groups has yet to be employed in subsequent enquiries into maternal deaths in the United Kingdom, although it was eventually adopted in the late 1990s by the Confidential Enquiries into Stillbirths and Deaths in Infancy.

Concerned that maternal mortality did not fall in England and Wales, the Ministry of Health and the Welsh Board of Health continued to monitor areas with high maternal mortality. In a further enquiry, launched in 1934, officials were sent to areas with high mortality and a sample of areas with low mortality, to review both maternity services and socio-economic conditions.[27,28] The reports of individual maternal deaths were studied in detail to investigate their care and social conditions. The reports again discussed abortion, as it was a major cause of maternal death, although the subject received more detailed consideration in the report of the Interdepartmental Committee on Abortion, published in 1939.[29]

The General Register Office contributed analyses of data from death registration, with a much more detailed breakdown by cause than was used in routine publications. The report for England also included a table prepared for the *Registrar General's Supplement on Occupational Mortality*, which showed a reverse social class gradient in maternal mortality. This suggested that that the care available to middle class women at this period was actually more dangerous than that available to less privileged women.[27,30]

There were no chapters specifically devoted to puerperal sepsis, but the report for England included a brief reference to a crucial development in the Colebrooks' research on the subject. 'Since early 1936 treatment of puerperal sepsis with Prontosil, a drug introduced by Domagk in Germany in 1935, has been carried out in Queen Charlotte's Hospital Isolation Block. This treatment has been used solely for patients infected by haemolytic streptococcus and the results have been very encouraging.'[27]

## Monitoring the mid-century fall in maternal mortality

The maternal mortality rate started to decrease in the early 1930s in Scotland and in the mid 1930s elsewhere in the United Kingdom. The figure shows how the marked decline in mortality attributed to puerperal sepsis contributed to the decrease in England and Wales. Data from death registration were used to monitor trends as they occurred[31-34] as well as to review them retrospectively later in the century.[35,36]

Not surprisingly, the decline in mortality is usually attributed to the introduction of sulphonamide drugs following the successful experimental studies at Queen Charlotte's Hospital, London. Slightly later, the availability of penicillin and of blood transfusions when women haemorrhaged contributed further to the dramatic fall in mortality. It was pointed out, however, that the decrease in the death rate from puerperal sepsis in England and Wales started in 1935[31,33] before 'Prontosil', the first sulphonamide, became generally available in the latter half of 1936. Mortality had also begun to fall in Scotland before this.[26] Similar points were also made about blood transfusions.[33]

Thus, it may be that sulphonamides and blood transfusions contributed to a fall which had started for other reasons. These could possibly include improvements in the organisation of maternity care and changes in practice in response to the various government reports on maternal mortality, recovery from the worst aspects of the depression, except in Scotland, or expansion of antenatal services. It is unlikely that these questions can ever be resolved in retrospect but, whatever the reasons, the decline in maternal mortality completely transformed the context of childbearing.

## Confidential Enquiries into Maternal Deaths in the second half of the 20th century

The system of confidential enquiries into maternal deaths, took its current form in England and Wales in 1952. The *Annual Report of the Chief Medical Officer* for that year commented that 'Under the old system the enquiries were often incomplete or had ceased in some areas'.[7] Of the new system, it commented that: 'Its prime purpose was to place the clinical enquiries and assessment of avoidable factors in the hands of practising consultant obstetricians'.[37]

The task of negotiating with the various organisations concerned and ensuring that confidentiality could be established and maintained fell to George Godber, who at the time was Deputy Chief Medical Officer at the Ministry of Health and later became Chief Medical Officer. Looking back from his retirement in the 1970s, he said that initially the Medical Officer of Health of each county and county borough was responsible for picking out maternal deaths from paper copies of death certificates for the area. The Medical Officer of Health then collated information from local authority services and general practice and passed it on to the local obstetricians who would obtain the full clinical information by personal enquiry and send the report to the regional assessor.[38]

George Godber observed that 'So far all this procedure was intended to secure improvement by the local review of cases, but it was soon apparent that avoidable factors were too often present in antenatal and intranatal care for the opportunity of central remedial action to be ignored'.[38] This led to the decision to publish free-standing reports at a national level.

He commented on the continuity of people's involvement with the new series of confidential enquiries and also mentioned Arnold Walker and GF Gibberd who, as young obstetricians, had acted as assessors for the Departmental Committee. As well as continuing to review maternal deaths from the 1930s onwards, they had advised on and taken part in the confidential enquiries established in 1952.

The first report, for the years 1952–54, covered 77% of all the registered 'true maternal deaths'. By 1976–78, 99.6% of registered deaths were included. Unlike the old system, 'associated deaths' were also included. Reports were issued triennially until 1982-84. From 1985–87 onwards, a single report has been published for the whole of the United Kingdom.

In Northern Ireland, a similar system was set up in 1956 and five reports were published. The first three covered the four-year periods 1956–59, 1960–63 and 1964–67. The fourth, published in 1982, covered the ten-year period 1968–77. Because the population is small and the maternal death rate was low, it was based on only 54 true maternal deaths and 34 deaths from associated conditions. The last report covered just 32 deaths in the years 1978–84.

Similar considerations applied in Scotland where a series of reports were published. The first dealt with the years 1965–71. The second, for the years 1972–75, covered 50 of the 51 known true maternal deaths in those years and all of the 42 deaths from associated conditions and the next report covered the years 1976–1980. Two further reports covered maternal and perinatal deaths in 1981–85 and 1986–92. The Scottish reports subdivided the deaths from associated conditions into 'associated' deaths and 'fortuitous' deaths. The definition of 'associated' deaths given in the Scottish reports is similar to the ICD ninth revision definition of 'indirect' deaths.

All these enquiries included deaths within one year of delivery or abortion. Thus, in the past, they included deaths which would not be classified as maternal or associated deaths by the ICD, which bases definitions on a period of six weeks. As the Northern Ireland report for 1968–77 pointed out, there is a risk that the association with pregnancy in some types of death outside the six-week period may be under-reported. It gave as an example, women with postnatal depression who commit suicide.[35]

## From 'avoidable factors' to 'substandard care'

Up to the three-year period 1976–78, attempts were made to follow the precedent of the earlier system and assess whether factors associated with the death were avoidable and to attribute responsibility for these factors. The subjective nature of the process was acknowledged in the report for England and Wales for 1976–78:

> 'Throughout the 27 years of history of these confidential enquiries the presence of avoidable factors has been recorded; there has been a rise in the generally accepted standards of satisfactory care which may have been partly as a consequence of the publication of these reports. It is therefore not surprising to find that the proportion of deaths associated with avoidable factors has not decreased as have the absolute numbers of deaths and the mortality rates. Indeed, the entry of new consultant advisers in obstetrics will bring fresh viewpoints and alter standards. In this report most of the avoidable factors concern failure to provide appropriate care.'

As the reports acknowledged, even if the 'avoidable' factors had been prevented, it is not possible to state with any certainty that death would not have occurred. It was for this reason that a different approach was used from 1979–81 onwards in England and Wales. In this report, the term 'substandard care' superseded 'avoidable factor' 'because the term was sometimes misinterpreted to mean that avoiding these factors would have prevented the death'.

## Lessons from history and the changing agenda

This account has quite deliberately devoted more space to the first half of the 20th century than to the second. One reason is that there are few people left who remember the enquiries in their earlier form. Another is that Alexander Turnbull reviewed the eleven enquiry reports for England and Wales in the last of that series, covering the years 1982–84. There is an intention to update this in the next report with a review of the first 50 years of confidential enquiries.

The methods used since 1952 are based largely on those developed from 1917 onwards for use in the 1920s and 1930s. Despite this, there is a marked difference in the scope and range of the reports written in the first half of the 20th century and the current series, which George Godber described in the 1970s as 'a limited study of clinical results'.[38] The earlier reports concluded that the major challenge was to improve maternity services and the training of doctors and midwives at a time when these were in the early stages of their development. In doing so, they still took account of mothers' social conditions, considered morbidity as well as mortality and used a range of other methods to complement the formal enquiry process.

The reports for the last two triennia of the 20th century have signalled a step towards a return to this wider agenda. In doing so, the return to a consideration of social factors has been helped by the technical change in processing death certificates in England and Wales from 1993 onwards, which has increased the ascertainment of associated maternal deaths. A European concerted action on maternal mortality and morbidity has developed an approach to ascertain some causes of severe morbidity and new data were collected in a project arising out of UK participation in this. At a time when mortality, in developed countries at least, is a tiny fraction of the early 20th century level, we can still learn from the wider approach taken during that era.

## References

1. Gordon A. *A Treatise on the Epidemic of Puerperal Fever of Aberdeen.* London; 1795.
2. Loudon I. *The Tragedy of Childbed Fever.* Oxford: Oxford University Press; 2000.
3. Macfarlane A, Mugford M. *Birth Counts: Statistics of Pregnancy and Childbirth. Volume 1, Text.* Second edition. London: TSO; 2000.
4. Loudon I. *Death in Childbirth. An International Study of Maternal Care and Maternal Mortality, 1800–1950.* Oxford: Oxford University Press; 1992.

5. Williams W. *Deaths in Childbed, a Preventable Mortality*. London: HK Lewis; 1904.

6. Local Government Board. *Report on Maternal Mortality in Connection with Childbearing and its Relation to Infant Mortality. Supplement to the Forty-fourth Report of the Medical Officer, 1914–1915*. Cd 8085. London: HMSO; 1916.

7. Local Government Board. *Report by the Medical Officer on Infant and Child Mortality. Supplement to the Thirty-ninth Annual Report of the Local Government Board, 1909–1910*. Cd 5312. London: HMSO; 1910.

8. Local Government Board. *Second Report by the Medical Officer on Infant and Child Mortality. Supplement to the Forty-second Annual Report of the Local Government Board, 1912–1913*. Cd 6909. London: HMSO; 1913.

9. Local Government Board. *Report by the Medical Officer on Infant and Child Mortality in Lancashire. Supplement to the Forty-third Annual Report of the Local Government Board,1913–14*. Cd 7511. London: HMSO; 1914.

10. Local Government Board. *Report on Child Mortality at Ages 0–5. Supplement to the forty-fifth Annual Report of the Local Government Board, 1915–16*. Cd 8496. London: HMSO; 1916.

11. Local Government Board. *Report of the Medical Officer. Supplement to the Forty-fourth Annual Report, 1914–1915*. Cd 8153. London: HMSO; 1916.

12. Davies ML, editor. *Maternity: Letters from Working Women Collected by the Women's Co-operative Guild*. London: G Bell and Sons; 1915.

13. Kinloch, JP, Smith J, Steven, JA. *Maternal Mortality. Report on Maternal Mortality in Aberdeen, 1918–1927, with Special Reference to Puerperal Sepsis*. Edinburgh: Scottish Board of Health; 1928.

14. Scottish Departmental Committee on Puerperal Morbidity. *Report*. Edinburgh: HMSO; 1924.

15. Ministry of Health. *Annual Report of the Chief Medical Officer for 1919–20*. London: HMSO; 1920.

16. Campbell JM. *Notes on the Arrangements for Teaching Obstetrics and Gynaecology in the Medical Schools. Reports on Public Health and Medical Subjects No. 15*. London: HMSO; 1923.

17. Campbell JM. *The Training of Midwives. Reports on Public Health and Medical Subjects No. 21*. London: HMSO; 1923.

18. Campbell, JM. *Maternal Mortality. Reports on Public Health and Medical Subjects No. 25*. London: HMSO; 1924.

19. Campbell, JM. *The Protection of Motherhood. Reports on Public Health and Medical Subjects No. 48*. London: HMSO; 1927.

20. Williams AS. *Women and Childbirth in the Twentieth Century: a History of the National Birthday Trust Fund, 1928–93*. Stroud: Sutton; 1997.

21. Ministry of Health. *Interim Report of the Departmental Committee on Maternal Mortality and Morbidity*. London: HMSO; 1930.

22. Ministry of Health. *Final Report of the Departmental Committee on Maternal Mortality and Morbidity*. London: HMSO; 1932.

23. Ministry of Health. *Annual Report of the Chief Medical Officer for 1932*. London: HMSO, 1933.

24. Campbell J, Cameron ID, Jones DM. *High Maternal Mortality in Certain Areas. Reports on Public Health and Medical Subjects No. 68*. London: HMSO; 1932.

25. Colebrook DC. *The Source of Infection in Puerperal Fever due to Haemolytic Streptococci. Medical Research Committee Special Report Series No. 205.* London: HMSO; 1933.

26. Douglas CA, McKinlay PL. *Report on Maternal Morbidity and Mortality in Scotland.* Edinburgh: HMSO; 1935.

27. Ministry of Health. *Report on an Investigation into Maternal Mortality.* Cmd 5422. London: HMSO; 1937.

28. Ministry of Health. *Report on Maternal Mortality in Wales.* Cmd 5423. London: HMSO, 1937.

29. Ministry of Health and Home Office. Report of the interdepartmental committee on abortion. London: HMSO; 1939.

30. General Register Office. *The Registrar General's Decennial Supplement for England and Wales, 1931. Vol. IIa: Occupational Mortality.* London: HMSO; 1938.

31. Titmuss RM. *Puerperal Mortality in England and Wales. Public Health 1939: LII: 353–355.*

32. Stocks P. Fifty years of progress as shown by vital statistics. *BMJ* 1950;1:54–7.

33. Webb J, Weston-Edwards P. Recent trends in maternal mortality. *The Medical Officer* 1951;86:201–4.

34. Taylor W, Dauncey M. Changing patterns of mortality in England and Wales. II: maternal mortality. *Br J Preventive Soc Med* 1954;8:172-5.

35. Winter JM. Infant mortality, maternal mortality and public health in Britain in the 1930s. *J Eur Hist* 1979;8(2):439–62.

36. Loudon I. Puerperal fever, the streptococcus and sulphonamides 1911–1945. *BMJ* 1987;295:485–90.

37. Ministry of Health. *Annual Report of the Chief Medical Officer for 1952.* Cmd 9009. London: HMSO; 1953.

38. Godber G. The Confidential Enquiry into Maternal Deaths. A limited study of clinical results. In: McGlachan G, editor. *A Question of Quality.* London: Nuffield Provincial Hospitals Trust; 1976.

## Reports of confidential enquiries

### England and Wales

Ministry of Health. *Report on Confidential Enquiries into Maternal Deaths in England and Wales, 1952–54. Reports on Public Health and Medical Subjects No. 97.* London: HMSO; 1957.

Ministry of Health. *Report on Confidential Enquiries into Maternal Deaths in England and Wales, 1955–57. Reports on Public Health and Medical Subjects No. 103.* London: HMSO; 1960.

Ministry of Health. *Report on Confidential Enquiries into Maternal Deaths in England and Wales, 1958–60. Reports on Public Health and Medical Subjects No. 108.* London: HMSO; 1963.

Ministry of Health. *Report on Confidential Enquiries into Maternal Deaths in England and Wales, 1961–1963. Reports on Public Health and Medical Subjects No. 115.* London: HMSO; 1966.

Ministry of Health. *Report on Confidential Enquiries into Maternal Deaths in England and Wales, 1964–66. Reports on Public Health and Medical Subjects No. 119.* London: HMSO; 1969.

Department of Health and Social Security. *Report on Confidential Enquiries into Maternal Deaths in England and Wales, 1967–69. Reports on Health and Social Subjects No. 1.* London: HMSO; 1972.

Department of Health and Social Security. *Report on Confidential Enquiries into Maternal Deaths in England and Wales, 1970–72. Reports on Health and Social Subjects No. 11.* London: HMSO; 1975.

Department of Health and Social Security. *Report on Confidential Enquiries into Maternal Deaths in England and Wales, 1973–1975. Reports on Health and Social Subjects No. 14.* London: HMSO; 1979.

Department of Health and Social Security. *Report on Confidential Enquiries into Maternal Deaths in England and Wales, 1976–1978. Reports on Health and Social Subjects No. 26.* London: HMSO; 1982.

Department of Health and Social Security. *Report on Confidential Enquiries into Maternal Deaths in England and Wales, 1979–81. Reports on Health and Social Subjects No. 29.* London: HMSO; 1986.

Department of Health and Social Security. *Report on Confidential Enquiries into Maternal Deaths in England and Wales, 1982–84. Reports on Health and Social Subjects No. 34.* London: HMSO; 1989.

### Scotland

Scottish Home and Health Department. *A Report on an Enquiry into Maternal Deaths in Scotland, 1965–1971.* Edinburgh: HMSO; 1974.

Scottish Home and Health Department. *A Report on an Enquiry into Maternal Deaths in Scotland, 1972–1975.* Edinburgh: HMSO; 1978.

Scottish Home and Health Department. *A Report on an Enquiry into Maternal Deaths in Scotland, 1976–1980.* Edinburgh: HMSO; 1987.

Scottish Home and Health Department. *Report on Maternal and Perinatal Deaths in Scotland, 1981–1985.* Edinburgh: HMSO; 1989.

Scottish Office Home and Health Department. *Report on Maternal and Perinatal Deaths in Scotland, 1986–1990.* Edinburgh: HMSO; 1994.

### Northern Ireland

Government of Northern Ireland, Ministry of Health and Local Government. *A Report on Maternal Deaths in Northern Ireland, 1956–69.* Belfast: HMSO; 1962.

Government of Northern Ireland, Ministry of Health and Social Services. *A Report on an Enquiry into Maternal Deaths in Northern Ireland, 1960–1963.* Belfast: HMSO; 1965.

Government of Northern Ireland, Ministry of Health and Social Services. *A Report on an Enquiry into Maternal Deaths in Northern Ireland, 1964–1967.* Belfast: HMSO; 1968.

Department of Health and Social Services, Northern Ireland. *A Report on an Enquiry into Maternal Deaths in Northern Ireland, 1968–1977.* Belfast: HMSO; 1982.

Department of Health and Social Services Northern Ireland. *A Report on an Enquiry into Maternal Deaths in Northern Ireland, 1978–1984*. Belfast: HMSO; 1988.

## United Kingdom

Department of Health, Welsh Office, Scottish Home and Health Department, Department of Health and Social Services, Northern Ireland. *Report on Confidential Enquiries into Maternal Deaths in the United Kingdom, 1985–87*. London: HMSO; 1991.

Department of Health, Welsh Office, Scottish Home and Health Department, Department of Health and Social Services, Northern Ireland. *Report on Confidential Enquiries into Maternal Deaths in the United Kingdom, 1988–1990*. London: HMSO; 1994.

Department of Health, Welsh Office, Scottish Home and Health Department, Department of Health and Social Services, Northern Ireland. *Report on Confidential Enquiries into Maternal Deaths in the United Kingdom, 1991–1993*. London: HMSO; 1996.

Department of Health, Welsh Office, Scottish Office Department of Health, Department of Health and Social Services, Northern Ireland. *Why Mothers Die. Report on Confidential Enquiries into Maternal Deaths in the United Kingdom, 1994–1996*. London: The Stationery Office; 1998.

# Acknowledgements

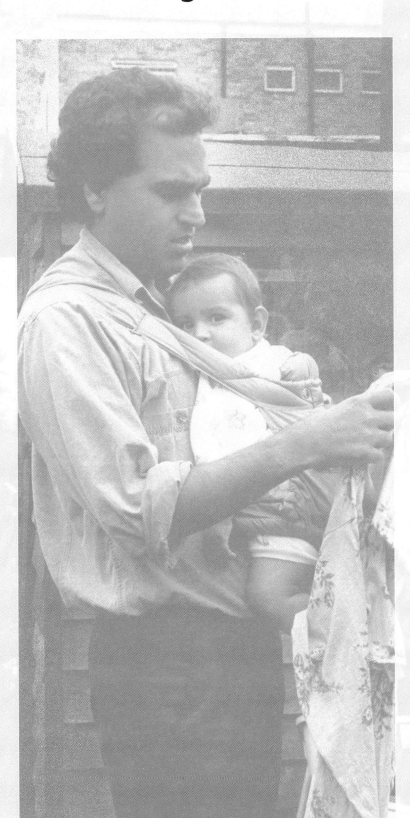

# Acknowledgements and lists of Assessors for the Enquiry 1997–99

This Report would not have been made possible without significant help from all the directors of public health in the United Kingdom, who initiated case reports and collected the information, and all those consultant obstetricians, anaesthetists, pathologists, psychiatrists, general practitioners and midwives who have supplied the detailed case records and autopsy reports.

Considerable assistance has also been given by procurators fiscal who have supplied copies of reports of autopsies, and by coroners who have supplied autopsy reports and occasionally inquest proceedings to the assessors.

The staff of the Medical Statistics Division of the Office of National Surveys in England have worked with their colleagues in Scotland, Wales and Northern Ireland to collate the statistical data and helped prepare some tables and figures.

## ENGLAND

### Central Assessors

| | |
|---|---|
| Obstetrics | Professor J Drife MD FRCOG FRCP (Ed) FRCS(Ed) |
| | Professor J Neilson MD FRCOG |
| Anaesthetics | Dr Griselda Cooper FRCA |
| | Dr Trevor Thomas MB ChB FRCA |
| Intensive Care | Dr S Willatts MD FRCA FRCP |
| Pathology | Dr GH Millward-Sadler FRCPath MHSM |
| Medicine | Professor Michael de Swiet MD FRCP |
| Midwifery | Ms Christine Carson RN RM PGDip MSc |
| | Ms Catherine McCormick RN RM |
| Psychiatry | Dr M Oates FRCPsych |

### Local Assessors in Obstetrics

| | |
|---|---|
| Northern | Professor JM Davidson MSc MD FRCOG |
| Yorkshire | Mr DM Hay FRCOG |
| Trent | Miss HJ Mellows FRCOG |
| East Anglia | Mr PJ Milton MA MD FRCOG |
| North West Thames | Mr HG Wagman FRCS(Ed) FRCOG |
| North East Thames | Mr ME Setchell FRCS FRCOG |
| South East Thames | Mr JA Elias FRCOG |
| South West Thames | Mr PM Coats MRCP FRCS FRCOG DCH |

| Oxford | Miss S Sellers MD FRCOG |
| South Western | Professor GM Stirrat MA MD FRCOG (until August 1999) |
| | Professor PW Soothill FRCOG (from August 1999) |
| West Midlands | Professor M Whittle MD FRCOG FRCP (Glas) |
| North West | Mr P Donnai MA FRCOG |
| Mersey | Miss A Garden FRCOG |
| Wessex | Mr CP Jardine Brown FRCS FRCOG |

## Local Assessors in Anaesthetics

| Northern | Dr MR Bryson FRCA |
| Yorkshire | Dr IF Russell FRCA |
| Trent | Dr D Bogod FRCA |
| East Anglia | Dr A Nicholl FRCA FFARCSI |
| North West Thames | Dr AP Rubin FRCA |
| North East Thames | Dr W Aveling FRCA DobsRCOG |
| South East Thames | Dr PB Hewitt FRCA (until 2000) |
| | Dr Phillipa Groves FRCA (from 2001) |
| South West Thames | Dr I Findlay MBchB DRCOG FRCA |
| Oxford | Dr MB Dobson MRCP FRCA |
| South West | Dr TA Thomas FRCA, (until 1999) |
| | Dr L Shutt FRCA (from 1999) |
| West Midlands | Dr M Lewis FRCA |
| North West | Dr E L Horsman MB ChB FRCA |
| Mersey | Dr RG Wilkes FRCA |
| Wessex | Dr D Brighouse BM MA FRCA |

## Local Assessors in Pathology

| Northern | Dr JN Bulmer PhD FRCPath |
| Yorkshire | Dr A Andrew FRCPath |
| Trent | Dr LJR Brown FRCPath |
| East Anglia | Dr PF Roberts FRCP FRCPath |
| North West Thames | Dr IA Lampert FRCPath |
| North East Thames | Dr J Crow FRCPath (until May 2000) |
| | Dr JE McLaughlin BSc BBS FRCPath (from May 2000) |
| South East Thames | Dr N Kirkham MD FRCPath |
| South West Thames | Dr M Hall FRCPath |
| Oxford | Dr W Gray FRCPath |
| South West | Professor PP Anthony FRCPath |
| West Midlands | Dr DI Rushton FRCPath, FRCPCH (until 2000) |
| | Dr T Rollason FRCPath |
| North West | Dr CH Buckley MD FRCPath (until May 2000) |
| | Dr G Wilson FRCPath (from May 2000) |
| Mersey | Dr IW McDicken MD FRCPath |
| Wessex | Dr A Hitchcock FRCPath (until May 2000) |
| | Dr L Hirschowitz FRCPath (from May 2000) |

## Local Assessors in Midwifery

Note: A new system for local midwifery assessment is under development and there are a number of vacancies pending which will be filled shortly. In the case of a vacancy, the midwifery assessments have been made by the English central midwifery assessors.

| | |
|---|---|
| Northern | Miss L Robson MA RN RM ADM PGCE |
| Yorkshire | Miss W Robinson RN RM QIDNS (until March 98) |
| | Mrs J Duerden MBa RN RM RSCN IHSM |
| | Mrs J Morris BA RN RM ONC DHSM |
| Trent | Miss E Bingham (until 2000) |
| | Miss JM Savage RN RM (from 2000) |
| East Anglia | Miss E Fern RGN RM MTD (until 2000) |
| | To be appointed |
| North West Thames | Miss C Nightingale BA RN RM RSCN DipN (Until 2000) |
| | Ms Suzanne Truttero MBA LLB ADM RN RM (from September 2001) |
| North East Thames | Ms M McKenna RM RN DPSM |
| South East Thames | Mrs I Bryan RN RM DMS |
| South West Thames | Mrs M Wheeler RN RM ADM BSc (Hons) |
| Oxford | Mrs C Osselton RN RM (until 2000) |
| | To be appointed |
| South West | Mrs V Beale RN RM Dip Man MSc |
| West Midlands | Mrs C McCalmont RN RM DPSM |
| North West | Miss J Bracken RGN RM MTD (until 2001) |
| | To be appointed |
| Mersey | Miss C Whewell RN RM ADM MTD |
| Wessex | Mrs M Elliott RN RM (until 2001) |
| | To be appointed |

## Department of Health

Dr Gwyneth Lewis MSc MRCGP FFPHM FRCOG

# SCOTLAND

## Chairman

Professor MH Hall MD FRCOG

## Obstetric Assessors

Professor MH Hall MD FRCOG
Dr WA Liston FRCOG
Dr HP McEwen FRCOG (until April 1999)
Dr CB Lunan FRCOG (from April 1999)

**Anaesthetic Assessor**

Dr JH McClure FRCA

**Pathology Assessor**

Dr ES Gray FRCPath

**Midwifery Assessor**

Mrs CS Docherty RN RMN RM ADM

**Medical Co-ordinator: Scottish Programme for Clinical Effectiveness in Reproductive Health**

Dr Gillian Penney FRCOG

**CMO's Representative: Scottish Executive Health Department**

Dr Ian Bashford MRCOG

## NORTHERN IRELAND

**Obstetric Assessor**

Professor W Thompson BSc MD FRCOG

**Anaesthetic Assessor**

Dr IM Bali MD Phd FFARCS

**Pathology Assessor**

Professor PG Toner DSc FRCPG FRCPath

**Midwifery Assessor**

Mrs E Millar RN RM NDNC MHSCert

**Department of Health and Social Services: Northern Ireland**

Dr Margaret Boyle (until July 2000)
Dr Miriam McCarthy (from July 2000)

# WALES

**Obstetric Assessor**

Professor RW Shaw MD FRCOG FRCS(Ed)

**Anaesthetic Assessor**

Professor M Harmer MD FRCA

**Pathology Assessor**

Dr R J Kellet FRCPath DMJ (Path) LLM

**Midwifery Assessor**

Ms K Isherwood RGN RM ADM

**National Assembly for Wales**

Dr Jane Ludlow FFPHM